T0296121

CAMBRIDGE PUBLIC HEALTH SERIES

UNDER THE EDITORSHIP OF

G. S. Graham-Smith, M.D. and J. E. Purvis, M.A.

University Lecturer in Hygiene and Secretary to the Sub-Syndicate for Tropical Medicine

University Lecturer in Chemistry and Physics in their application to Hygiene and Preventive Medicine, and Secretary to the State Medicine Syndicate

FLIES IN RELATION TO DISEASE

NON-BLOODSUCKING FLIES

FLIES IN RELATION TO DISEASE

NON-BLOODSUCKING FLIES

by

G. S. GRAHAM-SMITH, M.D.
University Lecturer in Hygiene, Cambridge

Cambridge:
at the University Press
1914

CAMBRIDGE
UNIVERSITY PRESS

32 Avenue of the Americas, New York NY 10013-2473, USA

Cambridge University Press is part of the University of Cambridge.

It furthers the University's mission by disseminating knowledge in the pursuit of education, learning and research at the highest international levels of excellence.

www.cambridge.org
Information on this title: www.cambridge.org/9781107458017

First edition 1913
First published 1913
Second edition 1914
First paperback edition 2014

A catalogue record for this publication is available from the British Library

ISBN 978-1-107-45801-7 Paperback

EDITORS' PREFACE

IN view of the increasing importance of the study of public hygiene and the recognition by doctors, teachers, administrators and members of Public Health and Hygiene Committees alike that the *salus populi* must rest, in part at least, upon a scientific basis, the Syndics of the Cambridge University Press have decided to publish a series of volumes dealing with the various subjects connected with Public Health.

The books included in the Series present in a useful and handy form the knowledge now available in many branches of the subject. They are written by experts, and the authors are occupied, or have been occupied, either in investigations connected with the various themes or in their application and administration. They include the latest scientific and practical information offered in a manner which is not too technical. The bibliographies contain references to the literature of each subject which will ensure their utility to the specialist.

It has been the desire of the editors to arrange that the books should appeal to various classes of readers: and it is hoped that they will be useful to the medical profession at home and abroad, to bacteriologists and laboratory students, to municipal engineers and architects, to medical officers of health and sanitary inspectors and to teachers and administrators.

Many of the volumes will contain material which will be suggestive and instructive to members of Public Health and Hygiene Committees; and it is intended that they shall seek to influence the large body of educated and intelligent public opinion interested in the problems of public health.

PREFACE

BY his historic observations on the development of *Filaria* in the mosquito Manson (1879) first directed attention to the possibility of flies transmitting disease, and the remarkable work of Bruce in 1895 and of Ross in 1898 conclusively demonstrated the parts played by bloodsucking flies of the genus Glossina in the spread of Tsetse fly disease, and by mosquitoes in the spread of malaria. Since that time it has been shown that bloodsucking flies are necessary factors in the transmission of several important human and animal diseases, most of them caused by protozoon, or animal, parasites, which undergo developmental changes within the flies. Consequently the distinguishing characters, life-histories, habits and distribution of many bloodsucking flies belonging to suspected genera have been extensively studied, and the modes of transmission of the parasites and the changes undergone by them within the flies investigated.

Little attention has, however, been paid to non-bloodsucking, or non-biting, flies. They have few opportunities of feeding on blood, and therefore are not common agents in transmitting diseases due to micro-organisms living in the circulating blood.

From time to time accounts of isolated observations have been published showing that under suitable conditions non-biting flies may transmit bacterial diseases by contaminating articles of food, wounds, etc., but few have attempted to study the subject systematically. In fact so little had the habits of the common house-fly (*M. domestica*) been studied that Hewitt (1912, p. vii) in his recently published book, *House-flies and how they spread disease*, says: "About eight years ago, on being asked for some information of a special kind regarding the house-fly, I was surprised to find, after looking into the matter, that our knowledge of the insect was of a most meagre character."

Since that time, however, the observations and experiments of Hewitt, Austen, Newstead, the investigators for the Local

Government Board and other workers in this country, and of Howard and other entomologists in America, have added greatly to our knowledge.

The work done up to the present has been mainly of a preliminary character. It has, however, established certain very important facts; that many of the non-biting flies found in houses frequently walk over and feed on decaying substances and excreta of all kinds, and that their larvae develop in them; that occasionally disease-producing bacteria may be present in these excreta; that flies can carry bacteria on their limbs and bodies for several hours, and internally for several days; that for some days they can infect substances, including human food materials, over which they walk or defæcate, and on which they feed; and that their habits are such that they constantly infect foods with the bacteria they carry. Further, the epidemiological evidence suggests that, when suitable conditions prevail, flies may be highly important factors in the spread of certain infectious diseases.

The conditions favourable for fly infection and subsequent human infection vary in different parts of the world, and even in different parts of the same country, or town, with the nature and distribution of the disease-producing organism, the habits and intelligence of the community, and the sanitary efficiency of the district.

Far-reaching conclusions founded on the insufficient data at present available can fulfil no useful purpose, and, if ultimately proved incorrect, may lead to the discredit by the public of well-established and important facts, such as the transmission of malaria by mosquitoes.

It may be justly claimed, however, that a very strong case has been made out for the thorough investigation of the relationship of non-biting flies to disease. Though the various aspects of the complex problems, which have been revealed, require for their elucidation careful, extensive and prolonged observations and experiments, it may be hoped that the time is not far distant when the exact part played by non-biting flies in the spread of infectious diseases, under the varied conditions presented in different parts of the world, will be thoroughly understood.

In order to determine with any degree of certainty the part really played by flies, we need more particularly a large amount of epidemiological evidence, such as would be afforded by changes in disease incidence following the control of the fly nuisance. At present there is very little of such evidence, and until recently there was none. Vague surmises have been plentiful, but trustworthy observations few.

Unfortunately the general tone of the medical profession in regard to the question is apathetic, if not actually antagonistic, and consequently the subject has received but scanty attention except from a few enthusiasts.

In this book an attempt has been made to collect the most important and reliable information available on the subject, and to arrange it in such a manner that all who are interested in its various aspects may be able to ascertain the present extent of our knowledge.

In order to meet the requirements of various classes of readers, those portions of the book which are devoted to matters of general interest and importance are printed in large type, and in them, as far as practicable, the use of technical terms has been avoided. The details of bacteriological experiments, essential to the formation of a correct judgment as to their value, and to the planning of future researches, and technical descriptions of important insects have been printed in smaller type, for the convenience of medical officers, bacteriologists and entomologists.

Opinions advanced without evidence have not been quoted.

The bibliography is by no means complete, since the titles of many locally printed, almost inaccessible, articles have been omitted, but it is hoped that all the important publications, containing original observations, have been included. For the assistance of those who are interested in special branches of the subject, the main aspect dealt with in each paper is indicated at the end of the reference.

I am greatly indebted to Mr G. C. Lamb for the loan of accurately identified specimens of all the flies illustrated in Plates II, III, IV, V, VI, VII, and IX, to Professor R. Newstead for very kindly lending specimens of *Pycnosoma* (Pl. XVII.

figs. 2 and 3), the Congo floor-maggot fly and its maggot, the screw-worm fly (Pl. XXI, figs. 1, 2 and 3), the screw-worm, and the tumbu fly (Pl. XXII, figs. 1 and 2) and to Dr L. Nicholls for specimens of *Oscinis pallipes*.

To Mr Edwin Wilson my special thanks are due for all the time and care he expended in producing extremely accurate illustrations of all the specimens, some of them very minute, submitted to him. These drawings are reproduced in Pls. I–IX, XVII, XXI and XXII, and figs. 1–4, 8–11, 24, 25, 27, 31, and 32.

For permission to reproduce illustrations, which had previously appeared in other publications, and for the loan of the original blocks, I am greatly indebted to the Controller of His Majesty's Stationery Office (Pls. XIV, XV, XVI, XVIII and figs. 13–16), to the Editors of *The Journal of Hygiene* (Pls. XII, XIII and figs. 20, 21, 22), to the Editors of *Parasitology* (figs. 28, 29, 30), to Professor R. Newstead (Pls. X, XI), to the Editors of the *Quarterly Journal of Microscopical Science* (figs. 5, 6, 7, 17), to Professor R. Hermes (fig. 12) and to Frederick A. Stokes Company (fig. 18).

Finally, I wish to acknowledge the very great assistance derived from the publications of Dr Howard, Dr Hewitt, Professor R. Newstead, and the Local Government Board.

G. S. G.-S.

CAMBRIDGE,
August 1913.

PREFACE TO THE SECOND EDITION

IN the first edition an attempt was made to collect, tabulate and examine critically the various facts and hypotheses relating to the life-histories, habits, and disease-carrying potentialities of non-bloodsucking flies, which had been published up to the end of the year 1912. Since that time much attention has been devoted to the subject, and several important contributions to our knowledge have been made.

In the present edition the work published during the year 1913 is treated in the same manner, and an account of some recent unpublished observations by the writer has been added.

In order to render it easy of access and as distinct and prominent as possible the description of the more recent work is contained in an Appendix, which also includes a summary of certain papers, which, the writer greatly regrets, were overlooked in preparing the first edition. Of these the most important was Bahr's work on *Dysentery in Fiji*. The subjects dealt with in the appendix are arranged in the same order as in the preceding chapters, and the reference to the page on which the subject was discussed previously is given in all cases.

The interest aroused by Niven's observations pointing to a relationship between the prevalence of flies and the mortality from summer diarrhœa has influenced the writer in devoting attention to the subject, and as a result of his study he now puts forward with some hesitation the suggestion that the annual diarrhœa epidemic in large cities is correlated in its time incidence, dimensions and severity with the weather conditions which influence the emergence, activities and numbers of flies. For the data relating to the meteorological conditions and diarrhœa mortalities in Birmingham and Manchester during a long series of years the writer is greatly indebted to Dr J. Robertson and Dr J. Niven, without whose generous assistance the mass of necessary information could not have been obtained. Mr Lynch very kindly placed the Cambridge weather records at the writer's disposal, and Dr A. J. Laird supplied the diarrhœa mortality notifications.

The writer is also very greatly indebted to Prof. J. M. R. Surcouf, of the National Museum of Natural History, Paris, for the loan of the excellent blocks from which the figures on Plate XXVII are reproduced.

G. S. G.-S.

CAMBRIDGE,
July 1914.

CONTENTS

LIST OF TEXT FIGURES

LIST OF PLATES

LIST OF CHARTS

CHAPTER I

INTRODUCTION

There would seem to have been a somewhat strong prejudice against flies as remotely as the time of the fourth plague of Moses, when "there came a grievous swarm of flies into the house of Pharaoh, and into his servants' houses, and into all the land of Egypt ; the land was corrupted by reason of the swarm of flies."

From time to time since that date various writers, usually without bringing forward any definite proofs, have connected swarms of flies with epidemics of various kinds, or with unhealthy seasons. Sydenham (1666), for example, remarked that if swarms of insects, especially house-flies, were abundant in summer, the succeeding autumn was unhealthy. Until recently, however, little trouble was taken to procure definite evidence in regard to their relationship to disease, practically nothing was known of their life-histories or habits, and many curious statements about them were unhesitatingly accepted. In 1824, for example, an interesting case of myiasis was reported in a lady, who after a prolonged course of earth eating, "became subject to constant vomiting, and produced a remarkable biological collection, in which, among many strange beasts, dipterous larvæ 'literally teemed,' larvæ, pupæ and imagines being ejected together. One realises the paucity of knowledge in the last century when one reads that it inspired 'a feeling of horror to see them (the larvæ) frisking along, occasionally expanding their jaws, and extending their talons,' and although the doctor himself witnessed the extrusion of these forms, it is impossible not to be a little sceptical of the patient's bona fides, when one reads that she invariably concluded by 'chanting the Litany at full length in a clear and beautiful voice'." (Lelean, 1904.)

The maggots of flies undoubtedly do useful work in devouring decaying matter of various kinds, but the flies themselves "do not display the sort of intelligence we appreciate, or the kind of beauty we admire, and as a few of the creatures somewhat annoy us, the whole Order is only too frequently included in the category of nuisances that we must submit to. It is therefore no wonder that flies are not popular and that few are willing to study them, or to collect them for observation." Thus wrote Sharp in 1899 (p. 439), but since that time many of the blood-sucking types, concerned in the transmission of protozoal diseases, have been accurately studied, and attention has been directed to some of the non-blood-sucking types. It has been proved that various species of the blood-sucking or *biting flies* are the necessary secondary hosts of the causative micro-organisms of various diseases affecting both men and animals. These diseases are due to protozoon (animal) parasites, which usually undergo developmental changes within the bodies of the flies, changes which are necessary for the completion of their life-cycles. Some of the most striking hygienic triumphs, as in making the Panama Canal Zone habitable and even healthy, have been due to the knowledge derived from the study of the habits of biting flies and their relation to disease.

Since non-biting flies cannot act as agents in spreading such diseases their study, until recently, has been neglected.

In this book an attempt has been made to place before the reader a summary of the more important experiments and observations which have been made, relating to the distribution of disease by *non-biting flies*.

During the latter part of the last century a number of papers were published dealing with this subject; a few contained accounts of careful observations, and a few produced evidence of an experimental nature, but the majority only offered surmises. Exact observations on the life-histories of flies, experiments on the ways in which they carry and distribute bacteria and the eggs of parasitic worms, and the collection of statistical data relating to their connection with disease have only been made within the last few years.

In 1895 Howard in the United States began to study the bionomics of the house-fly, and, soon recognizing its potentiality as a carrier of disease, has continued his observations up to the present time. The investigations relating to the outbreaks of typhoid fever in the military camps during the Spanish-American and South African wars further attracted attention to the subject in England and America. The work of Hewitt, Newstead and Austen, isolated observations by various writers at home and abroad, and the investigations carried out for the Local Government Board have added considerably to our knowledge and have helped to definitely establish some important facts.

Articles dealing with the disease carrying possibilities of the house-fly have been published recently in large numbers, and interest in the subject has spread to all parts of the world, so that we may hope within a few years to be in possession of accurate information relating to the connection between house-flies and the spread of various infectious diseases.

"In the United States a very active campaign is being waged on all sides against the house-fly, as it is considered to be a serious factor in the transmission of zymotic diseases, and as being synonymous with insanitary conditions. No small credit for this activity is due to the primary and continued efforts of Dr L. O. Howard, the Entomologist of the United States Department of Agriculture. As illustrating the popular feeling with regard to the fly campaign in the United States it may be mentioned that the Mayor of the capital of one of the States was elected almost solely on the strong stand which he had taken in advocating anti-fly measures. This sudden change of opinion, which has already affected and is reflected in the bye-laws relating to public health matters, is of more than ordinary interest, and is fully in keeping with the spirit of the age." (Hewitt, 1912, p. 4.) Howard (1911, p. xvi) has in fact proposed the name 'typhoid fly' as a substitute for the name 'house-fly,' now in general use. He admits that "strictly speaking the term 'typhoid fly' is open to some objection as conveying the erroneous idea that this fly is solely responsible for the spread of typhoid, but, considering that the creature is dangerous from every point of view, and that it is an important element in the spread of typhoid, it seems advisable to give it a name which is almost wholly justified and which conveys in itself the idea of serious disease. Another repulsive name that might be given to it is 'manure fly,' but recent researches have shown that it is not confined to manure as a breeding place, although perhaps the great majority of these flies are born in horse manure. For the end in view, 'typhoid fly' is considered the best name."

In the United States this name has been very generally adopted in the newspapers, and "it is undoubtedly true that people will fear and fight an insect bearing the name 'typhoid fly,' when they will ignore one called the 'house-fly,' which they have always considered a harmless insect."

Hewitt (1912, p. 106) states that "it has been proved that the house-fly plays an important part in the dissemination of certain of our most prevalent infectious diseases, when the necessary conditions are present," and Nuttall and Jepson (1909) regard the evidence relating to the spread of cholera and typhoid fever as "quite convincing."

Hitherto the house-fly (*Musca domestica*) has been mainly investigated since it occurs in all parts of the world, and is the species which is most commonly found in and round houses. Many other species, however, occasionally enter houses, or places where food is exposed for sale, and possibly act as carriers of disease. In regard to most of these little is known.

Up to the present the following facts have been definitely ascertained. The larvæ of many species of non-biting flies breed in human and animal excreta, or decaying animal and vegetable matter, and the adults frequent these substances and often feed upon them. Flies are therefore an indication of the presence of such insanitary substances in the neighbourhood of the houses in which they occur. They carry both in and on their bodies the putrefactive and fæcal bacteria acquired from the substances on which they feed, and, experimentally at least, can also carry and distribute many of the disease producing species of bacteria and the ova of parasitic worms. Since these bacteria and ova are present in the fæces of infected persons, flies *under suitable conditions*, mainly by infecting food substances, probably aid in the dissemination of the diseases these organisms produce.

It is scarcely necessary to point out that flies can only act as carriers of disease germs after they have come into contact with suitably infected materials, and that their opportunities for infecting themselves are in proportion to the care exercised by the community in removing such materials or rendering them harmless.

In military camps, where the conditions are often very favourable, typhoid fever seems to be disseminated by them, and the evidence relating to the part they may play in the spread of other diseases, such as infantile diarrhœa in temperate climates, and cholera, ophthalmia, and yaws in tropical countries, is very suggestive. Direct proof is, however, still almost lacking, and we have no reliable information concerning the extent to which they are responsible for the spread of any disease.

The larvæ of non-biting flies sometimes infest man, living under the skin or in wounds or natural cavities or in the intestinal canal.

It is certain that the house-fly is a potential disease carrier and a constant frequenter and disseminator of filth, but much remains to be done before Howard's name 'typhoid fly' or Hewitt's generalization can be completely justified. To both these investigators the greatest credit is due not only for the work they have done, but for the manner in which they have stimulated enquiry, by persistently bringing the subject to notice. Both, approaching the subject from the entomological standpoint, have based their conclusions in regard to disease mainly on evidence of an epidemiological character, and have apparently accepted the bacteriological evidence almost without criticism. From the bacteriological point of view, however, while the evidence relating to the carriage of pathogenic bacilli by experimentally infected flies is fairly conclusive, that relating to the presence of these micro-organisms in 'wild' flies is far from complete. The records are few, several of them are old, and only a small proportion reliable.

In the following chapters the information at present available on the habits and life-histories of non-biting flies, their capacity for carrying and distributing bacteria and parasitic ova, and their relation to various diseases is discussed, and the more important experimental evidence is given in detail. The reader can therefore make himself acquainted with the methods which have been adopted and the results which have been obtained, and perhaps gather some indications as to the lines on which future investigations should proceed.

Technical descriptions of species and details of bacteriological experiments are given in small type.

Several of the diseases, typhoid fever, cholera and infantile diarrhœa, which the house-fly is reputed to spread, are important ones. The problem of its relationship to such diseases can only be solved by the combined efforts of observers in various fields of work, and in different countries. Certain aspects of the problem must be left to specialists in entomology, bacteriology, mycology and helminthology, but sanitary officers, medical men and workers, who are not specialists in any of these branches of study, may render most important assistance. In every branch careful, prolonged and accurate study, with minute attention to details is necessary, but more particularly is this the case in regard to bacteriology. The difficulties attending the isolation and identification of pathogenic bacteria, particularly those belonging to the typhoid-colon group, from 'wild' flies are especially great, since allied, almost indistinguishable, types are frequently present in the intestines of flies. No diagnosis should therefore be accepted unless all the known tests for identification have been applied (see Chaps. XII, XIV).

With the knowledge now at our disposal of the habits of house-flies it should not be impossible to greatly diminish their numbers in some selected areas, where epidemic diarrhœa is usually prevalent, and thus definitely prove whether they are mainly responsible for the spread of this disease, or not. If they are proved to be responsible the application of suitable measures would save many thousands of lives annually.

Apart from the question of epidemic diarrhœa measures directed against flies and their breeding places would undoubtedly result in a vast improvement in the sanitary conditions of our towns and cities, and consequently in the health of the inhabitants.

The desirability of applying such measures in camps and temporary collections of dwellings, where large bodies of men are brought together, cannot be too strongly urged.

CHAPTER II

THE SPECIES OF NON-BLOOD-SUCKING FLIES FOUND IN HOUSES

In some tropical and subtropical countries house-flies (*Musca domestica*) are extraordinarily abundant, and the natives take so little notice of them that not only children but adults allow flies to settle in swarms about their eyes and seldom make any attempt to drive them away. Ophthalmia is common and under the conditions which prevail flies probably carry the germs directly from one person to another. In other parts of the world various species of flies appear to transmit the virus of yaws (Chapts. XVIII, XIX) in a similar manner. In temperate climates, however, the direct transference of disease germs from one individual to another cannot be so common, for the inhabitants of these countries have not acquired the same degree of indifference to the presence of flies on their persons. In these countries they are more likely to transmit disease by contaminating articles of food.

Since this book is mainly concerned with the danger from flies in temperate countries it has been thought best to consider first those species of non-biting flies which frequent houses and shops, where articles of food are exposed for sale.

The majority of non-biting flies, which at present appear to be of importance in the transmission of disease, belong to the Sub-order **Cyclorrhapha** of the Order **Diptera**, or two-winged flies.

The Order **Diptera** is composed of insects possessing two membranous, usually transparent, wings. Behind the wings is placed a pair of small stalk-like bodies terminating in small knobs—the halteres—frequently concealed beneath membranous hoods. The mouth parts are formed for sucking. The metamorphosis, or series of changes undergone during development, is very great, the larvæ or young forms which develop from eggs bearing no resemblance whatever to the perfect insects, being usually footless grubs or maggots.

The Order is divided into two Sub-orders, the **Cyclorrhapha** and the **Orthorrhapha.** The nature of the metamorphosis differentiates these two groups. In the **Cyclorrhapha** the larva does not escape from the larval skin at the last moult but shrinks within it, so that the larval skin, itself contracted and altered by an excretion of chitin, remains and forms a perfect protection for the enclosed organism or *pupa.* Such a pupa is described as *coarctate,* and the brown skin is called the *puparium.* This puparium, which is barrel shaped, has no marks except some faint circular rings and frequently a pair of projections from near one extremity. This sub-order is again divided into the **Aschiza,** in which the front of the head of the perfect fly shows no definite arched suture over the antennæ, and the **Schizophora** in most of which the frontal suture (see Fig. 2) is well marked and extends downwards along each side of the face, leaving a distinct *lunule* over the antennæ. Most of the important non-biting disease carrying flies belong to the latter group.

In the **Orthorrhapha** the pupa is a mummy-like object, or *pupa obtecta,* in which there is a crisp outer shell, formed in part by the adherent cases of the appendages of the future fly.

The external features of a fly.

In most of the flies considered in this book the body is composed of three easily recognizable divisions, termed respectively, head, thorax and abdomen.

The *head,* which is remarkable for its mobility, is connected with the thorax by a slender neck that permits the head to undergo semirotation, and carries the mouth parts, the visible portions being the *maxillary palps* and the *proboscis*, through which the fly sucks up the fluids on which it feeds. The upper part and sides of the head are mainly occupied by the large *compound eyes*. On the top of the head, in most of the flies with which we are dealing, the eyes are close together in the males and wider apart in the females, thus affording a ready means of distinguishing the sexes. During life the eyes are frequently of brilliant colours and variegate with stripes and spots; this condition disappears speedily after death, and it is uncertain

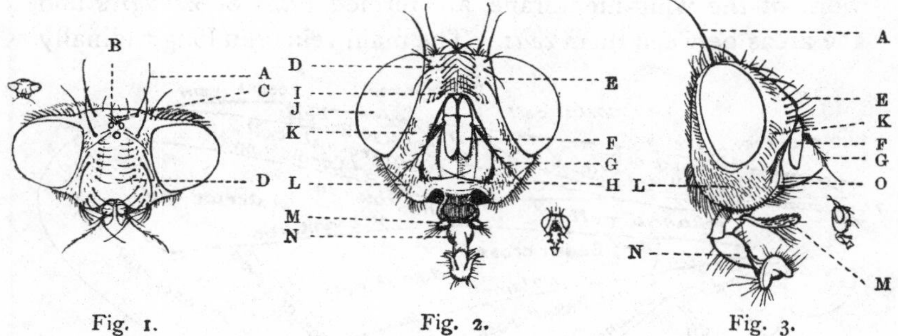

Fig. 1. Dorsal view.
Fig. 2. Front view.
Fig. 3. Side view of the head of the Flesh fly (*Sarcophaga carnaria*) (× 6). The actual sizes of the specimens are shown in the smaller figures.

A, vertical bristles; B, ocelli; C, vertex; D, frons, or front; E, fronto-orbital bristles; F, antenna (third segment); G, arista; H, face; I, frontal lunule (continued downwards on each side external to the antennæ to form a crescent-shaped scar); J, compound eye; K, cheek; L, jowl; M, maxillary palp; N, proboscis; O, vibrissa.

what the use of this colouration may be. In addition to the compound eyes many flies possess small *simple eyes*, or *ocelli*, which are usually three in number and set in a triangle, apex forwards, on the crown of the head. The *antennæ*, which are the principal means of classifying flies, are tactile and perhaps olfactory organs, generally placed between the eyes. They vary greatly in details of structure and may even differ in the sexes of the same species. The space between the eyes above the antennæ is the *front* or *frons*; that between the root of the antennæ and the upper margin of the mouth is the *face*; that behind and below the eye is the *cheek*[1].

In most of the flies here described each antenna consists of three dissimilar segments, the terminal one being much produced ventrally and bearing far back on its true upper surface a bristle or *arista*, which may be bare, or furnished with hairs variously arranged.

The *thorax*, or middle division of the body, consists of three segments firmly united together and carries the single pair of *wings*, the *halteres*, and the three pairs of *legs*. The dark lines running through the wings and forming the supporting framework of the wing-membrane, are termed *veins* or *nervures* and the areas between them *cells*. The main veins run longitudinally

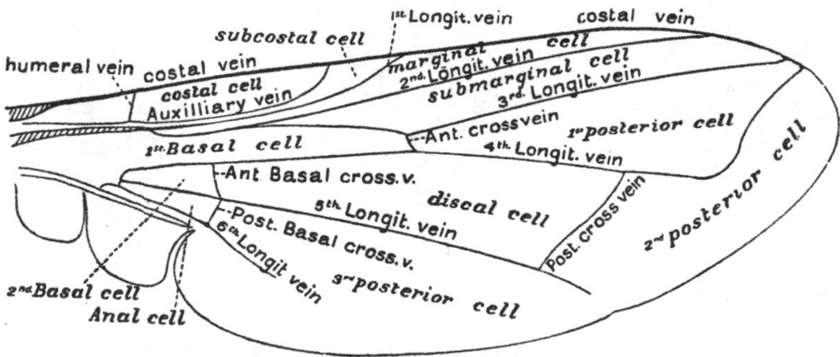

Fig. 4. Right wing of house-fly (*M. domestica*).

from the base to the tip of the wing, but there are also some cross veins, three being placed in the central part of the wing, one very short the others longer, which are clearly shown in the accompanying illustration, in which the small cross vein is seen to be about in the centre of the wing. The differences in the arrangements of the veins afford ready means of distinguishing the common house frequenting species. On the hind margin of the wing, near the base, there is often a more or less free lobe called the *alula*. Internal to the posterior lobule of the wing there are often placed one or two smaller membranous plates, known as the *squama* and *antisquama*. "The *squama* is thicker than the rest of the wing and is attached posteriorly to the

[1] Wingate (1906, p. 10) calls "the parts below the cheeks and the eyes," the *Jowls*.

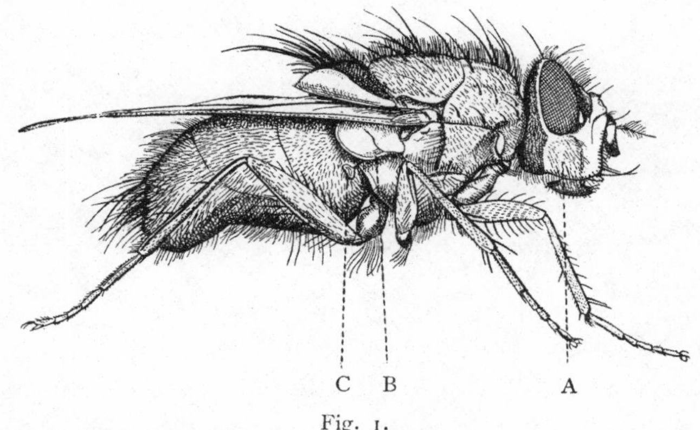

Fig. 1.

Side view of Blow-fly, *C. erythrocephala* (× 5). A, cheek (jowl); B, squama; C, halter.

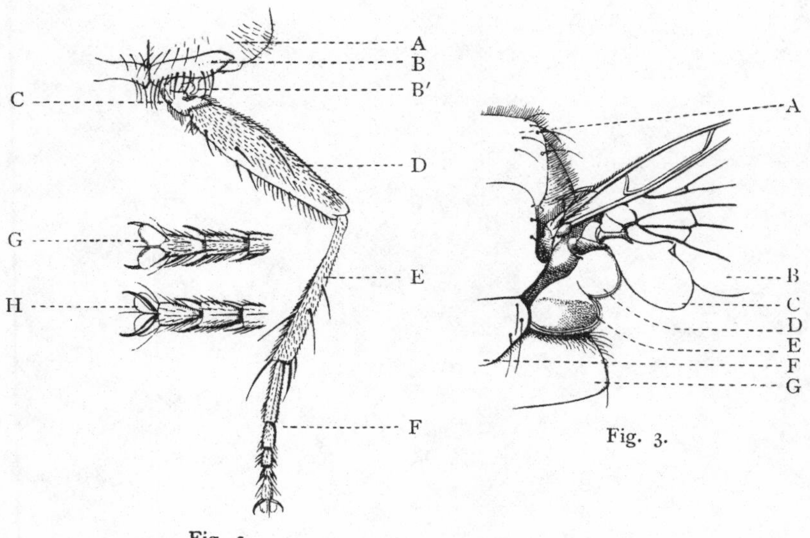

Fig. 2.

Fig. 3.

Fig. 2. Right middle leg of Flesh fly, *S. carnaria* (× 6). A, part of thorax; B, coxa; B′, chitinous spur fitting into groove in C, trochanter; D, femur; E, tibia; F, tarsus with five segments; G, under surface of terminal segments of tarsus showing pulvilli (× 12); H, upper surface showing claws.

Fig. 3. Right side of thorax and part of right wing of Blow-fly, *C. erythrocephala* (× 7). A, anterior part of thorax; B, anal angle of wing; C, alula; D, antisquama; E, squama; F, scutellum; G, abdomen.

wing root" (Hewitt, 1907, p. 412). "Possibly these facilitate the opening and closing of the wings" (Alcock, 1911, p. 37). Behind the wings the pair of *halteres*—commonly called balancers or poisers—is placed, the most characteristic of all the dipterous structures. They are believed to be the homologues of the hind wings, though their exact functions are far from clear. "Each consists of a conical base on which are a number of chordonotal sense-organs, and on this base is mounted a slender rod, at the end of which a small hemispherical knob is attached" (Hewitt, 1907, p. 413). They are provided with muscles at the base and can, like the wings, execute most rapid vibrations. In the *Muscidæ* the squama covers the halter like a hood. Notice should also be taken of the large bristles (if they exist) on the thorax as they are of importance in the classification of some groups.

Each *leg* consists of five segments—*coxa*, *trochanter*, *femur*, *tibia* and *tarsus*—the latter being composed of five segments The last tarsal segment carries a pair of *claws*, and below them there is usually a pair of membranous pads or *pulvilli*; between these there is often a small median appendix. "The pulvilli are covered on their ventral surfaces with innumerable, closely set, secreting hairs by means of which the fly is able to walk in any position on highly polished surfaces" (Hewitt, 1907, p. 414).

The *abdomen*, or hindmost division of the body, is composed of several segments, and generally shows lighter or darker markings, useful in distinguishing one species from another. "In the house-fly the total number of segments which compose the abdomen is eight in the male, and nine in the female. The visible portion consists apparently of four segments." Actually there are five segments but the first is much reduced and fused with the second. "The segments succeeding the fifth are greatly reduced in the male, and in the female form the

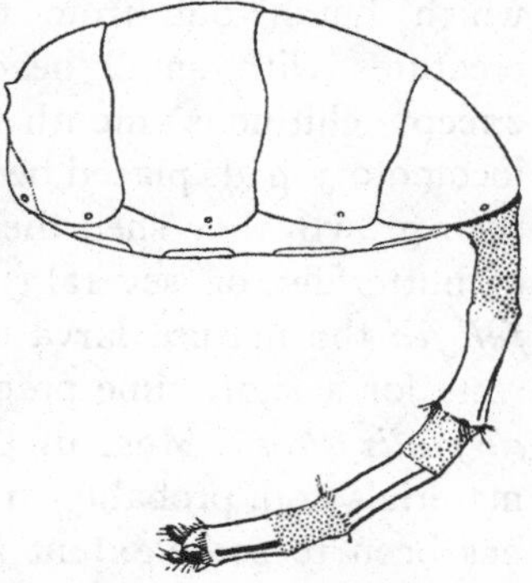

Fig. 5. Abdomen of female house-fly showing the extended ovipositor. (After Hewitt, 1907, Pl. XXIII, fig. 8.)

tubular *ovipositor*, which, in repose, is telescoped within the abdomen." The chitinous portions of the *male armature* are of great interest to the anatomist, and are of considerable importance in the classification of some groups of flies, but are too complex for consideration here.

Reproduction.

Most flies undergo a complete metamorphosis in which there are four well marked stages. These stages in the life-cycle are:

1. The egg.
2. The larva or maggot stage.
3. The pupa or chrysalis stage.
4. The imago or perfect fly.

"Most flies lay *eggs*, which are usually deposited, in a manner which simulates conscious foresight, in a medium or in a pabulum suitable to the future larva or maggot. The eggs are large and often sticky so as to adhere in masses. Some flies such as the flesh flies (*Sarcophaga*) give birth to small living larvæ" (Alcock, 1911, p. 41).

The *larvæ* of the principal group of flies under discussion, which hatch out from the eggs, are segmented worm-like creatures with small heads and without obvious appendages except chitinous mouth hooks. They move by means of locomotory pads placed beneath the posterior segments. During their growth they shed their skins or moult, like the caterpillars of butterflies, on several (three in house-flies) occasions. When *full-fed* the mature larva usually crawls to some dry place and rests for a short time preparatory to changing into the *pupal or chrysalis state*. Most of these larvæ feed on various decaying materials and, probably in consequence of this fact, their study has been to some extent neglected. Recent observations have shown that some of them are affected by the heat produced by the fermentation of the substance in which they are living, others by light, and others by the condition of the food supply.

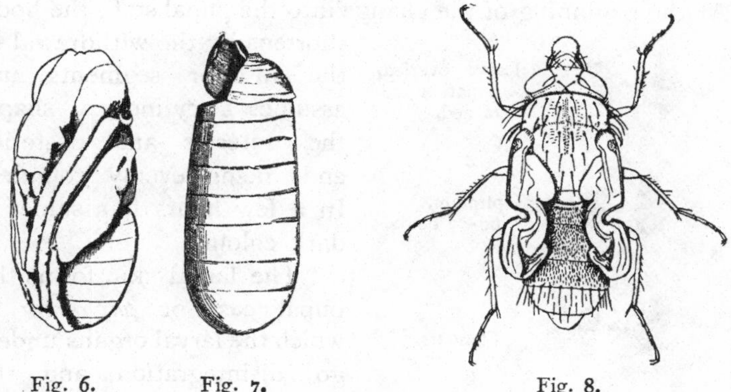

Fig. 6. Fig. 7. Fig. 8.

Fig. 6. 'Nymph' of *M. domestica* dissected out of pupal case about 30 hours after pupation. (After Hewitt, 1908, Pl. XXX, fig. 10.)

Fig. 7. Pupal case (puparium) of *M. domestica* from which the imago has emerged thus lifting off the anterior end or 'cap.' (After Hewitt, 1908, Pl. XXX, fig. 15.

Fig. 8. Blow-fly (*C. erythrocephala*) a short time after emerging from puparium showing unexpanded wings, and ptilinum protruding in front of the head.

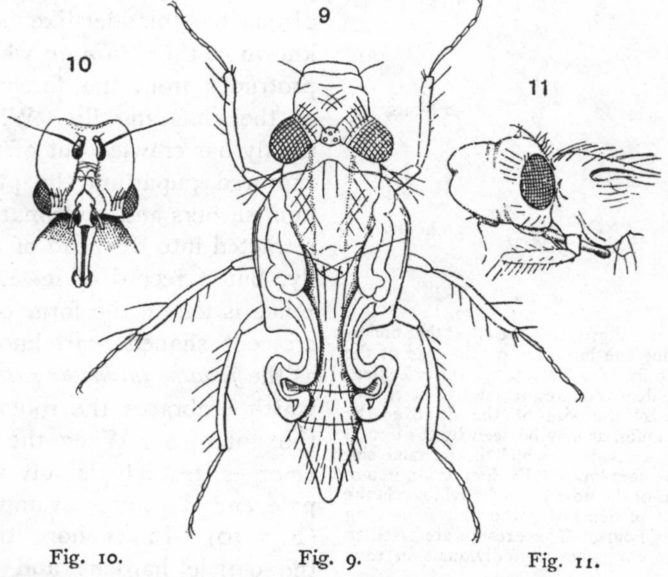

Fig. 10. Fig. 9. Fig. 11.

Fig. 9. An Anthomyid fly immediately after emerging from the puparium showing the greatly distended ptilinum and unexpanded wings.

Figs. 10 and 11. Ventral and side views of the head of the same fly.

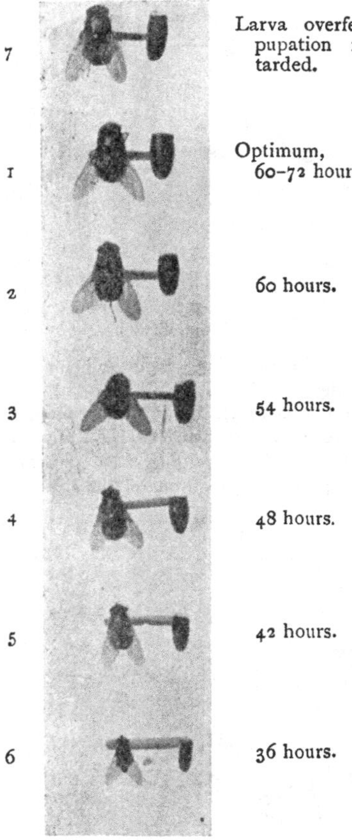

Fig. 12.—Illustrating the effect that underfeeding the larva has on the size of the adult fly (*Lucilia cæsar*). Overfeeding, if it does not result fatally, does not increase the size of the fly over the Optimum, as may be seen by the uppermost individual, which is the same size as the next lower individual or Optimum. Each of the next lower individuals is the result of decreasing the time of feeding by six hours. These results are based on a large number of individuals in each case.

At the beginning of the change into the pupal state the body shortens by the withdrawal of the anterior segments and assumes a cylindrical shape, the anterior and posterior ends being evenly rounded. In a few hours it assumes a dark colour.

"The larval skin forms the pupal case or *puparium* in which the larval organs undergo disintegration and the organs of the future fly are built up."

The mature fly or *imago* escapes from the puparium by pushing off the end of the puparium by means of a distensible bladder-like sac, known as the *ptilinum*, which protrudes from the forehead of the emerging fly. When the fly has crawled out of the ruptured puparium the ptilinum shrinks and is ultimately retracted into the head of the fly, but a record of its existence is left in the form of a crescent shaped scar, known as the *frontal lunule or suture*, which embraces the roots of the antennæ. When the fly emerges its body is soft and pale and its wings crumpled (Fig. 10). In a short time the cuticle hardens and the wings become fully expanded. After the cuticle has hardened the fly grows no more. Young flies are the same size as old flies. Occasionally flies are met with which are smaller than the normal individuals of the species. This is usually due to insufficient or unsuitable food during the larval stage. Hermes experimentally investigated this question and one of his plates is reproduced showing the effect of starvation and of overfeeding during the larval period[1].

Classification of house-frequenting flies.

In the following pages the adult forms, larvæ, life-histories, habits and distribution of the common house-frequenting non-biting flies will be very briefly described, but for the sake of reference their zoological classification is briefly given in the following table, the families and species being arranged in the apparent order of their hygienic importance.

Order **Diptera.**

Sub-order **Cyclorrhapha.**

Family	Genus and species	Common name
Muscidæ	*Musca domestica*	House-fly
	Musca corvina	Raven fly
	Calliphora erythrocephala	Blow-fly or blue-bottle
	,, *vomitoria*	,, ,, ,,
	Lucilia cæsar	Green-bottle
	Pollenia rudis	Cluster fly
	Muscina stabulans	
	**Stomoxys calcitrans*	Stable fly
Anthomyidæ	*Fannia canicularis*	Lesser house-fly
	,, *scalaris*	Latrine fly
	Anthomyia radicum	Root fly
Sarcophagidæ	*Sarcophaga carnaria*	Flesh fly
Sepsidæ	*Sepsis punctum*	Dung fly
	Piophila casei	Cheese fly
Cordyluridæ	*Scatophaga stercoraria*	Yellow dung fly
Drosophilidæ	*Drosophila fenestrarum*	Fruit fly

Sub-order **Orthorrhapha.**

Family	Genus and species	Common name
Psychodidæ	*Psychoda* sp.	Moth fly or Owl midge
Scenopinidæ	*Scenopinus fenestralis*	Window fly

* *Stomoxys calcitrans* is a blood-sucking fly and is included in this list because it is so often mistaken for the house-fly.

[1] It must be clearly understood that the foregoing account refers only to the muscid house-frequenting flies. For the life-histories of other dipterous insects the reader is referred to text-books on general entomology.

The relative frequency of different species of flies in houses.

During the last few years a number of workers have examined the flies caught in houses in fly traps or on fly papers, and have conclusively shown that the species most commonly caught is the house-fly (*M. domestica*). In considering such results it must be remembered several species are not attracted to traps or papers and are therefore not taken into consideration in such statistics. Most of these, however, are probably of little importance.

Hewitt (1910, p. 349) during a number of years made observations in town and suburban houses and country houses and cottages, and found that in the former *M. domestica* was by far the commonest fly. "But whereas *M. domestica* may be the only species in warm places where food is present, such as restaurants and kitchens, in other rooms of the house *F. canicularis*, the lesser house-fly, increases in proportion and often predominates. In country houses the proportions vary by the intrusion of *Stomoxys calcitrans*." In certain country houses *S. calcitrans* may form 50 % of all the flies, the rest being chiefly *F. canicularis* and *A. radicum*.

The following records are taken from a 'fly census' made by Hewitt in 1907, and may be taken as illustrative of the proportional abundance of the different species in different situations.

TABLE I.

Place	*M. domestica*	*F. canicularis*	Other species
Restaurant, Manchester	1869 (99 %)	14 (1 %)	2
Kitchen, suburban house, Manchester	682 (97 %)	7 (1 %)	14 (2 %)
,, ,, ,, Lancashire	581 (67 %)	265 (30 %)	14 (2 %)
Bedroom, suburban house	1 (3 %)	33 (87 %)	4 (10 %)
Stable ,, ,,	22 (12 %)	153 (81 %)	14 (7 %)
	3155 (85·8 %)	472 (12·8 %)	48 (1·3 %)

These figures are small and relate to different localities in the same neighbourhood, but larger figures are available of the collections formed by various workers in England and by Howard in the United States in houses and places where food is exposed. The results are recorded in the following table.

TABLE 2.

Place	Flies examined	*M. domestica*	*F. canicularis*	Other species	Observer
United States*	23,087	22,808 (98·8 %)	81 (·3 %)	198 (·8 %)	Howard (1912, p. 235)
London	35,000†	28,350‡ (82 %)	6950‡ (17 %)	700‡ (1 %)	Hamer
London	6,000§	3,540‡ (59 %)	1440‡ (24 %)	1020‡ (17 %)	,,
Manchester	8,553	8,196 (95 %)	293 (3 %)	64 (1 %)	Niven
Birmingham	24,562	22,360 (91 %)	1154 (4·7 %)	1058 (4·3 %)	Robertson (1909)
,,	43·430	30,325 (64 %)	9482 (21 %)	3623 (8 %)	,, (1910)
Manchester	3,856	3,374‡ (87·5 %)	443‡ (11·5 %)	38‡ (1 %)	Hewitt (1910, p. 350)
	144,488	118,953 (82 %)	19843 (14 %)	6701 (4 %)	

* These were collected on sticky fly papers in kitchens and pantries in the States of Massachusetts, New York, Pennsylvania, Virginia, Florida, Georgia, Louisiana, Nebraska, and California and examined in Washington by Mr Coquillet.

† Flies caught in London on four fly papers exposed in similar situations.

§ Flies caught in London in four fly traps.

‡ Figures calculated from the percentages given.

Of the whole total of flies examined by these workers 82 % were *M. domestica*. We have seen that the relative proportion of *M. domestica* to other species varies in different places in the same district and even in different rooms of the same house, and the two sets of figures given by Hamer seem to indicate that different results may be obtained by examining flies caught by different methods. Of the 35,000 flies caught by him on fly papers 82 % were *M. domestica*, whereas of the 6000 caught in balloon traps only 59 % belonged to this species.

Newstead (1907, p. 6) investigating the prevalence of different species says *M. domestica* "is by far the commonest species met with, and quite 90 % of the flies which infest houses in Liverpool are of this kind." Austen (1909, p. 4) examining flies caught in various centres in London also came to the conclusion that this was by far the commonest species.

All the records that are available emphasize the fact that at the height of the fly season *M. domestica* largely outnumbers all the other flies caught in traps or on fly papers in houses in towns, and by this means of obtaining statistics *F. canicularis* is the next most common, forming about 14 % of the flies caught.

In the earlier part of the year, however, *F. canicularis* is the most common species. For example Austen (1911, p. 12) records that in the kitchen of a house in Leeds fly papers in May, June and July caught 381 specimens of *F. canicularis* and only 48 specimens of *M. domestica.*

Descriptions of common house frequenting flies.

The figures illustrating each species have been very carefully drawn from accurately identified specimens so as to emphasize the principal features. In species showing marked sexual differences both males and females are illustrated. In the case of those species in which the sexes closely resemble each other, but can be easily differentiated by the space separating the compound eyes, a sketch of the head of the sex not figured is given also. In each species the antenna is illustrated as seen when the specimen is viewed from the side. In most cases the figure shows the fly magnified three times, but for the sake of clearness a life-sized sketch of the insect in the resting position is added.

In all cases the fly is described and illustrated as seen under a low power (F. 55) of a Zeiss binocular dissecting microscope with the head pointing towards the window. This uniform method has been adopted because in many species the markings appear totally different, when viewed from various directions.

No attempt has been made to give an exhaustive description of each insect, only the most important and characteristic features being mentioned. Moreover, those features, such as the venation of the wings, which can be clearly appreciated from the figures, have been omitted in the descriptions.

It is hoped that with the aid of the illustrations and descriptions the species mentioned may be approximately identified, but it should be clearly understood that the aid of an entomologist, interested in the Diptera, is necessary in order to make certain of identification, especially in doubtful cases.

Such of the habits of the adults as seem to be of interest and importance in relation to the possibility of the distribution of disease-producing bacteria are shortly described, and a brief account of the life-history is added in most cases. The larval habits of *F. canicularis*, *F. scalaris*, and *L. cæsar* are of special importance, and are more fully dealt with. In the case of *M. domestica* special chapters are devoted to the life-history and to the anatomy and habits of the adult.

It has been thought desirable to give, in later chapters, detailed descriptions of certain important species of foreign flies which cause myiasis or apparently spread disease, since it is difficult for observers to consult communications in journals and reports of societies.

Musca domestica L. The common house-fly.

The general colour is mouse grey. (Pl. II, fig. 1.)

Length. 6—7 mm.; span of wings 13—15 mm.

Head. In ♂ the eyes are separated by an area equal to one-fifth to one-fourth the width of the head, and in ♀ by an area equal to one-third. Frontal stripe dark velvety brown in ♂, velvety black with reddish tinge, narrow below and very broad above in ♀. Frontal margin of eye white in ♂, almost obliterated by frontal stripe in ♀. Cheeks and face silky white to yellow, 'shot' with brown. Antennæ brown; aristæ black and feathered. Palps black.

Thorax. Grey, marked by four equally broad dark longitudinal stripes, most clearly defined in front. Scutellum grey with blackish sides. Some long bristles on sides of thorax and scutellum.

Wings. Clear, but yellowish at base. The end of the 4th longitudinal vein bent sharply upwards so as nearly to meet the vein above it. Squamæ large, opaque, yellowish. Halteres yellow and covered by squamæ.

Legs. Blackish brown.

Abdomen. The sides of the basal half in ♂, and frequently in ♀, ochraceous buff, and somewhat transparent. The posterior segments brownish grey, with yellowish shimmer, and bearing a few slender bristles. A longitudinal brown band usually occupies the centre of the anterior segments. Looked at from the dorsal surface apparently four segments are visible. In reality the visible segments are five in number, but the first can only be detected with difficulty owing to its being much reduced in size and fused with the second. In the ♀ the long ovipositor formed by the posterior segments may sometimes be seen, but is usually telescoped in the abdomen.

Musca domestica is probably the most widely distributed insect to be found; the animal most commonly associated with man, whom it appears to have followed over the entire earth. It extends from the sub-polar regions to the tropics, where it occurs in enormous numbers.

Flies very closely resembling the house-fly.

Hewitt (1910, p. 352) states that "in India two species of flies closely allied to *M. domestica* are found—*Musca domestica* sub-sp. *determinata* Walker and *M. enteniata*, both of which, on account of their close resemblance to *M. domestica* and the similarity of their breeding habits, are frequently mistaken for it.

(1) *M. domestica* sub-sp. *determinata* Walker.

"This Indian variety of the house-fly was first described by Walker (1856) from the East Indies. His description is as follows:

'Black, with a hoary covering; head with a white covering; frontalia broad, black, narrower towards the feelers; eyes bare; palpi and feelers black; chest with four black stripes; abdomen cinereous, with a large tawny spot at each side at the base; legs black; wings slightly grey, with a tawny tinge at the base; præbranchial vein forming a very obtuse angle at its flexure, very slightly bent inwards from thence to the tip; lower cross vein almost straight; alulæ whitish, with pale yellow borders; halteres tawny.'

"In appearance and size it is very similar to *M. domestica.* Its breeding habits are also very similar. Aldridge (1904) states that at certain seasons of the year it is present in enormous numbers. The method of disposal of night-soil is to bury it in trenches about one foot or less in depth. From one-sixth of a cubic foot of soil taken from a trench at Meerut and placed in a cage 4042 flies were hatched. Lieut. Dwyer collected 500 from a cage covering three square feet of a trench at Mhow. Specimens in the British Museum collection were obtained from the hospital kitchens, and Smith found them in a ward at Benares."

(2) *Musca enteniata* Bigot.

This fly has a distribution somewhat similar to the last species, and like it has a marked resemblance to *M. domestica.*

Bigot (1887) says the frons is narrow but the eyes are well separated; antennæ and palps black; face white; thorax black with large longitudinal grey bands; sides greyish. Abdomen yellow with a dorsal black band; feet black. Fourth longitudinal vein bent with slightly rounded angle.

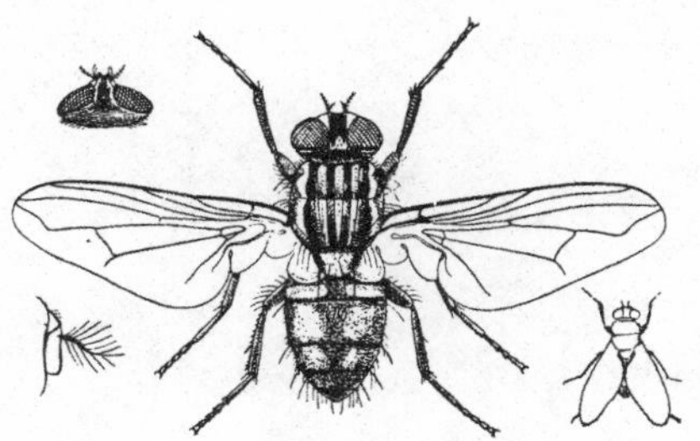

Fig. 1.

House-fly, *Musca domestica*, male (×3). Head of female, dorsal view. Antenna. Natural size, resting position.

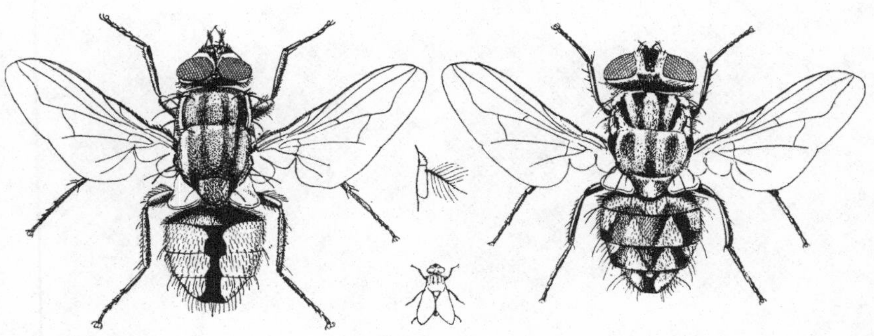

Fig. 2. Fig. 3.

Raven fly, *Musca corvina* (×5). Fig. 2. Male. Fig. 3. Female. Antenna. Natural size, resting position.

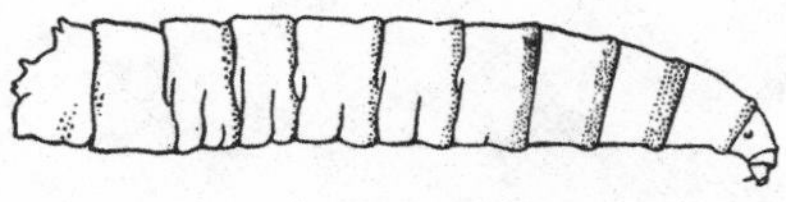

Fig. 4.

Full-grown larva of Blow-fly, *C. erythrocephala* (×3).

Hewitt says Smith obtained specimens from a hospital ward at Benares and bred it from human and cow fæces. Hewitt (1910, p. 353) received specimens from Aden, and Balfour (1908) in Khartoum bred it from human excrement and stable refuse.

Country flies closely resembling house-flies.

Though the house-fly sometimes occurs in large numbers away from the dwellings of man it is probable that the flies usually found under such conditions are not house-flies but species closely resembling it. Writing on this subject Howard (1912, p. 2) makes the following statement. "In the family Tachinidæ, a group composed almost entirely of species which lay their eggs upon other living insects, there are many species which almost precisely resemble the grey-and-black striped house-fly. In the family Dexidæ, of similar habits, there are also many species which closely resemble the house-fly. In the family Sarcophagidæ, which includes most of the so-called flesh flies, the species of which either live in carrion or excreta or in dead insects or in putrid matter, and are occasionally parasitic, as in the species which breed in the egg masses of grasshoppers, there are also many species hardly to be distinguished from Musca. There is another great family, the Anthomyidæ, which has many species which closely resemble the house-fly, and give rise to many mistakes in identity. Then too, in the family Muscidæ itself there are many genera of similar habits and similar appearance." He finally sums up by giving a simple method of differentiating these groups. "*Musca domestica* has four black lines on the back of its thorax. All Sarcophagidæ have three such black lines. Most Tachinidæ have four such lines, but the Tachinidæ have the bristle of the antenna smooth, whereas in *Musca domestica* this bristle is feathered. From all the Anthomyidæ, *Musca domestica* is at once separated by the bent vein near the tip of the wing. Moreover, *Musca domestica* has no bristles on the abdomen except at the tip which separates it from all others except some Tachinids and many Anthomyids, but from these it is separated by the characters given above."

Except certain species of the Anthomyidæ, which are easily

distinguished, very few members of the families mentioned, difficult to distinguish from *M. domestica,* enter houses. Consequently in collections from houses *M. domestica* can be identified fairly easily from other species.

Musca corvina F. The raven fly.

This fly closely resembles the house-fly (*M. domestica*) in general appearance, but the male has a yellow abdomen with a very distinct black longitudinal stripe, and the female a chequered abdomen. (Pl. II, figs. 2 and 3.)

Length. 6 mm.; span of wings 12 mm.

Head. In the ♂ the eyes almost meet, but in the ♀ are separated by an area equal to one-third of the diameter of the head. The frontal stripe is black, the frontal margins of the eyes, cheeks and face white. Antennæ dark. Arista feathered except the terminal one-fourth.

Thorax. In ♂ dark grey, with poorly marked darker longitudinal stripes; in ♀ lighter grey with the longitudinal darker stripes better marked, especially at the anterior part. There are long black bristles on the sides and on the scutellum.

Wings. Clear, but slightly yellow near the base. Squama whitish and more opaque. Halteres hidden under squama.

Legs. Black.

Abdomen. In ♂ bright yellow with a black median longitudinal band, of varying width; in ♀ dark and grey markings.

This fly frequently hibernates in country houses.

The larvæ live in excreta, especially horse manure. *M. corvina* only lays 24 eggs, which are larger than those of the house-fly, and the larvæ are said to develop very rapidly, so that the fly comes to maturity sooner than *M. domestica,* thus counterbalancing the low power of fecundity.

Calliphora erythrocephala Mg. The blow-fly or blue-bottle.

This is a large stoutly built fly, of metallic dark blue colour, which produces a loud buzzing sound during flight. (Pl. III, fig. 1.)

Length. 12 mm.; span of wings 25 mm.

Head. The eyes, which are red, are close together in the ♂ being separated by an area equal to one-tenth of the diameter of the head. In the ♀ they are separated by an area equal to one-third of the diameter of the head. The frontal stripe is black, the frontal margins of the eyes and upper parts of the cheeks whitish. The

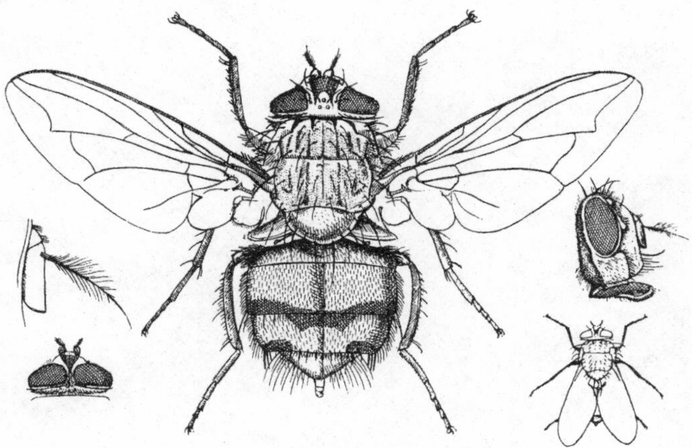

Fig. 1.

Blow-fly or Blue-bottle, *Calliphora erythrocephala*, female (× 3). Antenna. Male head, dorsal view. Side view of head. Natural size, resting position.

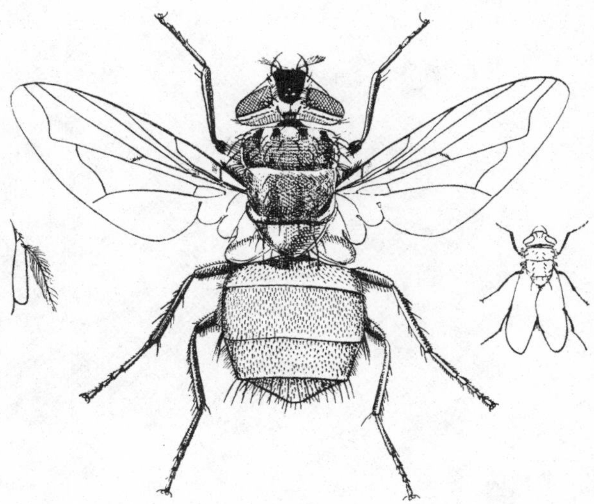

Fig. 2.

Blow-fly or Blue-bottle, *Calliphora vomitoria*, female (× 3). Antenna. Natural size, resting position.

jowls reddish with black hairs. The upper portion of the antenna dark grey, the lower joint and arista black. The upper portion of the arista is feathered, but the terminal one-fourth bare.

Thorax. Bluish grey, with indistinct darker blue longitudinal markings, and covered with numerous short black hairs, and longer black bristles. The longest of these are situated on the scutellum (see Pl. I, fig. 1).

Wings. Clear; squama opaque, yellowish white, and covers the halteres which are rather small.

Legs. Black, and covered with hairs and bristles. Pulvilli prominent.

Abdomen. Paler blue than thorax with darker blue, indistinct markings especially on second and third segments. The anterior three-quarters of each segment is covered by white pubescence.

According to Hermes (1911), this fly is not greatly attracted to light. It frequently enters houses, and is apt to lay its eggs on cold meat and other substances and to walk over any foods which may be exposed, stopping at intervals to suck the fluid parts. Outside the house it frequents decaying animal and vegetable matter and excrement on which it feeds and lays its eggs, and often visits fruit and meat exposed for sale. According to Porchinsky the female fly lays from 450 to 600 eggs.

The *egg* measures 1·4 to 1·5 mm. in length, "and has the form of an elongated ellipsoid, which is smaller at its anterior and broader at its posterior end. Its long axis is slightly curved, so that its ventral surface is convex and its dorsal surface flat, or even slightly concave" (Lowne, 1895, p. 678).

The *larva* when full-grown measures 18 mm. and "is a soft-skinned, cylindrical, wedge shaped worm, gradually increasing in diameter from before backwards, and truncated behind obliquely, so that the posterior extremity exhibits a concave surface, which looks upwards and backwards, within which the great posterior spiracles are situated" (Lowne, p. 32). There are twelve well marked visible segments, the fourth to the tenth showing foot-pads beneath. "Each segment has a thickened anterior border, covered by short recurved spines and sensory papillæ. The spines apparently prevent a retrograde movement in burrowing." The posterior end is surrounded by six pairs of tubercles, and a seventh pair is situated on the ventral surface posterior to the anus. Pl. II, fig. 4. Before pupating the larva ceases to feed, generally seeks a place of safety, and becomes languid and motionless. Before resting they often burrow a short distance into the ground. The *pupæ* are barrel shaped and dull red in colour.

According to Hewitt (1912, p. 48) the eggs hatch out "from eight to twenty hours after deposition"; the larval life, composed of three stages, the first and second lasting twenty-four hours and the third six days, is passed in seven and a half to eight days, and the pupal stage lasts fourteen days.

Calliphora vomitoria L. Blue-bottle.

This fly very closely resembles *C. erythrocephala* in size, general shape and colouration. Only the points of difference will therefore be recorded. (Pl. III, fig. 2.)

Head. Frontal stripe black with reddish tinge. *Jowls black or dark grey with red hairs.*

Thorax. Dark blue with very indistinct markings except near the head, where there are three lighter patches.

Abdomen. Dark metallic blue without distinct markings.

The habits of this species are similar to those of *C. erythrocephala*, but the fly is not nearly so abundant. Both these flies may be attracted into dark places by odours.

Both *C. erythrocephala* and *C. vomitoria* occasionally deposit their eggs in wounds in living animals, and more rarely in the nostrils (see Chapter XXII).

According to Howard (1911, p. 254) a smaller species *Phormio terrænovæ* Desv. is widespread in the United States, and is occasionally found in houses.

Lucilia cæsar L. Green-bottle.

This is a stoutly built fly resembling the blow-fly in general shape, but it is smaller, and its colour is shining metallic green. (Pl. IV, fig. 1.)

Length. 10 mm. Span of wings 18 mm.

Head. In ♂ the eyes, which are reddish, nearly meet below the vertex, but in the ♀ are separated by an area equal to one-third of the width of the head. Frontal stripe black, frontal margin of eye and cheeks silvery white. Vibrissæ large. Antennæ black; arista feathered, black.

Thorax. Metallic green, without markings, but covered with numerous very short black hairs; long black bristles especially at the sides, and at the posterior end of the scutellum.

Wings. Clear; squama opaque and yellowish white. Halteres small and covered by squama.

Legs. Black; pulvilli well marked.

Abdomen. Metallic green, and covered with small black hairs; many long black bristles on terminal segments, especially on their posterior edges.

This fly, which is the type of a common and widely distributed family characterized by its shining metallic green or blue colour, is not very frequently found in houses.

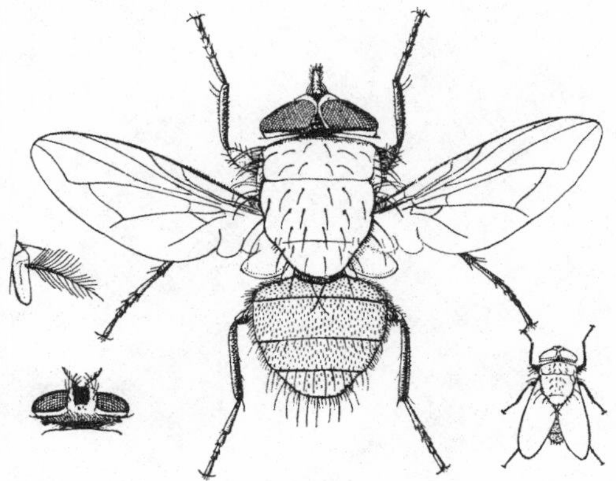

Fig. 1.

Green-bottle, *Lucilia cæsar*, male (× 3). Antenna. Female head, dorsal view. Natural size, resting position.

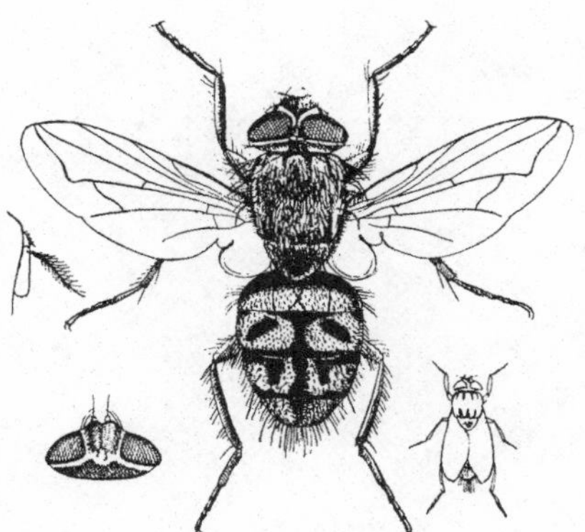

Fig. 2.

Cluster fly, *Pollenia rudis*, male (× 3). Antenna. Female head, dorsal view. Natural size, resting position.

Hermes (1911), who very carefully observed these flies, and made numerous experiments with them, came to the conclusion that they are more strongly attracted to light than many of the allied species, and hence if by chance one of these flies finds its way into the house, it soon escapes through an open window.

Flies of this family are very commonly found about dead animals, especially stale fish, excreta and other decomposing substances.

The *eggs* are "cylindrical, rounded at both ends and slightly curved, smooth and white." Hermes states that they are deposited in irregular masses on the softer portions of decaying fish, etc., e.g. around the eyes, around the anus and nostrils, and on abrasions, and on the under sides of carcases. "This is due to the presence of much liquid food at these particular portions, which the adults suck up while depositing the eggs." The eggs are also laid on excreta and decaying matter of all kinds. Hewitt (1910, p. 361) says: "The chief breeding place on which I have found it in this country is on the backs of sheep. It is one of the destructive species of 'maggots' of sheep."

Larvæ hatch in from 8—18 hours. When the eggs have been laid on carcases "the young larvæ at once eat into the softer parts, attacking the viscera, and later consuming the muscular portions." For example an exposed "fish is eaten clean to skin and bone, the skin remaining as a mere shell; this too would be eaten to the scales were the entire surface sufficiently moist. This is evident because the portion of skin nearest the earth, where it is moist, is invariably eaten away, leaving a hole on the under side, which incidentally allows a concealed means of escape during migration." The actual feeding period varies, according to Hermes (p. 54), from two to two and a half days and over. When full fed the larvæ measure 10—11 mm. and very closely resemble those of *C. erythrocephala* in size and general appearance.

Hermes, studying the larvæ living under natural conditions on dead fish cast up on the shore, states that before pupating the larvæ migrate from the carcase on which they have been feeding.

"Migrating wholly depends on the food supply. If the fish is large enough, and the number of larvæ is not too great, migration takes place in from one and a half to three days, during which time the larvæ have reached their full growth. If the number of larvæ is large in proportion to the fish, migration takes place earlier."

"On leaving the remains, the larvæ immediately burrow into the sand below or close to the fish. The great majority burrow just beneath, going down two to six inches into the sand and remaining there temporarily. This migration may take place at any time during the day or night, though the tactics vary for these periods. Burrowing temporarily just beneath the fish carcase during the day not only affords protection from the intense heat of the sun, but also from birds. On cloudy days when migration sometimes takes place away from the fish, the sandpipers, in numbers, feed on the plump migrating larvæ......During the night, or when the sand is cooled, migration from beneath the remains takes place, and it is then that the larvæ travel a greater distance—fifteen, twenty feet or over—and then again burrow. Larvæ that were kept indoors in boxes were observed to repeat this performance several nights in succession, each time burrowing for the day. The sand in the laboratory was not heated by the sun, yet the larvæ followed the normal habit and were characteristically active at night."

The interval between migration and pupation varies from two to four days or over. "With individuals reared indoors this interval varies with the degree of moisture—extreme moisture retarding pupation, as also does extreme dryness......Temperature probably also affects this stage."

"The actual period of pupation is more constant—about eight days." "In the region studied all the periods are generally quite regular, so that we may consider the period of development from the egg to the imago as covering about fifteen days, varying a day either way."

"The emergence of the imagines from their pupal cases is interesting. With the great blister-like frontal sac, not unlike a tiny balloon attached to their heads, the case is burst and gradually the body is withdrawn much as a person might extricate himself from a closely fitting tube. All the while the sand particles are thrown aside by the rhythmically inflated sac. Slowly, pull after pull, the imago passes upwards through the sand, and emerges at the surface. After a moment of rest, it starts for the nearest grass stem; up which it crawls in apparent haste and there it remains to unfold its wings."

Hermes also made a number of observations on larvæ which fed either naturally or under artificial conditions for varying times, and found that there was an optimum period. "From this point either way the chances for pupation and emergence of adults diminish, most rapidly of course, at the extremes. The pupa cases of optimum forms and beyond are very chitinous, making a comparatively rigid shell, which affords the optimum of protection. On the other hand, the further below the optimum, the less rigid the case, until at the lowest extreme it is a mere flimsy covering. This shows that here the least possible energy is expended, while the greatest amount possible is stored up for the trying transformation from larva to imago."

The optimum feeding period is 60—72 hours. After 54 hours' feeding "pupation takes place readily and promptly and adults emerge in time, but are short of weight and small in size." After 48 or 42 hours' feeding the adults are still smaller. With 36 hours' feeding adults were small, and many died before the wings expanded. With less than 36 hours' feeding adults could not be raised (see Fig. 12, p. 14).

As yet no comparable observations have been made on the habits of these larvæ in places away from shores.

This fly has been known to lay its eggs in neglected wounds in human beings. Under these conditions extensive sores, with great loss of tissue, may be caused by the larvæ (see Chapter XXII).

"*L. sericata* Mg., is the well-known 'Sheep maggot fly,' which in summer months is often a pest to farmers and flock-masters."

Pollenia rudis Fabr. The cluster fly.

This is a rather sluggish stoutly built fly of reddish grey colour, a little larger than the house-fly, and often mistaken for it. The male is distinctly smaller than the female. (Pl. IV, fig. 2.)

Length. 8 mm.; span of wings 18 mm.
Head. In the ♂ the eyes almost meet, but are separated in the ♀ by an area equal to one-fourth of the diameter of the head. The frontal stripe is black and the frontal margins of the eyes and cheeks grey. Antennæ with upper joints yellow and terminal joint dark grey. Arista black and feathered.
Thorax. Clothed with a thick layer of fine reddish yellow hair of considerable length giving it a velvety appearance. Numerous black bristles are also present.
Wings. Clear, with slight smoky tinge. Squama opaque and whitish.
Legs. Black.
Abdomen. Dark grey, with irregular lighter patches, altering with the angle of view. When at rest the wings are folded more closely together over the back than is the case with the house-fly.

This fly frequents houses especially in the spring and autumn, and is apt to collect in clusters in corners and crevices especially in rooms seldom occupied. Owing to their slow movements they are driven out of the house with difficulty, and are said to emit an odour like honey when crushed.

Very little seems to be known about the larvæ of this fly. Howard (p. 239) thinks they live in excreta and decomposing matter, but Keilin states that they are parasitic in certain earth worms.

Muscina (*Cyrtoneura*) *stabulans* Fallen.

A broad, stoutly built fly resembling the house-fly and frequently mistaken for it. It is, however, larger and more robust in appearance. General colour grey. (Pl. V, fig. 1.)

Length. 8 mm.; span of wings 16 mm.
Head. The eyes in the ♂ are close together, being separated by an area equal to one-ninth of the diameter of the head. In the ♀ they are separated by an area equal to one-third of the diameter of the head. Frontal stripe in ♂ black, in ♀ blackish brown. Ocellar triangle black with a lighter area round it. Frontal margins of eyes white, and cheeks grey. Upper segments of antennæ yellowish, terminal segment black. Arista black with bristles above and below. The general colour of the head is whitish grey, with a 'shot' appearance.
Thorax. Grey, marked with two median moderately distinct black stripes, and two lateral indistinct stripes. Scutellum grey. The thorax bears marked bristles, which are larger on the scutellum.
Wings. Clear; the 4th longitudinal vein gradually bends upwards towards the third. Squama opaque, white. Halteres yellow.
Legs. Rather slender and variable in colour ranging from "reddish gold to dirty orange and black in colour."
Abdomen. Very dark grey with lighter markings.

This fly is usually found near houses in the early summer, before the house-fly appears in great numbers. It is common throughout Europe and the United States. It is not very common in houses, Howard (1911, p. 248) only finding 37 amongst 23,087 flies collected in dining rooms and kitchens in different parts of the United States.

Howard (p. 249) thinks "this fly is one of the dangerous occasional inhabitants of houses, not only because it may breed in human excreta, but because it is greatly attracted to this substance when it chances to be deposited in the open."

The full-grown *larva* is 11 mm. long and creamy white. "The anterior spiracular processes are five lobed and are like hands from which the fingers have been amputated at the first joint. The posterior spiracles are round and enclose three triangular shaped areas, each containing a slit-like aperture" (Hewitt, 1910). The life-cycle occupies from five to six weeks.

The larvæ live in all kinds of decaying vegetable matter and also in growing vegetables. They have also been found in excrement and in the remains of insects. They occasionally cause intestinal myiasis in man.

Stomoxys calcitrans. The stable fly or biting house-fly.

This fly is grey in colour, about the size of the house-fly, and is very frequently mistaken for it. It is more stoutly built, and may be easily distinguished by the appearance of its proboscis, which is modified into an awl-like structure, adapted for piercing and sucking. In the resting position the wings are held rather widely apart. It has only been included in this list because it is so commonly mistaken for the house-fly, which is therefore often accused of being able to bite. (Pl. V, fig. 2.)

Length. 7 mm.; span of wings 16 mm.

Head. The eyes in the ♂ are separated by an area equal to one-quarter the diameter of the head, and in the ♀ by an area equal to one-third. The frontal stripe is black, and the frontal margins of the orbit and cheeks silvery white. The proboscis is black and slender and projects horizontally in front of the head, being visible from above when the fly is at rest. The antennæ are black, and the aristæ bear bristles on the upper side only.

Thorax. Dark grey, marked by four conspicuous blackish longitudinal stripes. The scutellum is paler, but has a small dark transverse patch on its upper border. There are many long bristles on the thorax and scutellum.

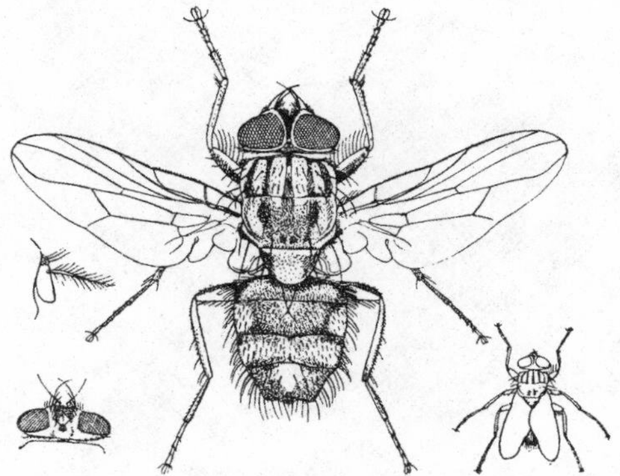

Fig. 1.

Muscina stabulans, male (× 3). Antenna. Female head, dorsal view. Natural size, resting position.

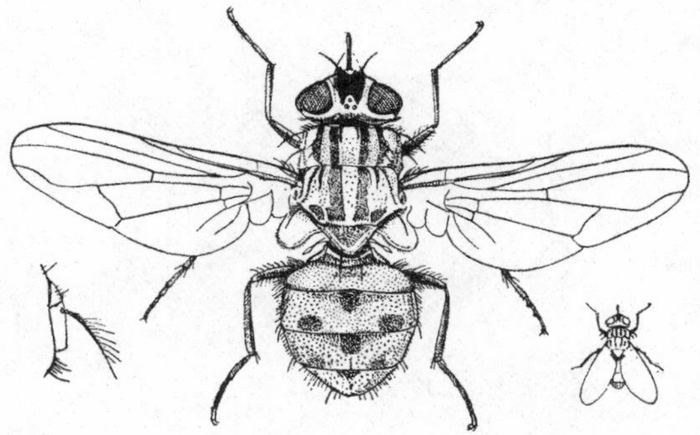

Fig. 2.

Stable fly, *Stomoxys calcitrans* (× 5). Antenna. Natural size, resting position.

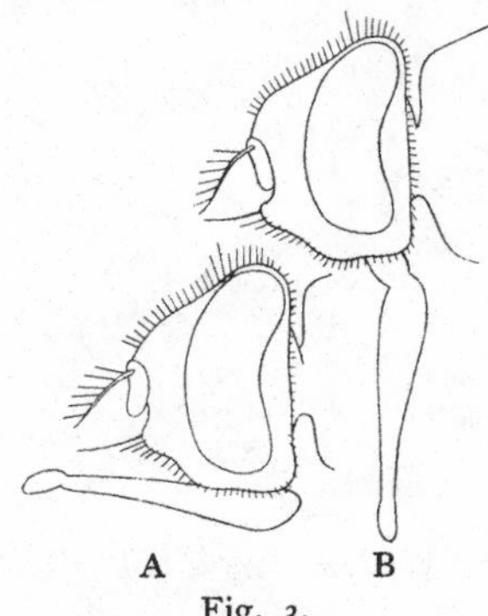

Fig. 3.

Side view of head of Stable fly; A, proboscis in resting position; B, proboscis extended.

Wings. Clear. The end of the 4th longitudinal vein is bent up, but not so sharply as in the house-fly, so that its termination is distinctly separated from that of the vein above it. Squama opaque, white. Halteres rather long and partly covered by the squamæ.

Legs. Black. Pulvilli rather marked.

Abdomen. Grey, and without ochraceous-buff patches, but spotted with clove brown, the spots being usually more conspicuous in the ♀. There are three conspicuous spots, one median and two lateral, on the second and third segments, and one median spot on the fourth.

This fly is very widely distributed, being found in Europe, North, Central and South America, and parts of Asia and Africa. It is an outdoor fly which loves the sun, and may often be seen resting on doors, paling, etc., exposed to its full glare. Both sexes suck blood and attack both men and animals. It is very common in stables and cow sheds, and is not infrequently found in country houses in the summer and autumn, especially in wet weather, but is not attracted to food. Although it frequents stable manure, it is probably not an important agent in distributing the organisms of intestinal diseases.

The *egg* is like that of the house-fly and is 1 mm. in length. The eggs are usually laid in irregular heaps, and the average number deposited is about sixty.

The *larvæ* are very like those of the house-fly, but can be distinguished "by the plates on the posterior end of the body bearing respiratory apertures being much smaller and circular (instead of the inner side of each plate being straight), and from four to six times as far apart, with the openings straight instead of sinuous."

The *pupa* is chestnut brown, barrel shaped, with the front end somewhat pointed; "precisely similar in general appearance to pupa of *M. domestica*, but can be distinguished by size and distance between posterior respiratory plates of larva which are still visible" (Austen, 1909).

The eggs hatch out in two to three days, and the larvæ, which usually live on horse manure, are full-fed in fourteen to twenty-one days under favourable conditions. According to Newstead the absence of excessive moisture and the admission of a little light materially retard development, which then extends over a period of thirty-one to seventy-eight days. The pupal stage lasts nine to thirteen days. The development of this species is therefore slower than that of the house-fly. Newstead is of opinion that the winter is passed chiefly in the pupal condition.

Fannia (*Homalomyia*) *canicularis* L. The lesser house-fly.

This fly in general appearance closely resembles the house-fly (*M. domestica*), but is smaller and more slender in build, and can be easily distinguished by the fact that the 4th longitudinal vein of the wing does not bend upwards towards the 3rd vein, but runs straight to the edge of the wing. (Pl. VI, fig. 1.)

Length. 6 mm.; span of wings 12 mm.

Head. In the ♂ the eyes, which are reddish, are close together, being separated by a space equal to one-seventh of the diameter of the head. In the ♀ they are separated by an area equal to one-third the diameter of the head. The frontal stripe is black, but the frontal margins of the eyes and cheeks are silvery white in the ♂, and grey in the ♀. The antennæ are blackish grey, with non-feathered aristæ. The palps are black.

Thorax. Blackish grey, with three plainly marked longitudinal black stripes in the ♀. In the ♂ these stripes are indistinct. The scutellum is grey and bears long bristles.

Wings. Clear. The end of the 4th longitudinal vein is parallel to the vein above it, not bent up. In the resting position the tips of the wings are closer together than in the house-fly, thus increasing the narrower appearance of the insect. Squama large and white; halteres yellow.

Legs. Black. The femora of the *middle* legs bear comb-like bristles beneath (Fig. 14).

Abdomen. Five segments visible. Narrow and tapering, dark brown in colour, and has ochraceous-buff patches on each side of the basal half in the ♂, but in the ♀ is generally uniformly greenish. In the ♂ the buff areas when seen against the light, as on a window-pane, are transparent. In the ♀ the abdomen is more pyriform than in the ♂.

This fly, which is common in Europe and in America, appears in the house before the true house-fly and may be found in May and June. Later it is displaced by the house-fly. "The males accompanied by a varying number of females may frequently be observed flying round chandeliers, etc., in the living rooms and bedrooms of houses, in a characteristic, jerky and hovering manner" (Hewitt, 1912, p. 40). Next to the house-fly, it is the fly most commonly found in houses.

Food brought into a room does not greatly attract these insects, which often continue to fly about near the ceiling without making any attempt to settle on it.

Although this fly is undoubtedly capable of carrying disease germs, and frequents excrement, it is from its indoor habits probably much less dangerous than the house-fly or blow-fly.

Proportion of sexes. "Great disparity in the proportion of males to females is found in this species as it occurs in houses. Hamer showed in 1909 that the males constitute from 75 to 85 per cent. of the total flies of this species caught in balloon traps and on fly papers. This, however, does not indicate a disparity in the proportion of males to females in the species, as I have found that the females are more common out-of-doors, especially in the neighbourhood of the breeding places" (Hewitt, IX, 1912, p. 163).

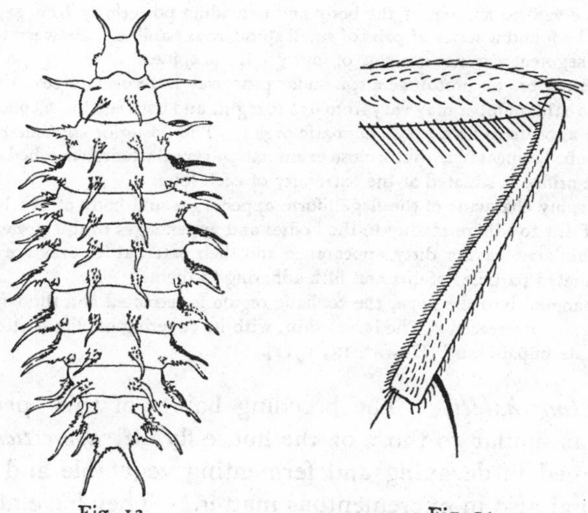

Fig. 13. Fig. 14.

Fig. 13. Larva of *F. canicularis*. (From Hewitt, *Report to Local Government Board*, 1912, reduced by one-half.)

Fig. 14. Part of right middle femur and tibia of *F. canicularis*. (From Hewitt, 1912.)

The *eggs* are white and cylindrically oval.

"The *larva* is wholly different from that of *M. domestica*; its body being provided with a number of appendages or spiniferous processes. These are arranged in three pairs of longitudinal series and there are in addition two pairs of series of smaller processes.

"The body is compressed dorso-ventrally and the surface is roughened in character and in places spiniferous. It consists of twelve segments, of which the first, or pseudo-cephalic segment, is often withdrawn into the second or prothoracic segment. The posterior end of the body is very obliquely truncate. The full-grown larva measures 5 to 6 mm. in length. The three series of pairs of spiniferous flagelliform processes, or appendages, are arranged as follows: A dorsal series consisting of ten pairs of processes commencing with an antenna-like pair of processes at the anterior border of the prothoracic segment (segment II) and slightly increasing in size posteriorly. A latero-dorsal series of ten pairs of processes which commences on segment III and is continued to the posterior end of the body. A latero-ventral series, which commences on segment III and is continued posteriorly. These flagelliform processes are spiniferous, the spines being well developed at the bases of the processes and gradually decreasing in size distally. The twelfth or anal segment is provided with three pairs of these processes of unequal size; the anterior pair is the longest on the body and the intermediate pair is shorter.

"There is a series of pairs of small, almost sessile branched appendages near and slightly posterior to the bases of the latero-dorsal appendages. Each of these processes has three or four branches, and they carry a small nucleiform organ, which Chevril (1909) has also described.

"On the ventral surface of the body and extending posteriorly from segment III there is to be found a series of pairs of small spiniferous papillæ. Between these there is on each segment a transverse row of four groups of spines.

"The anterior, or prothoracic spiracular processes have usually seven finger-like lobes, though the number may vary from five to eight, and between the second and third lobes there appears to be a small stigmatic organ. The posterior spiracular processes have a tri-lobed appearance, but a close examination reveals their four-lobed character; a stigmatic orifice is situated at the extremity of each lobe.

"The spiny character of the flagelliform appendages and body of the larva cause particles of dirt to adhere readily to the bodies and appendages of the larvæ. In consequence the larvæ have a dirty appearance and their external features are hidden by the accumulated particles of dirt and filth adhering to them."

"In changing into the *pupa*, the cephalic region is retracted and the length of the larva is thereby decreased. The larval skin, with its covering of dirt particles, forms the co-arctate pupal case" (Hewitt, IX, 1912).

Breeding habits. "The breeding habits of this species are somewhat similar to those of the house-fly, *M. domestica.* The larvæ breed in decaying and fermenting vegetable and animal matter and also in excrementous matter." They have also been found in caterpillars, snails, old cheese, humble-bees' nests, and pigeon nests, and on sugar beet and stalks of rape. They are also not infrequently found in rotting grass. Occasionally they cause intestinal myiasis in man (Chapter XXII).

"The larval period may extend over a week or it may last for three or four weeks, if the substances in which the larvæ are feeding become rather dry." "The pupal stage extends over a period of seven to twenty-one days or longer" and it is not unlikely that the winter is passed in the pupal state.

The larval stages may be found between May and October.

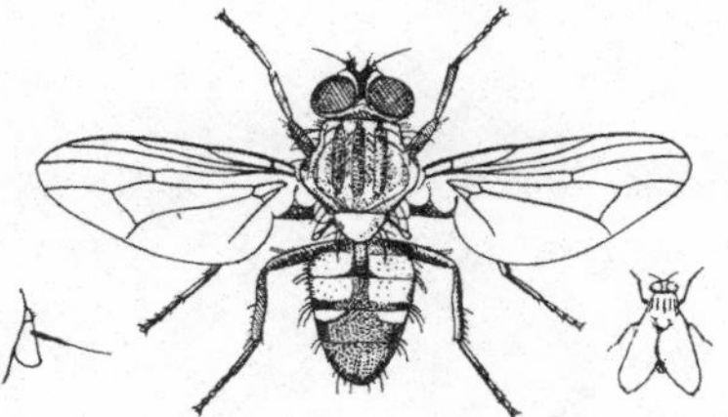

Fig. 1.

Lesser house-fly, *Fannia canicularis*, male (× 3). Antenna. Natural size, resting position.

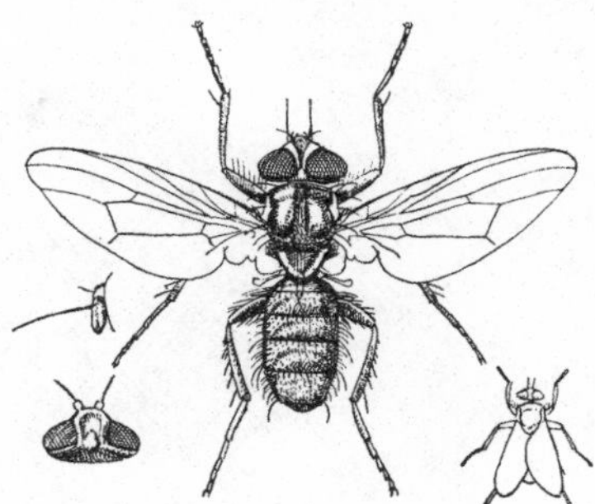

Fig. 2.

Latrine fly, *Fannia scalaris*, male (× 3). Antenna. Head of female, dorsal view. Natural size, resting position.

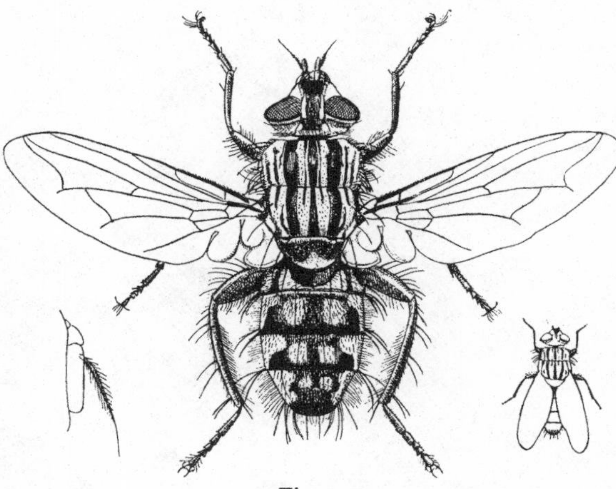

Fig. 3.

Flesh fly, *Sarcophaga carnaria*, female (× 3). Antenna. Natural size, resting position.

Fannia (*Homalomyia*) *scalaris* Fab. The latrine fly.

This species very closely resembles the lesser house-fly, and is probably often mistaken for it. "The abdomens of both species are conical, but the basal segments of the abdomen of *F. canicularis* are partially translucent and the abdomen of *F. scalaris* is black overspread with bluish grey; the mid-tibiæ of the latter species bear a distinct tubercle which is not found in *F. canicularis*" (Hewitt, IX, 1912, p. 162). (Pl. VI, fig. 2.)

Length. 6 mm.; span of wings 12 mm.

Head. In the ♂ the eyes almost meet, but in the ♀ are separated by an area equal to one-third of the diameter of the head. The frontal stripe is dark brown and the orbital margins and cheeks white. The antennæ are blackish grey, with non-Weathered arista.

Thorax. Dark grey with indistinct darker longitudinal stripes in the ♂. In the ♀ the stripes are moderately distinct. The thorax and scutellum bear long bristles.

Wings. Clear, and similar to those of *F. canicularis.*

Legs. Black. The middle femur is swollen ventrally, and bears on its broader side a group of brush-like bristles. The middle tibia bears a distinct tubercle. (Fig. 16.)

Alaomen. In the ♂ it is very dark and has a darker median longitudinal band. In the ♀ it is almost uniform dark brown. Yellow transparent patches are not piesent in either sex.

"The habits of this species are very similar to those of *F. canicularis,* but it prefers excrementous matter as a nidus for the eggs and is very commonly found breeding in human excrement." The larvæ are often found in privies when the excrement is in a semi-liquid condition and on rubbish tips when it is mixed with ashes and clinker. They have also been found in mushrooms and in rotting fungus. Occasionally they are the cause of intestinal myiasis in man (Chapter XXII).

The *eggs* are white and cylindrically oval.

"The *larva* of this species has a general resemblance to that of *F. canicularis*, but a closer examination will reveal very marked differences and a number of distinguishing characters. In shape it is very similar to the larva of *F. canicularis*, being compressed dorso-ventrally. The appendages or processes, however, are very different. The pair of antenna-like processes at the anterior and upper edge of the prothoracic (second) segment are much shorter than those of *F. canicularis*, as will be seen from the figure (15), where they are shown dorsal to the oral lobes. On the dorsal side of the larva, from segment III to segment XI, is a series of nine pairs of short and somewhat thick processes of a very spiny character; the first two pairs being little more than spinous tubercles. As the processes of the third segment differ from the succeeding segment, they may be mentioned separately. There is a pair of latero-dorsal processes bearing spines. Ventral and slightly anterior to the base of each of these processes is a small spiniferous papilla. A short spinous latero-ventral appendage is situated slightly more posteriorly. Viewed from above the larva is seen to be surrounded by a fringe of feather-like processes. Segments IV to XI are each provided with a pair of pinnate latero-dorsal processes which gradually increase in size posteriorly. Three pairs of these pinnate processes surround the obliquely truncate dorsal surface of the twelfth segment. Situated laterally and ventral to the series of pinnate processes is a series of latero-ventral processes which are spinous, but much less pinnate and shorter than the latero-ventral series. The latero-ventral processes of segment XII are situated more ventrally than those of the preceding segments and their usual place is taken by a small group of spines. Posterior to the base of each of the latero-dorsal processes of segments V to XI is a small branched process.

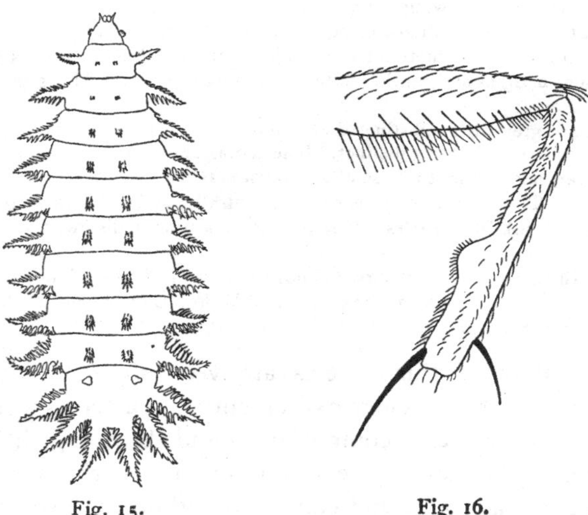

Fig. 15. Fig. 16.

Fig. 15. Larva of *F. scalaris*. (From Hewitt, *Report to Local Government Board*, 1912, reduced by one-half.)

Fig. 16. Part of right middle femur and tibia of *F. scalaris*. (From Hewitt, 1912.)

"On the ventral side of the larva, extending from segments VI to XI there is a series of pairs of small spiniferous papillæ, each of which is situated at the end of a transverse row of spines. Posterior to this transverse row of spines there is a shorter row of spines, divided into four groups. The anterior, or prothoracic, spiracular processes are six or eight lobed; the usual number of lobes being seven. The posterior spiracular processes are very similar to those of *F. canicularis*.

"The feathery character of the processes of *F. scalaris* is probably associated with the fact that the larvæ usually live in substances of a semi-liquid character when such processes will be more advantageous than those of *F. canicularis* for life in such a medium" (Hewitt, IX, 1912).

"Prior to *pupation* the larva leaves the moist situation for one of a drier character, and the pupation is similar to that of *F. canicularis*."

The larvæ emerge about eighteen hours after the eggs are deposited and become full-fed in six to twelve days. The pupal stage lasts nine days or more.

Anthomyia radicum. The root fly.

Many species of the Anthomyidæ occasionally find their way into houses. They are mostly dull, obscurely marked flies about the size of *F. canicularis,* with non-feathered arista and straight 4th longitudinal veins. The larvæ feed on vegetable matter or excrement and the adults frequent these substances. One of the commonest is *A. radicum.*

Sarcophaga carnaria L. The flesh fly.

A large hairy, thick-set but relatively rather elongated fly, with thick legs; about the size of a blow-fly, but having a grey striped and chequered appearance. (Pl. VI, fig. 3.)

Length. 13 mm.; span of wings 22 mm.

Head. Viewed from above has a triangular appearance. The eyes reddish, in the ♂ separated by one-fifth and in the ♀ by one-fourth the diameter of the head. Frontal stripe black. Frontal margins of eyes shining white or slightly yellow. Cheeks and face white. Antennæ black.

Thorax. Grey with three well-marked broad longitudinal dark stripes. At each side of the middle stripe is a very narrow dark stripe. Numerous long black bristles on the thorax and scutellum.

Wings. Transparent. Squama large, opaque, white. Halteres small.

Legs. Black, thick and with numerous bristles. Pulvilli very marked.

Abdomen. Grey and black with distinct chequered appearance, the marking varying when the insect is viewed in different lights. All segments, but especially the last two, have well-marked black bristles on their posterior margins.

The whole body has a very hairy appearance.

This species is widespread and common in Europe and Australia, and is not infrequently found in houses. It does not occur in the United States. In the United States two other species are common, a large one, *S. sarraceniæ* Riley, and a smaller one, *S. assidua* Walker, about the size of a house-fly. These flies detect the presence of food in a remarkably short time "and this can only be accounted for on the assumption of a very acute sense of smell. Comparatively fresh fish were exposed, on the shore of L. Erie, N. America, and in ten or fifteen minutes many flies were hovering about the food and some eggs had already been deposited. That the compound eyes so prominent in the *Sarcophagidæ* are of importance in orientation we are reasonably certain. If these insects were deprived of their eyesight, food would probably be found with difficulty. In several cases the eyes of *Sarcophaga sarraceniæ* were painted with India ink, affecting the flies in a manner similar to that of animals whose semicircular canals are disturbed. Orientation was almost completely lost for a time. On placing the individuals on their backs they were barely able to right themselves after frantically using both legs and wings. They crawled about on the table in an aimless manner, or on the writer's fingers. After a few minutes they flew slowly away, buzzing noisily, passing over several pieces of fish placed on the table. Their flight was directed towards a window which they struck with a thud. From this it would seem that light was not perfectly excluded. No doubt much of the disturbance was due to the penetration of the India ink" (Hermes, 1, 1907, p. 49).

Many species of the *Sarcophagidæ* are viviparous, producing numerous small maggots at birth. The larvæ live in filth and carrion of all kinds, and have also been found in wounds and in the nasal passages and intestines of man. They resemble the larvæ of *Chrysomyia* (Chap. XXII), the segments being separated by well-marked constrictions, but the spines on the segments are very minute.

The flies are greatly attracted to putrefying animal remains and excreta, and frequently settle on food, which they may infect occasionally with disease producing bacteria.

Sepsis punctum Meig. Dung fly.

A small glistening black or violet, slender fly, resembling the cheese fly. (Pl. VII, fig. 1.)

Length. 4—5 mm.; span of wings 8 mm.

Head. Round, deep violet in colour, and as broad as the thorax. The eyes are separated by an area equal to half the diameter of the head. There are strong bristles on the vertex. Cheeks and face dark yellow. Antennæ dark yellow, with the terminal joint swollen and the arista bare.

Thorax. Brighter coloured than head, with three longitudinal lines produced by rows of minute hairs; strong laterally directed bristles on thorax and scutellum.

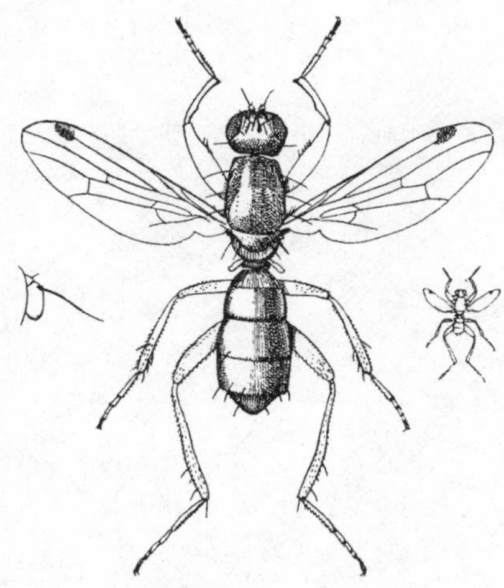

Fig. 1.

Dung fly, *Sepsis punctum* (×6). Antenna. Natural size.

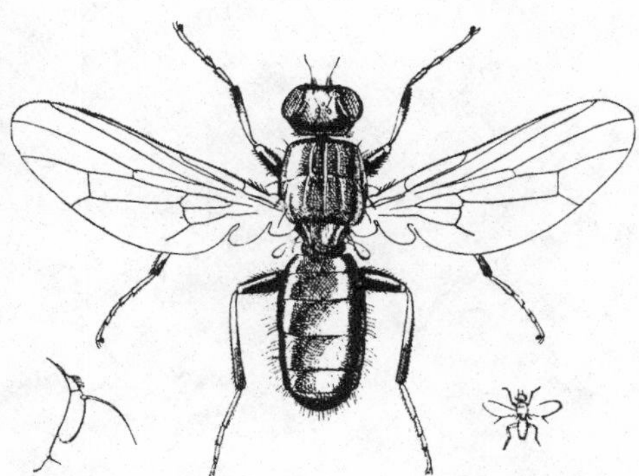

Fig. 2.

Cheese fly, *Piophila casei* (×8). Antenna. Natural size.

Wings. Clear, with smoky patch near the tip. Squama small. Halteres relatively large and knob flattened dorso-ventrally.

Legs. Yellow, but last joint of tarsus black. Tibiæ show several stout spines.

Abdomen. Shining violet, with four distinct visible segments. One pair of marked dorso-lateral bristles on second and fourth segments, and two pairs on third segment.

This fly is not infrequently found in houses, but as a rule stays on the windows and is not attracted to food. It breeds in excreta of various kinds.

Piophila casei L. The cheese fly.

A small, shining black, elongated fly, with transparent iridescent wings. (Pl. VII, fig. 2.)

Length. 4 mm.; span of wings 8 mm.

Head. Globular, eyes separated by an area equal to half the diameter of the head. Frons and vertex black, cheeks and face yellow. Antennæ yellow with black non-feathered aristæ.

Thorax. Black with a few bristles.

Wings. Very transparent. Squama small and rather more opaque.

Legs. Femur dark, tibia proximal part yellow, distal portion black, tarsus yellow except two terminal joints which are dark.

Abdomen. Very dark, with well-marked segments.

The fly is not uncommonly found in houses. It runs actively and is quick of flight.

"The larvæ, commonly called cheese-skippers, live in cheese, ham, bacon, and any fatty material and do much damage. The cheese fly, under ordinary circumstances, is not a dangerous species, but it is well to remember that not only has it been reared from dead bodies, but that it is also attracted to excreta of all kinds" (Howard, 1911, p. 251). Austen records a case of myiasis of the nasal cavity due to the larvæ of this fly (1912, p. 13).

Scatophaga stercoraria L. The yellow dung fly.

This is an active, rather slender fly. The male is bright yellow and the female dull brownish yellow. (Pl. VIII.)

Length. 8 mm.; span of wings 18 mm.

Head. Globular, eyes brown and separated in both sexes by an area equal to half the width of the head. Frontal stripe rich yellowish brown in ♂, dull yellow in ♀. Frontal margins of orbits, cheeks and face yellow. Facial bristles very marked. Antennæ dark brown, arista bare except the upper third which is slightly feathered.

Thorax. In ♂ yellowish brown, marked with longitudinal stripes. Below the wings are numerous bright yellow hairs, and on the dorsal side and scutellum many long black bristles. In ♀ colour darker, stripes more plainly marked, and hair below wings absent.

Wings. Clear, but slightly yellow; anterior cross vein very distinct, with slight smoky colouration round it. Squama small. Halteres long and distinct and not covered by squama.

Legs. Femur brownish yellow, and covered with long yellow hair; other parts yellow and not hairy in ♂. In ♀ femur dark and clothed with a few dark hairs.

Abdomen. In ♂ bright yellow and very hairy. The most prominent hairs are arranged in fringes on the posterior margins of the segments. In ♀ yellowish brown, and not hairy.

This fly may often be seen in large numbers on animal excreta, especially cow dung. It also frequents flowers, and is predaceous, attacking various species of flies. It is rarely found in town houses, but very frequently finds its way into country houses and farm buildings.

The larvæ live in animal excreta, and the pupæ are also found in this material. Probably this insect, which is not attracted to food, plays little or no part in the spread of disease producing bacteria.

Drosophila fenestrarum. Fruit fly.

A very small pale yellow fly. (Pl. IX, fig. 1.)

Length. 2 mm.; span of wings 6 mm.

Head. Round and as broad as thorax. Eyes reddish. Frons, cheeks and face pale yellow. Bristles on vertex and frontal margin of orbit very marked. Antenna yellow, terminal joint swollen, and arista with upper and lower bristles.

Thorax. Darker yellow, with lines of very minute hairs; some bristles laterally and on scutellum.

Wings. Clear, with peculiar venation. Halteres large and broadly expanded.

Legs. Pale yellow.

Abdomen. Pale yellow, with some bristles of medium length.

"The species of this family are always small, seldom exceeding a length of 5 to 6 mm., and usually from one to three; of rather plump appearance, giving a feeling of coldness to the fingers when grasped. The bristles of the front are usually conspicuous, but the body is without hairs" (Williston, 1908, p. 299).

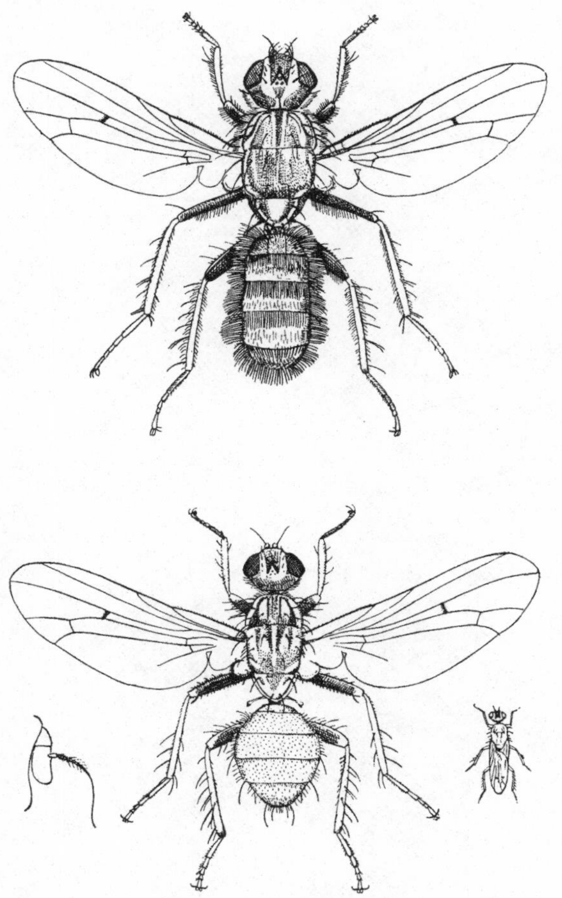

Yellow dung fly, *Scatophaga stercoraria* (× 4).
Upper figure male, lower female. Antenna. Natural size, resting position.

Flies of this family are greatly attracted to fruit and jam, and are often found in great numbers round cider-presses and packing houses and in orchards. Barrows (1907) tested the reaction of these flies, particularly *D. ampelophila* Lœw., to substances commonly found in fermenting fruits, such as ethyl alcohol, acetic and lactic acids, acetic ether and mixtures of them. "The intensity of concentration was known in each, an important consideration in such work. It was found that the optimum strength of ethyl alcohol and acetic acid was 20 and 5 per cent. respectively. It was further ascertained that cider vinegar, fermented cider and California sherry contain alcohol and acetic acid in per cents. very close to the optimum strength. By experiment it was next determined that the sense of smell, by means of which the food is found, is located in the terminal segment of the fly's antenna."

The larvæ of most species feed on decaying vegetation, but "they are nearly all attracted to excreta, and some of them breed in human excrement" (Howard, 1911, p. 252). Consequently these small flies may at times carry dangerous bacteria and contaminate foods.

Psychodidæ. Owl midges or moth flies.

Minute moth-like flies, very commonly found on windows in houses. The wings are very large and broad in proportion to the size of the body, and when the insect is at rest slope in a roof-like manner. (Pl. IX, fig. 2.)

In the species illustrated the ground colour is dark grey with lighter patches. Body and wings covered with long fine hairs.

Length. 2·3 mm.; span of wings 6 mm.

Head. Eyes nearly meeting below vertex. There is a tuft of long white hairs below the antennæ, which are as long as the body, and consist of twelve well-marked oval joints clothed with hair.

Thorax. Covered with greyish white hairs, especially at the sides.

Wings. With peculiar straight venation, covered with grey and black hairs arranged in double rows along the veins. The borders are also very hairy.

Legs. Clothed with black and white hairs arranged in bands.

Abdomen. The segments are well marked and clothed with long hairs.

Some of these flies of the genus *Phlebotomus* occurring in Southern Europe are blood-suckers and transmit a disease known as "Three-day fever," but the species found in this country are non-biting flies. Newstead (1907, p. 22) states that in Liverpool the larva of *P. phalænoides* "was common in human fæces and many examples of the flies were bred from this material. It is also common in putrid sewage matter."

The flies are common in houses from March onwards, and judging from their habits may occasionally carry disease producing bacteria.

Scenopinus fenestralis L. The window fly.

This is a long, narrow, black fly with a hump-backed appearance. The abdomen is relatively very long and flattened, and shows well-marked segments. It is often found on windows, especially in out-houses, and is not very active. (Pl. IX, fig. 3.)

Length. 6 mm.; span of wings 10 mm.

Head. Semicircular, and well separated from thorax. The frons and vertex are almost flush with the eyes, or so slightly sunk that the eyes cannot be termed bulging. The eyes in the ♂ are almost touching, in the ♀ separated by an area equal to one-fifth the width of the head. Cheeks and face, which is very broad but short, are quite bare, and very dark grey in colour. Antennæ are three jointed, and close together at the base. The basal joints are short, but the third joint is elongated and bent downwards and bears no distinct arista.

Thorax. Dull black, almost shagreened, and has no bristles. It is flattened on the surface, but the insect appears hump-backed because the head is depressed.

Wings. Clear, but slightly yellow, with peculiar simple venation. Squama small. Halteres very long and with an oval knobbed termination, which is very variable in colour "being sometimes all clear white, but often white on the under side of the knob" or dark grey.

Legs. Yellowish, sometimes with dark markings. The terminal joints of the tarsus dark.

Abdomen. Shining black and flattened, with seven well-marked segments, each of which has a transverse channel across its middle. The second segment bears peculiar oval pitted areas. Ovipositor in ♀ concealed.

"The larva is long, white, and snake-like in shape with a dark head. It apparently has many segments to the body, since each of the abdominal segments is divided by a strong constriction" (Howard, 1911, p. 260).

"The larva was at one time supposed to feed on stable clothing and old carpets, especially when thrown into a heap and neglected, whence the perfect insect obtained the name of 'carpet fly.' It is now however known to be predaceous and to feed on the larvæ of the clothes moth (*Tinea pellionella*) or of

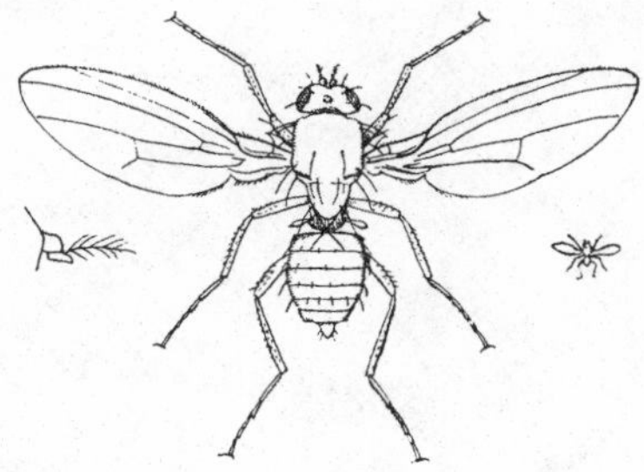

Fig. 1.

Fruit fly, *Drosophila fenestrarum* (× 8). Antenna. Natural size.

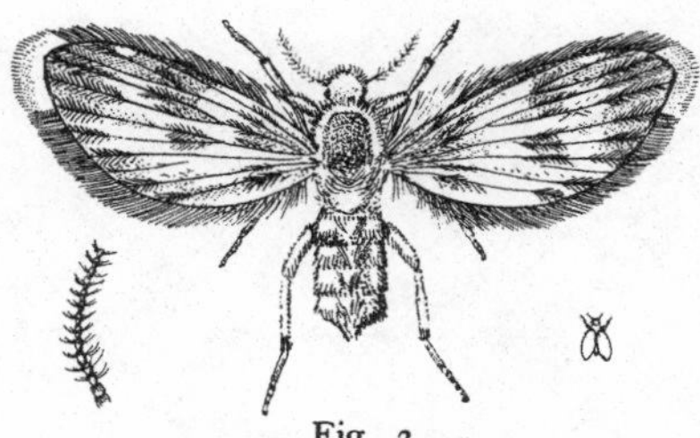

Fig. 2.

Owl midge or moth fly, *Psychoda* sp. (× 8). Antenna. Natural size, resting position.

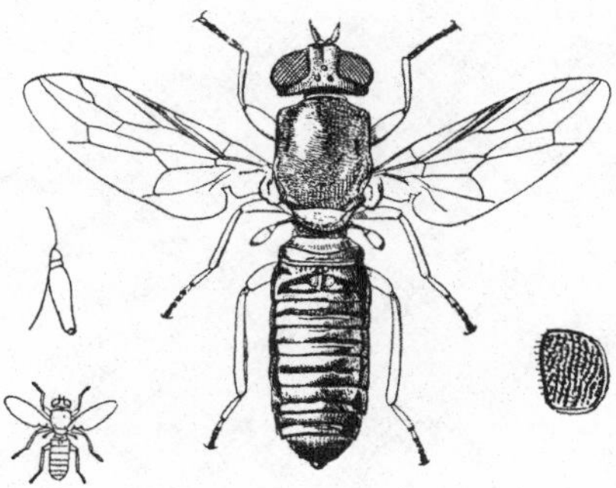

Fig. 3.

Window fly, *Scenopinus fenestralis*, female (× 5). Antenna. Natural size. Oval pitted area on second abdominal segment (× 30).

the *Pulicidæ* (fleas) which are the real culprits, and consequently it is a benefactor instead of being injurious" (Verrall, 1909, p. 600).

From its habits it is very unlikely that this fly transmits disease.

The larvæ of all the species mentioned except *P. rudis* and *S. fenestralis* feed on animal and human excreta, carrion and decaying vegetable matter, and the flies frequent these substances, and consequently carry putrefactive and fæcal bacteria both in and on their bodies.

Further information on the relation of the sexes to the materials mentioned is given in Chapter VII, and a list of the species which breed in or frequent human excrement in Chapter XXVI.

CHAPTER III

LIFE-HISTORY OF THE HOUSE-FLY (*M. DOMESTICA*)

The description of the life-history of the house-fly given in this chapter is mainly taken from Newstead's (1907) account of his very careful study of the subject in the city of Liverpool.

"The *eggs* are laid in small irregular clusters, or in large collective masses consisting of many thousands of individual eggs. They are almost invariably on or in such substances as will provide food for the larvæ or maggots. They are usually placed in narrow crevices near the surface, but, occasionally, also at a distance of four to six inches below the surface, the *favourite spots* in all cases being fermenting vegetable matter or the refuse lying immediately over such materials, or in refuse that is likely to ferment. They are often laid, however, on materials which do not ferment, and in all such cases (in this country at least) the developmental cycle is greatly prolonged."

"The eggs are pure white, and present a highly polished

surface due to the clear, viscous substance with which they are coated." Each egg is about 1 mm. ($\frac{1}{25}$ inch) in length, cylindrically oval, and slightly curved in its long axis, and somewhat broader at one end than at the other (anterior end). The extremities are rounded, and along the concave dorsal side run two distinct, nearly parallel, rib-like thickenings. Under a high power of the microscope the polished surface appears to be covered with minute hexagonal markings.

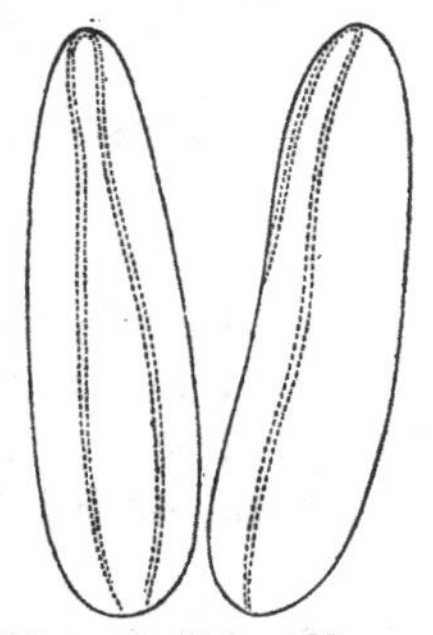

Fig. 17. Eggs of house-fly, greatly enlarged. (After Hewitt, 1908.)

"The number of eggs laid by a single fly averages from 120 to 140. More than one batch may be laid during the life of the fly." Howard (1911, p. 18) says that as many as four batches may be laid.

"The larvæ or maggots hatch out from the eggs in periods varying from eight hours to three or four days; the average time may be given as twelve hours, but when laid in fermenting materials the incubation period is reduced to a minimum of eight to twelve hours."

"The time of hatching varies according to the temperature. With a temperature of 25° C. to 35° C. the larvæ hatch out in 8—12 hours after the deposition of the eggs; at a temperature of 15—20° C. it takes 24 hours, and if kept as low as 10° C. two or three days elapse before the larvæ emerge."

Hewitt (1908, p. 506) has carefully observed the hatching of the eggs and described the process as follows: "A minute split appeared at the anterior end of the dorsal side to the outside of one of the ribs; this split was continued posteriorly and the larva crawled out, the walls of the chorion (egg-shell) collapsing after its emergence."

"The young larva as it issues from the egg is a slender creature tapering from the blunt, round hinder end to the pointed head end. It is glistening white in colour and only about 2 mm. ($\frac{1}{14}$ inch) in length. It is extremely active and burrows at once into the substance upon which the egg from which it has been hatched had been laid, rapidly disappearing from sight. In the

Plate X

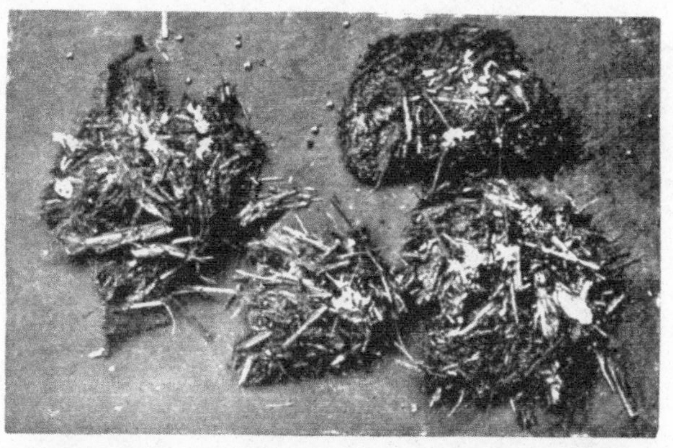

Fig. 1.

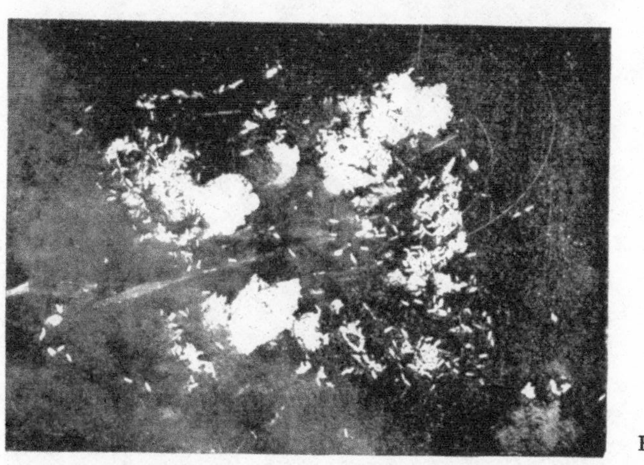

Fig. 2.

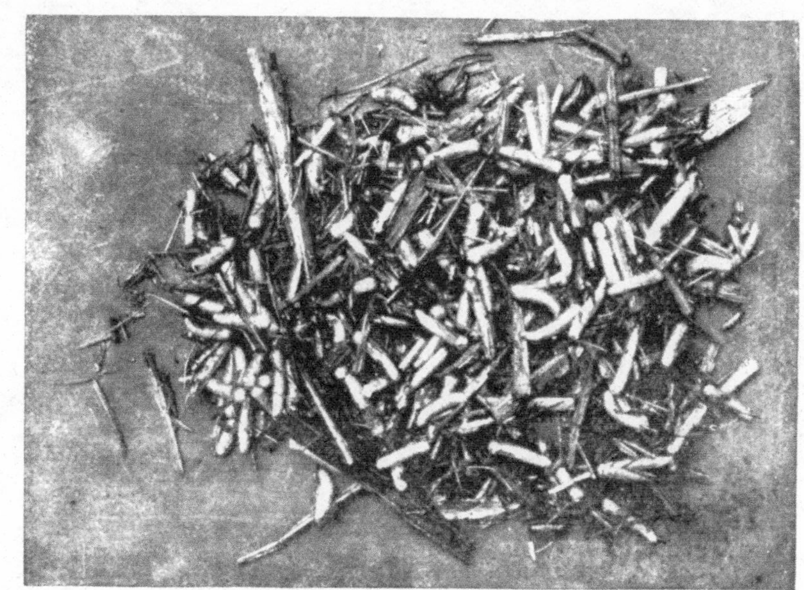

Fig. 3.

Fig. 1. Four batches of eggs of house-fly on manure. Natural size.
Fig. 2. Collective batches of eggs in stable manure, numbering about 1,500. Natural size.
Fig. 3. Mass of larvæ in stable manure. Natural size.

(From Newstead, *Report to City of Liverpool*, 1907.)

course of its growth it casts its skin twice, and therefore passes through three distinct stages of growth. In the first stage the anal spiracles, or breathing holes, on the last segment, are contained in a heart-shaped aperture. After the first molt these spiracles issue in two slits, and after the second molt there are three winding slits" (Howard, 1911, p. 20).

The first stage usually occupies 24 to 36 hours, but may last as long as three or four days. The second stage lasts between 24 hours and several days.

"The full-grown larva is a creamy white legless maggot measuring 12 mm. (½ inch) in length. It is slender and tapering

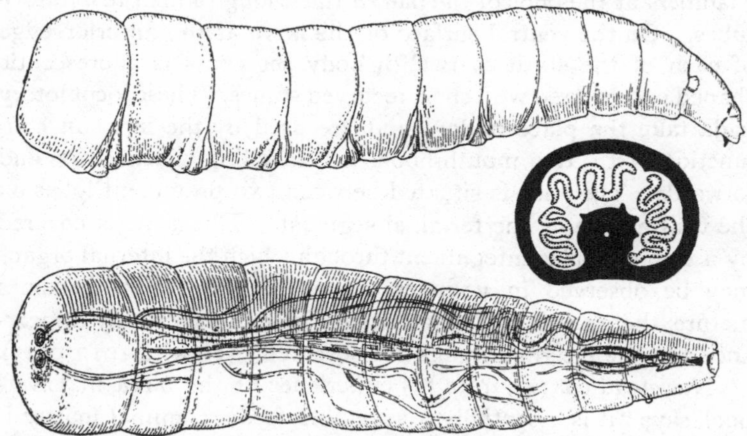

Fig. 18. Full-grown larva of house-fly; greatly enlarged; upper figure, side view; lower, view of under surface; middle figure, anal spiracle still more enlarged. (From Howard, 1911, Fig. 7, p. 22.)

in front, large and terminating bluntly behind. Twelve distinct segments can be recognized; in reality there are thirteen, the second segment being of a double nature" (Hewitt, 1912, p. 22). The body gradually tapers off from the middle to the anterior end where it terminates in a pair of oral lobes, each of which bears two small sensory tubercles. The mouth opens on the under side of and between the oral lobes, which can be withdrawn into the succeeding segment. Above the orifice of the mouth there projects from between the oral lobes a black hook-shaped process. "This is part of the skeleton of the larval head, and is used in locomotion, and also in tearing up the food which is absorbed in a semi-fluid form, the solid portions, such as small pieces of straw, etc., not being taken into the mouth. At the sides of the second segment is seen a pair of golden fan-shaped organs, each having six to eight lobes or rays. These are the anterior spiracles, through which air is taken into the respiratory tubes of the larva."

"A second pair of eye-like spiracles, the posterior spiracles, is found in the middle of the obliquely blunt posterior end of the larva. Each of these consists of a black chitinous ring enclosing three sinuous slits through which air passes into small chambers at the ends of the pair of thick longitudinal respiratory tubes. On the ventral surface of the larva at the anterior edge of each of the sixth to twelfth body segments is a crescentic shaped pad covered with short recurved spines. These locomotory pads take the place of legs and are used by the larva in conjunction with the mouth-hook in travelling backwards and forwards. The anus is situated between two prominent lobes on the ventral side of the terminal segment. The larva is covered by a thin cuticular integument through which the internal organs may be observed in younger larvæ. As the larva becomes mature, the growth of the fat tissues gives it a creamy appearance and the internal organs are obscured" (Hewitt, 1912, p. 23).

Newstead (p. 14), from his experience of the larva in Liverpool, says "it is essentially a vegetable feeder; animal matter is eaten only, so far as one has been able to gather, when in the form of human fæces. It was never found feeding on the carcases of dead cats and dogs, or on bird and fish remains." Hewitt (1908, p. 499) however successfully reared larvæ in "horse-manure, cow-dung, fowl-dung, both as isolated fæces and in ashes containing or contaminated with excrement obtained from ash-pits attached to privy-middens, and such as is sometimes tipped on public tips. I found that horse-manure is preferred by the female flies for oviposition to all other substances, and that it is in this that the great majority of larvæ are reared in nature; manure heaps in stable yards sometimes swarm with the larvæ of *M. domestica.* It was also found that the larvæ feed on paper and textile fabrics, such as woollen and cotton garments

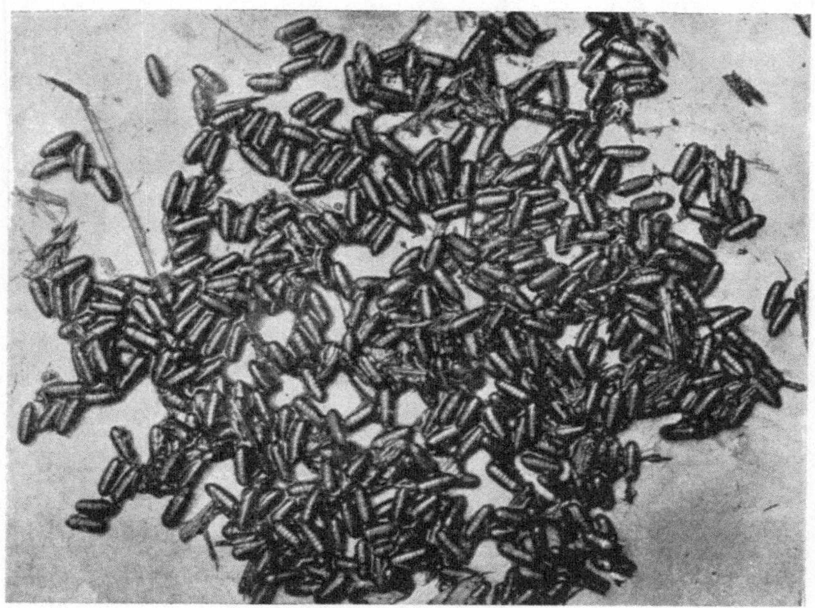

Fig. 1. Mass of pupæ separated from stable manure. Natural size.

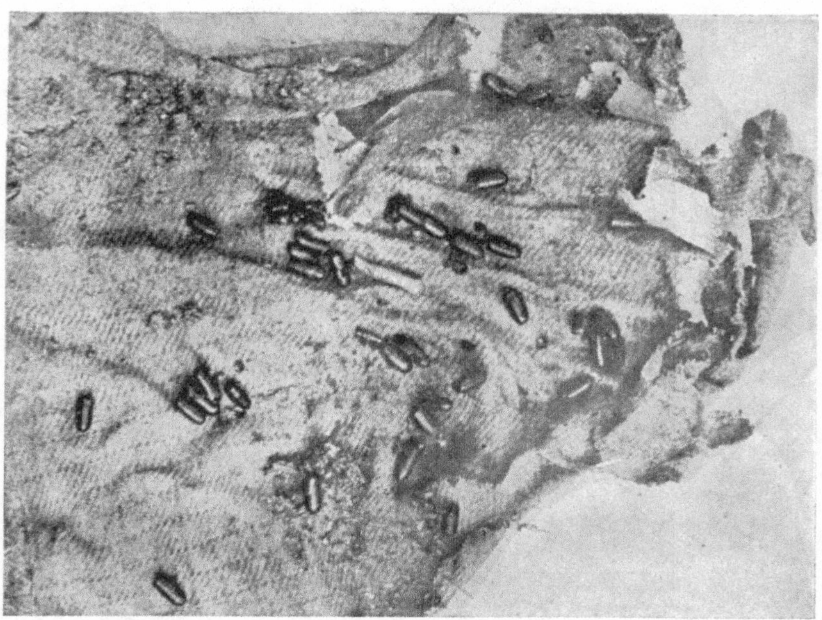

Fig. 2. Larvæ and pupæ in old rags (ash-pit refuse). Natural size.
(From Newstead, *Report to City of Liverpool*, 1907.)

and sacking, which are fouled with excremental products, if they are kept moist and at a suitable temperature. They were also reared on decaying vegetables thrown away as kitchen refuse, and on such fruits as bananas, apricots, cherries, plums and peaches, which were mixed, when in a rotting condition with earth to make a solid mass."

In India the breeding of *M. domestica* and allied species in large numbers in night soil has been noticed by numerous observers.

During their whole lives the larvæ shun the light, but according to the experiments of Felt (1910, p. 34), although flies crawl into dark crevices of manure to lay their eggs, they will not lay them freely in dark places.

The larvæ "thrive and mature most rapidly, and are always most abundant in fermenting materials; but they can also mature in non-fermenting substances during warm weather, though under such conditions they do so very slowly. In stable manure they are generally most numerous a few inches below the surface, and undoubtedly work their way upwards day by day into the fresh material a few hours (five or six) after it has been added to the previous accumulation. This marked habit is evidently due to the excessive heat which is engendered in the lower strata of the manure."

"Under the most favourable conditions as to temperature and food supply they mature in five to eight days; but when fermentation does not take place, this stage, even in hot weather, may be prolonged to several weeks (six to eight)."

"In midden steads the fully matured larvæ crawl away to the sides or to the top of the wall or framework of the receptacle; in ash-pits they locate themselves in various materials as well as ashes, but are evidently partial to old bedding, paper, rags, usually in or near the centre of fermentation" (Newstead, p. 15).

In any case the larva leaves, if possible, the more or less moist situation and crawls away sometimes several yards in search of some dry and sheltered spot.

After a short resting stage during which the alimentary canal is emptied of organic matter pupation occurs.

At the beginning of this change the body contracts by the

withdrawal of the anterior segments, and assumes a cylindrical shape, the ends being evenly rounded. The larva now retracts from the outer skin, which remains outside as the barrel-shaped puparium, and its organs after undergoing disintegration are built up into those of the future fly. Within twenty-four hours most of the parts of the future fly can be distinguished although sheathed in a protecting nymphal membrane. The pupa, or more properly the puparium, is at first of a pale yellow colour, but rapidly changes to bright red and finally to a dark chestnut colour. It is barrel-shaped, the posterior portion being slightly larger in diameter than the anterior, and both ends equally rounded. At the posterior end are two minute processes corresponding to the larval spiracles and "the locomotory pads can still be recognized as roughened areas on the ventral side of the pupa" (Hewitt, 1912, p. 25). The pupa varies in length from 6—8 mm. ($\frac{1}{6}$ to $\frac{1}{4}$ inch). "Small examples are found when the temperature has been low or excessively hot and somewhat dry. Large examples invariably occur in fermented materials, more especially so in stable manure" (Newstead, p. 15). Lack of moisture and consequently of available semi-liquid food seems to be the principal cause of dwarfing and retarded growth.

"In stable-middens the pupæ occur chiefly at the sides or at the top of the wall or framework of the receptacle, where the temperature is lowest. In such situations they were often found packed together in large masses numbering many hundreds. The flies emerge from the pupæ, under the most favourable conditions, in five to seven days. In ash-pits they occur in the positions already indicated, and if similar conditions as to heat prevail, the period is approximately the same; but in all cases when heat is not produced by fermentation, the pupal stage may last from 14 to 28 days, or even considerably more" (Newstead, p. 15).

The fly escapes from the puparium by pushing off the anterior end of the pupal case in its "dorsal and ventral portions by means of the inflated frontal sac, which may be seen extruded in front of the head above the bases of the antennæ. The splitting of the anterior end of the pupal case is quite regular, a circular split is formed in a line below the remains of the anterior spiracular processes of the larva. The fly levers itself out of the barrel-shaped pupa and leaves the nymphal sheath" (Hewitt, 1908, p. 510). By the successive inflation and deflation of the sac the fly is able to make its way upwards through the manure pile, etc., to the open air. Once liberated the wings, which have hitherto been crumpled, expand, the integument hardens, and within an hour or two the fly takes wing (see Figs. 8, 9).

No further growth ever takes place after the wings have once developed.

The flies become sexually mature in ten to fourteen days after emergence from the pupal state, and four days after mating they are able to deposit eggs.

From these observations "it may be seen that in very hot weather the progeny of a fly may be laying eggs in about three weeks after the eggs from which they were hatched had been deposited. As a single fly lays from 120 to 140 eggs at a time and may deposit five or six batches of eggs during its life, it is not difficult to account for the enormous swarms of flies that occur in certain localities during the hot summer months, and algebraical calculations are not required to more vividly impress the fact" (Hewitt, 1908, p. 504).

CHAPTER IV

THE INTERNAL ANATOMY OF THE HOUSE-FLY

The two most important contributions to the internal anatomy of non-biting muscid flies published in the English language have been Lowne's (1895) monograph on the blow-fly and Hewitt's (1907—10) papers on the house-fly. Both deal very thoroughly with the anatomy of the species under consideration, and for detailed accounts of the various internal organs of these insects the reader is referred to these works and to the various papers dealing with special organs, which have been published from time to time by other workers. In this chapter most of the systems are described very briefly, since they are not concerned in the transmission of bacteria. The alimentary system, which is of the greatest importance in this connection is more fully described. The chief external features have already been described (pp. 8—12) and the structure and function of the proboscis is discussed in Chapter V, and the function of the crop and proventriculus in Chapter VI.

Externally the integument (skin) of the fly consists of a hard chitinous layer, with softer portions at the joints, which acts as a skeleton or supporting framework, for the attachment of muscles and other structures.

In these insects the *muscular system* is particularly well developed, the thoracic muscles being enormous and almost filling the thorax. They are arranged in two series. The *dorsales* (Fig. 19, G) arranged in six pairs of muscle bands, on each side of the median line, run longitudinally, and the *sterno-dorsales*, which are arranged vertically and external to the dorsales, are arranged in three bundles on each side. The former depress and the latter lift the wing. There are also muscles controlling the proboscis, roots of the wings, legs, halteres, etc.

The *nervous system* is remarkable for its concentration. In the head is placed a large mass of nervous tissue, the *cephalic ganglion* or brain (Fig. 19, E), perforated by a small opening for the passage of the œsophagus, and in the thorax a very large mass the compound *thoracic ganglion*. These two masses are connected by a median ventral nerve cord. From the main ganglia nerves run to the various organs and limbs.

The only definite organ belonging to the *vascular system* is the *heart*, a long vessel which lies immediately below the dorsal surface of the abdomen, and extends from its posterior to its anterior end. It has four large chambers corresponding to the four visible abdominal segments, and is continued anteriorly as a narrow tube along the dorsal side of the ventriculus. By the rhythmic contractions of the heart the colourless blood is circulated through the body-cavity, which forms a closed chamber, so that all the organs are bathed in blood. "Associated with the blood system is a diffuse structure known as the *fat-body* which consists of a large number of very large cells. The size of the fat-body varies considerably; just before hibernation it seems to fill almost the whole abdominal cavity, and after hibernation it is found to have shrunk to almost nothing" (Hewitt).

The *respiratory* or *tracheal system* is developed to a very great extent in the fly and occupies more space than any other anatomical structure. By means of the *tracheæ*, which are thin-walled branching tubes, supported by chitinous rings, air is distributed to every organ of the body, in most of which very minute ramifications run in all directions. The system consists of *tracheal sacs* of varying size having extremely thin walls and the *tracheæ*, which arise from the sacs, or, in the case of the abdominal tracheæ, independently from *spiracles*. The anterior thoracic spiracles are very large vertical openings in the thorax above the anterior legs. They supply the head, legs and most of the thorax, and a large part of the abdominal viscera. The posterior thoracic spiracles are situated in the posterior margin of the thorax, and only supply part of the thorax. According to Hewitt there are seven pairs of abdominal spiracles in the male, and only five pairs in the female. These communicate with tracheæ which ramify among the abdominal viscera, but are not connected with sacs.

The *reproductive system* is very greatly developed in the *female*, the two *ovaries* being very large and almost filling the whole abdomen. Each ovary contains about seventy "strings of eggs" in various stages of development. They open into two ducts, which unite and form one central duct which passes into the *ovipositor* (Fig. 5). "Connected with this central oviduct are certain glands and a set of small vesicles which store the spermatozoa received from the male during coitus. The long telescopic *oviduct* is composed of the last four segments of the abdomen, which can be retracted entirely within the abdomen. When the fly lays its eggs the ovipositor is extended, and when fully extended is as long as the abdomen. The possession of an extensile ovipositor is of great importance as the fly is thereby enabled to deposit its eggs in the crevices of the substance chosen as a nidus for the larvæ" (Hewitt, 1912, p. 17).

"The internal reproductive organs of the *male* consist of a pair of small brown pear-shaped *testes*, which open by fine ducts

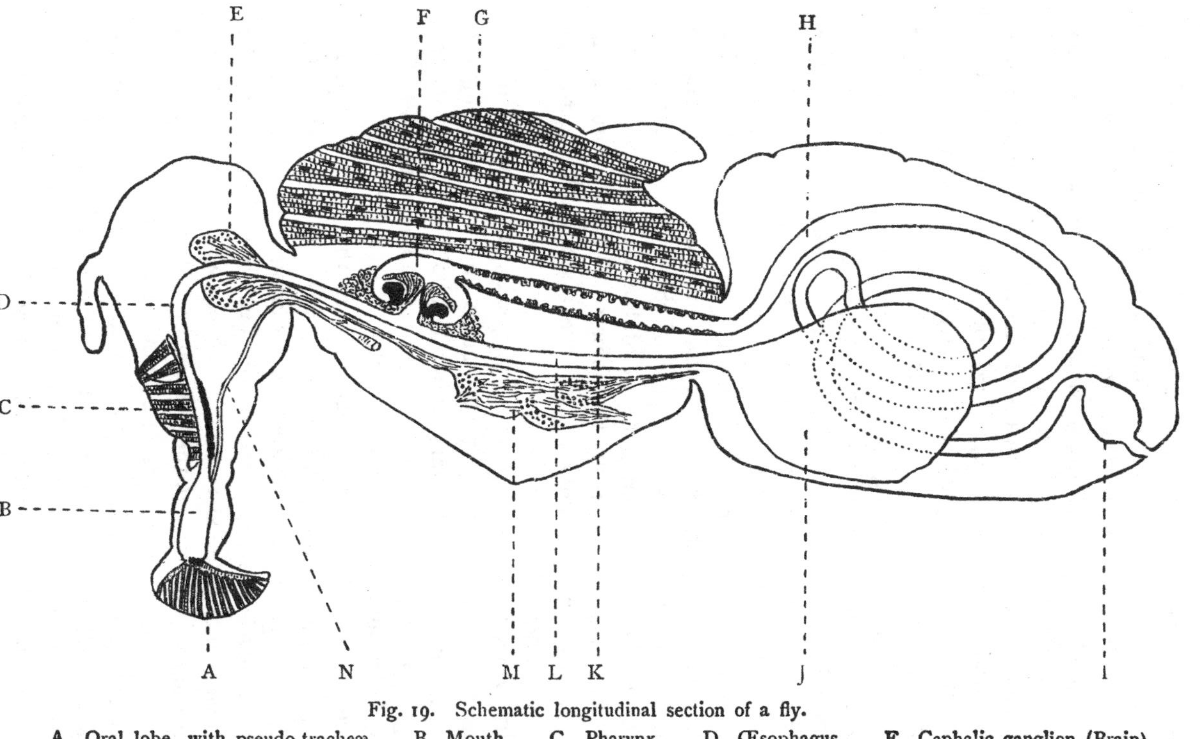

Fig. 19. Schematic longitudinal section of a fly.

A. Oral lobe, with pseudo-tracheæ. B. Mouth. C. Pharynx. D. Œsophagus. E. Cephalic ganglion (Brain). F. Proventriculus. G. Thoracic muscles (Dorsales). H. Proximal intestine. I. Rectal valve. J. Crop. K. Ventriculus. L. Crop duct. M. Thoracic ganglion. N. Salivary duct.

into a common ejaculatory duct. The external organs consist of a chitinous penis and accessory plates." The male armature is of considerable importance in the classification of certain groups of flies, but need not be considered in detail here.

The *alimentary system* commences at the *mouth* (Fig. 19, B), which is a cylindrical tube occupying the first half of the proboscis, and passes into the sucking organ or *pharynx* (Fig. 19, C), which is supplied with strong muscles and occupies most of the upper third of the proboscis. From the pharynx a thin-walled tube, the *œsophagus*, runs upwards into the head, through the cephalic ganglion and neck into the thorax (Fig. 19, D). At the junction of the anterior and middle thirds of the thorax it divides. One branch, the *crop duct* (Fig. 19, L), is continued backwards into the *crop* (Fig. 19, J and Pl. XV), and the other passes into the *proventriculus* (Fig. 19, F), which is situated immediately above the bifurcation. The crop is a bilobed sac, capable of considerable distension, which when greatly distended loses its bilobed shape, and occupies a large portion of the antero-ventral region of the abdomen. Its walls exhibit unstriped muscle fibres. The proventriculus, into which one branch of the œsophagus passes, is a curious circular organ, flattened dorso-ventrally, and is described by Hewitt (1907, p. 421) in the following way: "In the middle of the ventral side it opens into the œsophagus, and on the dorsal side the outer wall is continued as the wall of the ventriculus. The interior is almost filled up by a thick circular plug of cells, which have a fibrillar structure, and it is pierced through the centre by the œsophagus. The neck of the plug is surrounded by a collar of elongated cells, external to which the wall of the proventriculus begins, and, enclosing the plug at the sides and above, it merges into the wall of the ventriculus." Beyond the proventriculus the alimentary canal is continued as the *ventriculus* or *chyle stomach* (Fig. 19, K), the walls of which are thrown into a number of transverse folds, with saculi between them. The ventriculus passes into the abdomen to become the *proximal intestine* (Fig. 19, H) which begins at the anterior end of the abdomen and after a number of turns and bends passes into the *distal intestine.* The junction is marked by the entrance of the ducts of the two *malpighian tubes.* Each malpighian tube shortly divides into two tubules, which are very long and convoluted and internately bound up with the fat-body, which occupies the space not taken up by the intestine and other organs. The malpighian tubes are excretory in function. The distal intestine runs into the *rectum*, from which it is separated by a cone-shaped dilatation, the *rectal valve* (Fig. 19, I). The rectum finally opens at the *anus*.

In connection with the alimentary system mention must be made of the two pairs of *salivary glands*, the lingual and the labial. The *lingual salivary glands* are of great length, and consist of blind-ended tubes. From the blind ends, which are situated near the posterior part of the abdomen the glands pass forwards into the thorax, and run along the ventriculus, when they are much convoluted. Thence they run forwards along the sides of the œsophagus, losing their glandular structure, and becoming ducts in the neck region. Finally in the neck they unite below the œsophagus and the single duct runs direct to the end of the hypostome, where it opens (Fig. 19, N). The *labial salivary glands* lie at the base of the oral lobes of the proboscis and their ducts open into the oral pits.

In order to explain the process of feeding it is necessary to give in the succeeding chapters a detailed account of the structure and function of the proboscis and of the functions of the crop and proventriculus.

CHAPTER V

THE STRUCTURE AND FUNCTION OF THE PROBOSCIS

In the course of a long series of experiments carried out by the writer (Graham-Smith, 1910—11) on the distribution of bacteria by non-biting flies (*Musca domestica* and *C. erythrocephala*) it became evident that such flies are able to filter off and reject the larger particles contained in the fluids on which they feed. This fact seems to have escaped the notice of most

Plate XII

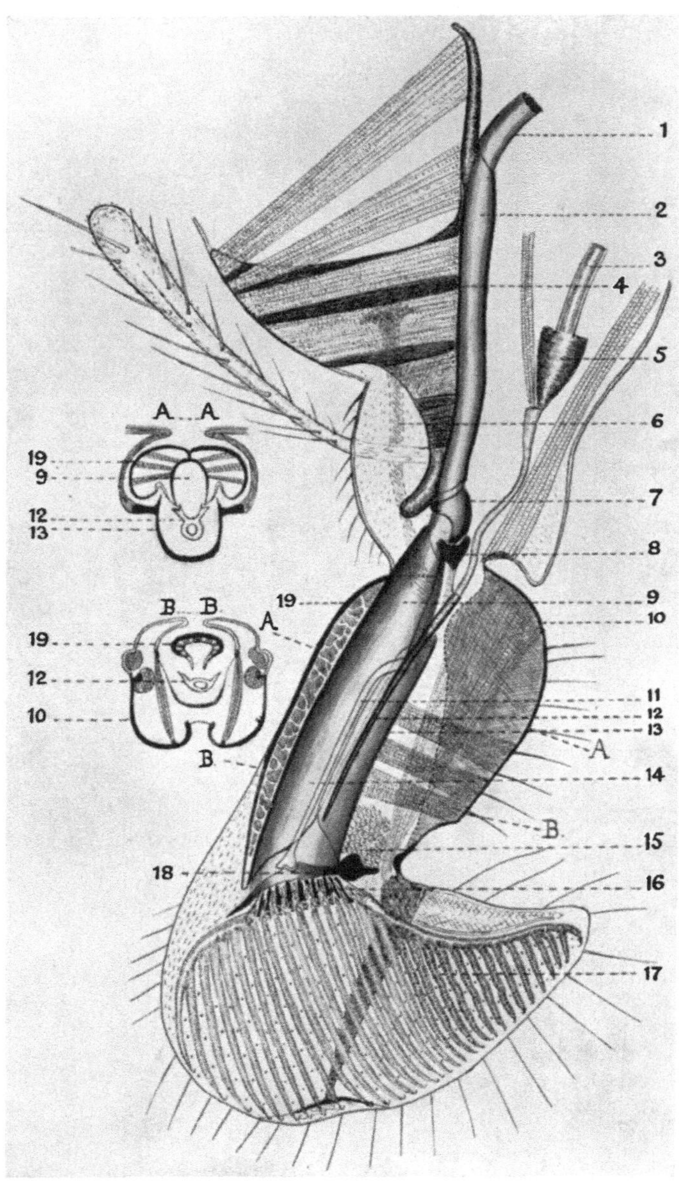
1
2
3
4
5
6
7
8
9
10
11
12
13
A
14
B
15
16
17
18
19
A
B
A A
19
9
12
13
B B
19
12
10

observers, and although the proboscis of the blow-fly has been a favourite subject of study for many years no observations appear to have been recorded which throw any light on the means by which the filtration is effected. In order to ascertain the mechanism by which the filtration is accomplished the writer (Graham-Smith, 1911, p. 390) made a large number of dissections of the proboscis of the blow-fly, and carried out experiments on the living fly to test the degree of its efficiency.

The following account is reproduced from his paper.

(A) *The anatomy of the distal end of the proboscis of the blow-fly.*

The proboscis of the blow-fly has been carefully described by Lowne (1895) and others, and consequently there is no necessity to describe in detail the principal parts of the structure.

Briefly the proboscis of the blow-fly consists of two parts, a proximal conical portion, the rostrum, and a distal half, the proboscis proper, or haustellum, which bears the oral sucker. The relationship of the structures, which compose the main portions of this organ, may be seen by reference to Pl. XII, which represents a schematic longitudinal section through the proboscis, constructed from drawings made from numerous dissections and serial sections which were studied in order to ascertain whether any valvular structures exist in the proboscis. These observations failed to reveal any valve-like structures.

EXPLANATION OF PLATE XII.

The right lateral half of the proboscis of the blow-fly divided in the middle line, and seen from the cut surface. The diagram has been reconstructed from dissections and serial sections. The mouth, prepharyngeal tube and pharynx are shaded.

1. Œsophagus. 2. Pharyngeal tube. 3. Salivary duct. 4. Fulcrum (with pharyngeal muscles). 5. Salivary valve. 6. Apodéme of the labrum. 7. Hyoid sclerite. 8. Flange at proximal end of ligula. 9. Cavity of prelabrum (passing up to prepharyngeal tube). 10. Thyroid sclerite and contained muscles. 11. Paraphysis. 12. Ligula. 13. Hypoglossal sclerite. 14. Cavity of prelabrum. 15. Salivary gland of oral disc. 16. Prestomal teeth and prestomal cavity. 17. Labellum showing pseudo-tracheæ, the anterior and posterior sets opening into common collecting channels. The epifurca can be seen running downwards behind the pseudo-tracheæ. 18. Lateral plate of discal sclerite with nodulus (black). 19. Anterior portion of prelabrum with contained muscles.

The smaller figures are transverse sections at *A—A* and *B—B*, and are numbered as in the larger figure. (From Graham-Smith, *Journal of Hygiene*, 1911, Pl. IV.)

The filtering mechanism is situated in the oral sucker or suctorial disc which is described by Lowne (1895, p. 136) as "a fleshy oval disc, deeply cleft at its anterior margin. The edges of the cleft are continuous with the margins of the groove in the theca, and are united as far as the edge of the disc by a remarkable bead and channel joint. The thick edge of one lobe, or labellum, of the disc fits into a corresponding cylindrical channel in the other. The distal or oral surface of the disc is channelled by the well-known pseudo-tracheæ. In the centre is a deep longitudinal fissure, which extends into the tubular mouth situated between the labrum and the theca. The proximal or aboral surface of the sucker is convex and covered by setæ; those near its margin are very long and form a fringe."

EXPLANATION OF PLATE XIII.

Fig. 1 represents a dissection of a portion of a pseudo-trachea. On the right-hand side the integument of the oral surface of the labellum has been removed so as to show a portion of the pseudo-trachea with the alternate bifid and flattened extremities of the chitinous rings and the membrane lining the interior of the tube stretching between them. On the left-hand lower portion the appearance of the surface integument is represented. Two interbifid grooves leading to their interbifid spaces are shown. Between the spaces are elevated masses, each of which is produced by a fold of the integument enclosing the flattened end of a ring and the extremities of the adjacent forks on each side. In the left-hand upper portion of the diagram is shown the appearance of these structures as seen by transmitted light so as to indicate more clearly the relationship of the integument to the rings.

Fig. 2 is a photograph (× 340) of part of the oral surface of the labellum, treated with potash, showing portions of four pseudo-tracheæ. The flattened and bifid extremities of alternate pseudo-tracheal rings are well seen.

Fig. 3 is a photograph (× 700) of ten consecutive chitinous pseudo-tracheal rings treated with potash and compressed, showing their alternate flattened and bifid extremities.

Fig. 4 is a photograph (× 600) of a transverse section of part of the oral surface of a labellum. Four complete pseudo-tracheæ are included in the section. In each case the chitinous ring and the opening of the longitudinal fissure is very distinct. It happens that in each case the bifid extremity is situated on the left side of the pseudo-trachea. The point of bifurcation is indicated by a dark spot above which the forks are curved inwards. From the point of bifurcation a distinct line, which represents the reflection of the cuticle at the base of the interbifid groove, passes obliquely upwards and outwards to the surface of the integument (see Fig. 6).

Fig. 5 is a photograph (× 600) of a longitudinal section through a pseudo-trachea slightly to one side of the median line. The interbifid spaces and the manner in which the integument passes over and binds together the flattened extremities of the rings and the contiguous forks of the adjacent rings on each side can be clearly seen. (From Graham-Smith, *Journal of Hygiene*, 1911.)

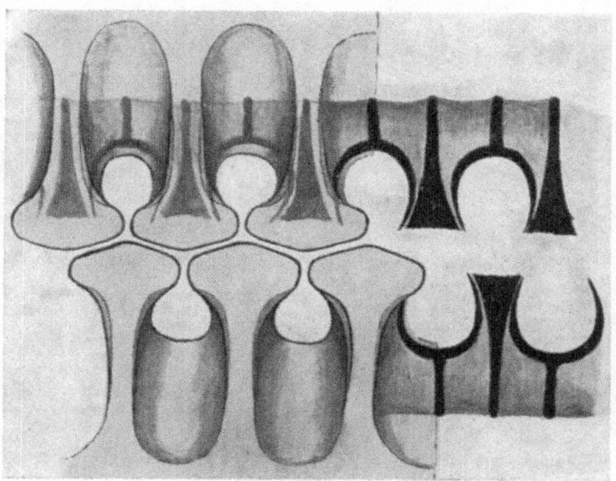

Fig. 1.

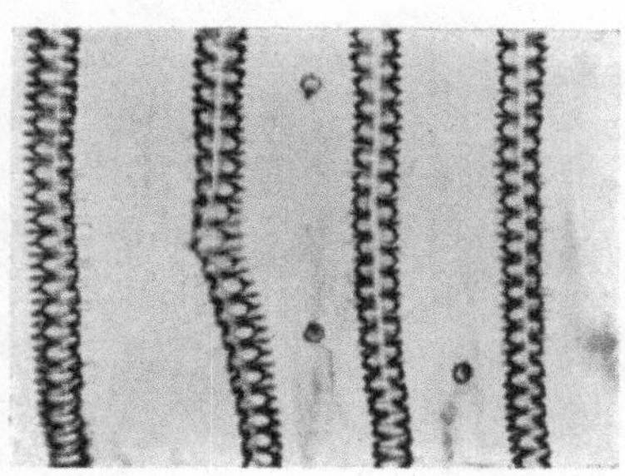

Fig. 2.

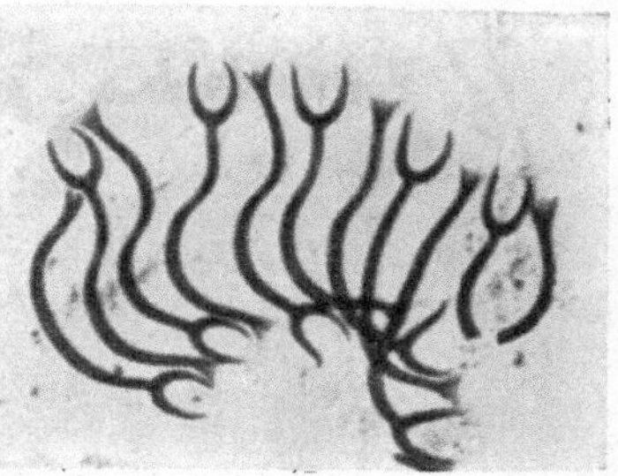

Fig. 3.

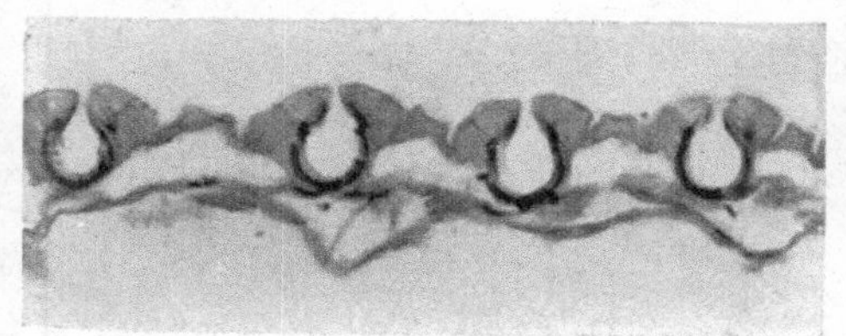

Fig. 4.

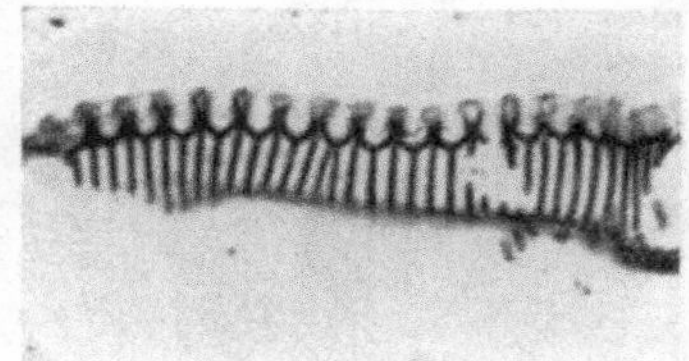

Fig. 5.

Lowne (p. 390) describes the mouth as "a cylindrical tube extending from the thecal (or discal) sclerites to the prepharyngeal tube, which may be regarded as its posterior limit or isthmus faucium." The deep cleft between the two lateral halves of the oval disc into which the mouth opens he terms the prestomum (p. 143).

The dissections and feeding experiments described later show that the liquid food is sucked into the pseudo-tracheæ and drawn through the collecting channels and along the gutters of the prestomum into the mouth, and it seems probable that crop contents and saliva may be forced at will in the reverse direction for distribution over solid food which has to be moistened and dissolved. In order to explain the process of sucking food into the mouth the structures involved, namely the oral surface of the suctorial disc, the pseudo-tracheæ, and the prestomal cleft, must be described in detail.

The pseudo-tracheæ, varying in number between 28 and 32, run transversely across the labellum or lobe of the oral sucker. They form three sets. The seven anterior pseudo-tracheæ run into a common longitudinal collecting channel which opens into the prestomum between the first and second prestomal teeth, and the posterior eight to twelve in the same way run into a common posterior collecting channel, which opens into the prestomum at its shallow posterior extremity. The central pseudo-tracheæ terminate in short channels which run directly into the prestomum without the intervention of common collecting channels. By this arrangement all the pseudo-tracheæ are made to converge to the prestomum. The arrangement of the pseudo-tracheæ is clearly shown in Pl. XIV, fig. 1, which is a photograph of the oral surface of the expanded suctorial disc of a blow-fly with 30 pairs of pseudo-tracheæ. On each side the anterior eight run into a common anterior collecting channel, and the posterior twelve into a common posterior collecting channel, while the ten central pseudo-tracheæ are continued separately into the prestomum.

From the points at which they cease to be tubular in structure the collecting channels are continued along the prestomal cavity to the mouth as grooves or gutters, whose lateral walls are formed by the prestomal teeth.

The pseudo-tracheæ.

The pseudo-tracheæ are deep furrows or incomplete membranous tubes embedded, more or less deeply according to the degree of its inflation, in the substance of the oral surface of the labellum, but under any conditions projecting sufficiently to produce distinct ridges. Along the apex of the ridge the wall of the pseudo-trachea is lacking so that the interior of the tube is in communication with the oral surface of the disc through a very narrow zigzag fissure. The lumen of the tube is kept open by means of incomplete chitinous rings running transversely

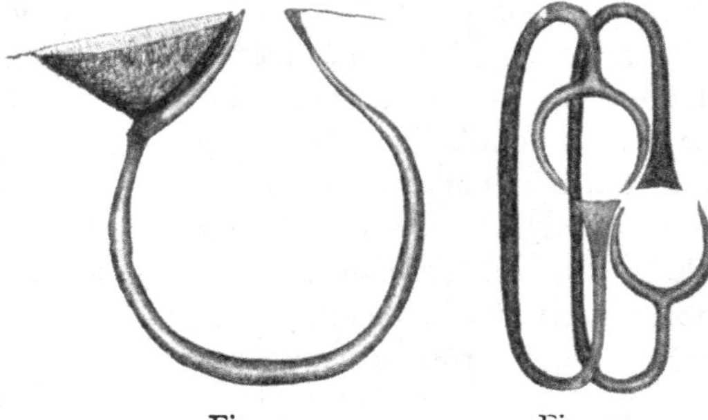

Fig. 20. Fig. 21.

Fig. 20 is a side view of a pseudo-tracheal ring. At its right-hand end the ring has a flattened expanded extremity; at its left-hand end a bifid extremity. The opening of the longitudinal fissure is seen between the flattened end of the ring and the tips of the forks. The arrangement of the fold of integument forming the interbifid groove is indicated by means of shading. (From Graham-Smith, *Journal of Hygiene*, 1911.)

Fig. 21 represents two consecutive pseudo-tracheal rings, showing the relationship of their bifid and flattened extremities, as seen from the oral surface of the disc.

round the tube, each of which has one fork-like bifid extremity, enclosing a rounded space between the prongs, and one extremity slightly expanded and flattened so as to resemble the tail of a fish. The rings are arranged in such a manner that along each side of the central fissure the bifid extremity of one ring alternates with the expanded extremity of the next ring. In consequence of this arrangement, which is very clearly seen in preparations treated with potash for the purpose of demonstrating the chitinous structures, the margin of the pseudo-trachea at each side of the central fissure has a deeply indented or scalloped appearance.

The really effective entrances into the pseudo-tracheæ are through the spaces between the bifid extremities of the rings and not through the narrow continuous zigzag fissure, which is at any time extremely narrow and is probably closed during the act of feeding, as will be explained later.

The pseudo-tracheæ gradually diminish in diameter as they approach the margins of the disc, and the size of the forked extremities of the rings and consequently of the spaces between them also diminishes though not to a corresponding degree.

The term 'interbifid space' is used to indicate the area enclosed between the forks of the bifid extremity of a ring.

Fig. 21 illustrates two consecutive rings with their bifid and flattened extremities, and Fig. 20 illustrates a side view of one of these rings. Pl. XIII, fig. 3, is a photograph of several consecutive pseudo-tracheal rings which have been treated with potash and compressed. The terminations of the consecutive rings are well shown. Pl. XIII, fig. 2, is a photograph of the oral surface of the disc of a blow-fly after treatment with potash showing portions of four pseudo-tracheæ. The longitudinal fissures of the pseudo-tracheæ and the forked extremities of the rings and interbifid spaces can be clearly seen. Pl. XIII, fig. 4, is a photograph of a section of the disc showing four pseudo-tracheæ cut transversely. The chitinous rings, the openings of the longitudinal fissures and the ridges caused by the projection of the tubes above the surface are clearly shown.

The pseudo-tracheæ of several of the common non-biting flies closely resemble each other, though they exhibit slight and apparently unimportant differences in their structure. The average measurements of the various parts in six common species are as follows.

	Pseudo-tracheæ		Interbifid spaces	
	Diameter at proximal end	Diameter at distal end	Diameter near the proximal ends of the pseudo-tracheæ	Diameter near the distal ends of the pseudo-tracheæ
Calliphora erythrocephala	·02	·01	·006	·004 mm.
Sarcophaga carnaria ...	·02	·01	·005	·004 mm.
Lucilia cæsar	·02	·01	·006	·004 mm.
Fannia (*Homalomyia*) *canicularis*	·016	·008	·006	·004 mm.
Ophyra anthrax ...	·016	·008	·006	·004 mm.
Musca domestica ...	·016	·008	·004	·003 mm.

The cuticle lining the oral surface of the labellum dips down into the pseudo-tracheæ through the longitudinal fissure and also forms the lining of these tubes, as may be seen by reference to Pl. XIII, fig. 4. In passing downwards into a pseudo-trachea the cuticle accurately follows its chitinous margins, being closely adherent not only to the chitinous sides of the interbifid spaces but also to the intervening elevations between them produced by the projection of the expanded ends of the alternate rings, and the application to them of the adjacent forks of the neighbouring rings on either side.

Owing to this arrangement a remarkable series of folds is produced in the cuticle forming channels or grooves leading into the interbifid spaces. If the cuticle is traced along the edge of the longitudinal fissure from the bottom of one interbifid space to the bottom of the next it can be observed to be very closely attached to the chitin along the base of an interbifid space and up the side of a fork to its pointed extremity. It then passes over the expanded portion of the alternate ring and down the adjacent fork of the next ring, binding the two forks mentioned and the expanded portion of the intermediate ring into an elevated mass which lies between the deep depressions of the interbifid spaces. The arrangement described can be most easily understood by reference to Pl. XIII, fig. 5, a longitudinal section through a pseudo-trachea just to one side of the central fissure. The depressions caused by the cuticle adhering to the bases of the interbifid spaces are continued outwards as folds or grooves in the cuticle for a considerable distance which are gradually lost on the surface of the labellum. Each 'interbifid groove' thus forms a well-defined channel leading into the pseudo-trachea through the interbifid space with its long axis at right angles to the line of the pseudo-trachea. The deepest part of the groove is at its entrance into the pseudo-trachea, and at this point it loses its groove-like character and becomes a tunnel, though still communicating with the surface by a very narrow slit. When the proboscis is erected by slight pressure on the head and the oral sucker viewed with a microscope these grooves can be easily seen as regularly placed channels running at right angles to each pseudo-trachea.

Though difficult to describe the arrangement can be easily understood by reference to Pl. XIII, fig. 1, representing a dissection of a portion of a pseudo-trachea. On the right-hand side the integument of the oral surface of the labellum has been removed so as to show a portion of the pseudo-trachea with the alternate bifid and flattened extremities of the chitinous rings and the membrane lining the interior of the tube stretching between them. On the left-hand lower portion the appearance of the surface integument is represented. Two interbifid grooves leading to their interbifid spaces are shown. Between the interbifid spaces are elevated masses, each of which is produced by a fold of the integument enclosing the flattened end of a ring and the extremities of the adjacent forks on each side. In the left-hand upper portion of the diagram is shown the appearance of these structures as seen by transmitted light so as to indicate the relationship of the integument to the rings.

In Pl. XIII, fig. 4, illustrating transverse sections of four pseudo-tracheæ the interbifid groove is indicated on the left side of each pseudo-trachea, but is perhaps best seen in the central ones. In each case the point of bifurcation of the chitinous ring is indicated by a dark spot above which the forks are curved inwards. From the point of bifurcation a distinct line, which represents the reflection of the cuticle at the base of the interbifid groove, passes obliquely upwards and outwards to the surface of the integument. Fig. 20 illustrates diagrammatically the condition seen in transverse sections.

Anthony (1874), Wright (1884) and Lowne (1895, p. 395) all regarded the interbifid grooves as suckers. The latter figured them as blind sacs attached to the forks of the rings with openings into the pseudo-tracheæ only. None of these authors seemed to regard them as channels leading into the pseudo-tracheæ.

The fact that these interbifid grooves are really channels leading into the pseudo-tracheæ can be demonstrated however by a very simple experiment. If the proboscis of a blow-fly is placed in alcohol, formalin or other preserving agent, and the suctorial disc is later mounted in water under a cover-glass and examined with the aid of a microscope the grooves can be clearly seen. As the specimen begins to dry air bubbles often form in the slight depressions on the oral surface of the disc between the pseudo-tracheæ. As the drying continues the bubbles run into the interbifid grooves and through them into the pseudo-tracheæ, clearly showing that the grooves lead into the pseudo-tracheæ.

The collecting channels.

It has already been stated that the anterior and posterior sets of pseudo-tracheæ run into common collecting channels, and that the central pseudo-tracheæ also run into separate closed channels. These channels, which are kept open by incomplete chitinous rings without bifid extremities, communicate with the exterior by narrow fissures which are continuations of the longitudinal fissures of the pseudo-tracheæ. Since there are no interbifid spaces there are no interbifid grooves or other openings into these channels. Each channel opens into its corresponding gutter between the prestomal teeth in a remarkable manner, the more deeply situated portions of the proximal rings being expanded and prolonged towards the prestomum, so as to form a spout-like opening to the channel.

The posterior common collecting channel of one labellum has ten pseudo-tracheæ opening into it. Throughout the greater part of its length the extremities of the rings are either quite plane, or slightly expanded, or possess only the rudiments of forks. Consequently the channel opens to the exterior by a longitudinal fissure only. At its proximal end the chitinous bars representing the rings are elongated and form a shallow groove leading towards the discal sclerite which forms the side of the entrance of the mouth. The central pseudo-tracheæ open through their own collecting channels into gutters between the prestomal teeth. In Fig. 22 the proximal portions of three of the central pseudo-tracheæ with their collecting channels terminating in spout-like openings are illustrated.

When at rest the oral surfaces of the labellæ or oral lobes are in apposition, but during feeding they are spread out over the surface of the food so as to form an oval disc. In order to attain this position that part of the oral surface of the labellum adjoining the prestomum, which is situated just external to the

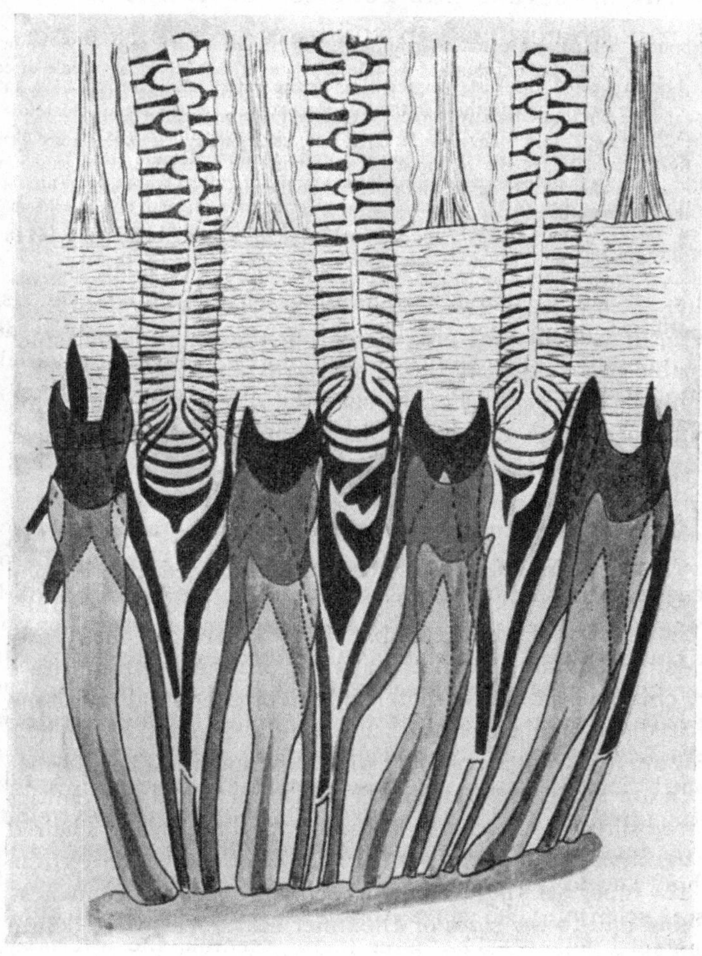

Fig. 22 represents four rows of prestomal teeth and the corresponding portion of the labellum seen from the oral surface. In the upper part of the figure three of the central pseudo-tracheæ, showing the alternate bifid and flattened ends of their rings and the longitudinal fissures, are represented. Each passes into a collecting tube with non-bifid rings which terminates by a spout-like opening between the distal extremities of two rows of prestomal teeth. The inner, shortest set of teeth are lightly shaded. They are unbranched and articulate with the lateral plate of the discal sclerite by their strong proximal extremities. The teeth of the intermediate set, which are more darkly shaded, branch behind the distal extremities of the inner set. The branches diverge to each side of the corresponding inner teeth to articulate with the lateral wall of the discal sclerite. The teeth of the outer set are most darkly shaded. The two central teeth of this set branch behind the distal extremities of the intermediate set. The branches diverge widely behind those of the intermediate set, but do not articulate directly with the discal sclerite. At each side of the figure this set is represented by separate chitinous bars which do not unite to form definite teeth.

The teeth of the inner set form the side walls of gutters whose floors are formed by the branches of the intermediate and outer sets of teeth and the integument covering them. Fluids drawn through the collecting tubes pass along the gutters into the mouth.

The tendinous chords described by Lowne (p. 395) are indicated between the pseudo-tracheæ. (From Graham-Smith, *Journal of Hygiene*, 1911.)

teeth, in fact all that area bordering the longitudinal sulcus, is capable of being bent through a right angle. It is over these highly flexible regions of the suctorial disc, which are invariably bent during the act of feeding, that the pseudo-tracheæ are converted into closed collecting channels.

The prestomal teeth.

On each side of the prestomum is arranged a series of rows of chitinous teeth, usually ten in number. The central rows each consist of three teeth. The innermost teeth are the strongest and are articulated at their proximal extremities on to the chitinous side of the lateral plate of the discal sclerite, while their distal free extremities are bifid. Except at their bases they are free from investment with integument. The intermediate teeth are longer than the inner and their distal extremities are placed directly external to those of the inner set. Their distal extremities are bifid. Immediately behind the free extremities of the inner set these teeth branch, and the two branches pass behind and to the sides of the inner set to be inserted into the discal sclerite. The upper thirds only of these teeth are free from integument. The outer teeth resemble the intermediate set in their general shape and disposition, but are longer. Their distal extremities are bifid, but their proximal branched extremities are not inserted into the discal sclerite, but seem to articulate with it indirectly through the intervention of plates of chitin. Only the distal ends of the outer set are free from integument.

The arrangement of these teeth will be best understood by reference to Fig. 22 which represents the teeth as seen from the oral aspect.

The spaces between the rows of teeth form the gutters, leading into the prestomum, which have already been mentioned. The gutter is bordered by the teeth of the inner set, whilst its floor is formed by the branches of the intermediate and outer sets of teeth, and the integument investing these structures.

The arrangement described is only found near the centre of the prestomum. On either side of the two or three central pseudo-tracheæ each tooth of the outer set is represented by two bars of chitin, which are not united at their distal extremities (see Fig. 22). Still further from the centre the outer set is lacking, while at either end of the series both the outer and intermediate sets are lacking.

The arrangement of the teeth varies greatly in different species. *C. erythrocephala* has as described three teeth in each row, *S. carnaria* has four, and *L. cæsar* has three. In *M. domestica*, *F. canicularis* and *O. anthrax* there seems to be only one definite series corresponding to the inner set of *C. erythrocephala*. In these species the sets which are lacking seem to be represented by modified plates of chitin.

When fluid food is being taken the teeth merely aid the conveyance of the fluid into the mouth by assisting in the formation of the gutters. They may be used however under suitable conditions in scraping the surfaces of hard substances to render their solution more easy. In order to bring the teeth into action as scrapers the lobes of the suctorial disc have to be more widely separated than they usually are when liquid food is being taken. When the teeth are in action as scrapers the prestomal cavity is open to the surface, and if sucking efforts are made probably large particles can pass into the mouth.

(B) *Feeding experiments.*

If hungry flies are fed on drops of syrup or other fluids they rapidly suck up large quantities. The general behaviour of flies during the act of feeding is described later. In all cases the suctorial disc is inflated and the lobes spread out so that the oral surfaces of the labellæ are nearly in one plane. If viewed from its oral surface the disc presents the appearance seen in Pl. XIV, fig. 1, the adjacent sides of the lobes being pressed together so that the prestomal cavity is almost completely closed.

If the flies are fed on shallow drying drops of somewhat concentrated syrup containing finely ground Indian ink deposited on glass, proboscis marks, recognizable as white areas where the ink deposit has been removed, can frequently be observed (Pl. XIV, fig. 2). These areas correspond with the shape of the inflated proboscis showing that the margins, and probably the greater part, of the suctorial disc are closely applied. The firmer the application of the disc to the surface supporting the food the more completely are the walls of the prestomal cavity pressed against one another. Hence under these circumstances no material can enter directly into the mouth but has to be conveyed into it through the agency of the pseudo-tracheæ and collecting channels.

If the head of a blow-fly is removed and the proboscis erected by slight pressure on the head and fixed in that condition with plasticine it is possible to obtain an excellent view of the expanded disc. In this position each lobe of the disc is convex in its transverse diameter and the entrance to the prestomal cavity is recognizable as a logitudinal sulcus slightly expanded near its centre. By applying a cover-glass to the oral surface of the disc it can be readily shown how pressure exerted on the disc closes the prestomal cavity in proportion to the degree of the pressure.

Under natural conditions flies probably seldom have the opportunity of feeding on large drops but suck up thin films of moisture and consequently feed with their proboscides so closely applied that the longitudinal prestomal sulcus as well as the longitudinal fissures of the pseudo-tracheæ are to a great extent obliterated. Under these conditions it seems impossible that food should enter the mouth except through the interbifid grooves, and that this is actually the case can be proved by experiments with suitable fluids. If flies are allowed to suck at films of partially dried Indian ink they often remove from the glass only those portions which lie immediately under the interbifid grooves. In such cases beautiful patterns like gratings are left on the glass. Pl. XIV, fig. 3, is a photograph of a portion of one of these patterns. The fly has applied the proboscis firmly to

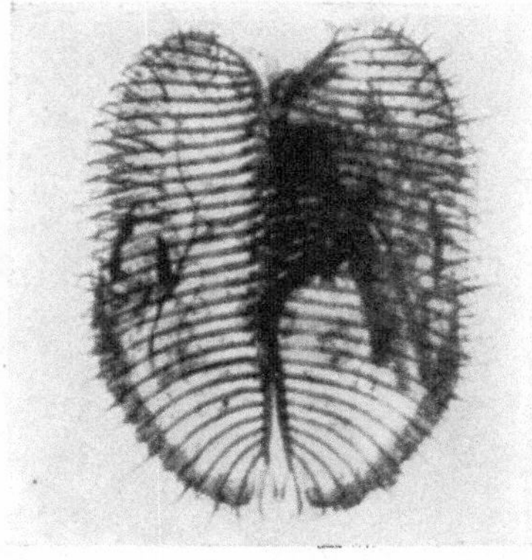

Fig. 1.

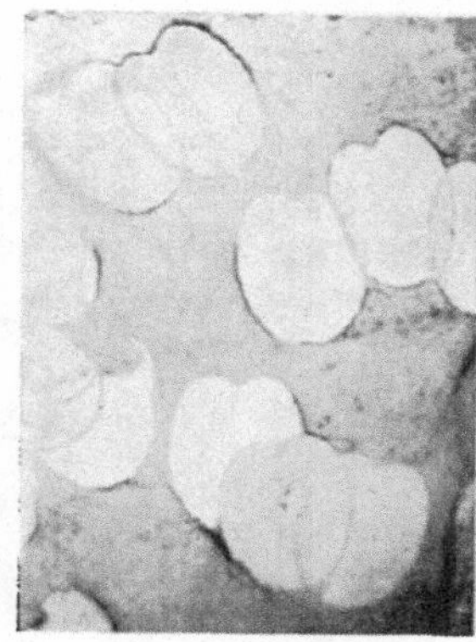

Fig. 2.

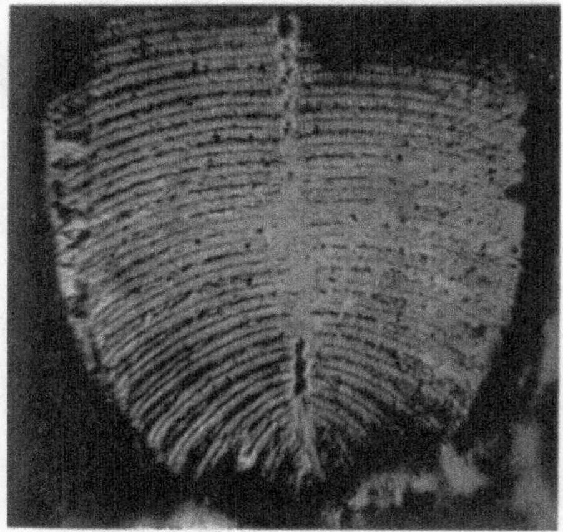

Fig. 3.

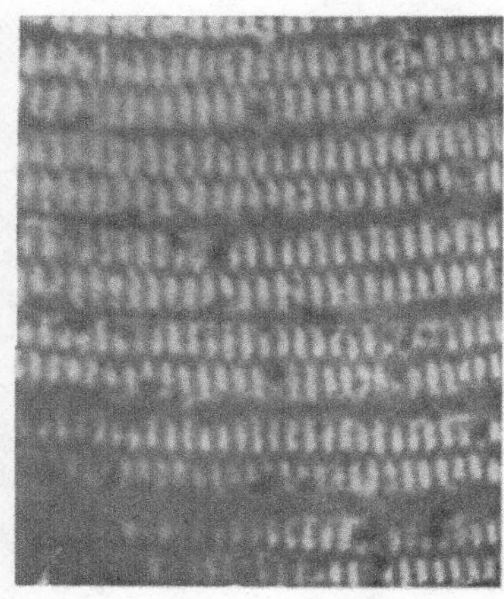

Fig. 4.

Fig. 1 is a photograph (×66) of the oral surface of the erected suctorial disc of a blow-fly. The pseudo-tracheæ and anterior and posterior common collecting channels are well seen.

Fig. 2 is a photograph of proboscis marks produced by a fly feeding on a thin layer of Indian ink spread on glass. The position of the anterior cleft is indicated in every proboscis mark. The marks show that in each case the proboscis has been firmly and evenly applied.

Fig. 3 is a photograph (×77) of a portion of a proboscis mark left by a fly attempting to suck up a layer of partially dried Indian ink deposited on glass. The outline of the suctorial disc is clearly shown. The marks indicating the position of the longitudinal sulcus are very narrow, showing that the prestomal cavity was almost completely closed. The lines of the pseudo-tracheæ are marked by double rows of regularly placed clear oval areas, separated by thin black lines. Each of these areas, from which the pigment has been removed by suction, represents the space covered by an interbifid groove.

Fig. 4 is a photograph of part of a proboscis mark similar to that shown in Fig. 3, more highly magnified (×770). The longitudinal axis of each pseudo-trachea is marked by a zigzag black line, showing that the longitudinal fissure was closed. On each side of the zigzag black line are clear areas produced by the removal of the pigment through the interbifid grooves. Their shapes are very clearly defined. The way in which this pattern is produced can be readily comprehended by reference to Pl. XIII, Fig. 1 (left-hand side). The broad black lines, separating the clear areas, represent the inter-pseudo-tracheal plane areas of the disc.

(From Graham-Smith, *Journal of Hygiene*, 1911.)

the surface so that the outline of the disc is clearly visible. It may also be seen that the longitudinal prestomal sulcus was almost completely closed. The lines of the pseudo-tracheæ are marked by double parallel rows of regularly placed clear oral areas separated by thin black lines. Each of these areas from which the pigment has been removed by suction represents the space covered by an interbifid groove. Pl. XIV, fig. 4, is a photograph of a portion of a similar pattern more highly magnified. It will be noticed that no traces of the zigzag fissures running longitudinally along the pseudo-tracheæ can be seen. These fissures are entirely obliterated by the pressure of the proboscis on the surface causing the free ends of the rings to meet, as can be readily understood by reference to Pl. XIII, fig. 4.

The longitudinal axis of each pseudo-trachea is marked by a zigzag black line. On each side of this line are clear areas caused by the removal of pigment through the interbifid grooves. The way in which this pattern is produced is best understood by reference to Pl. XIII, fig. 1 (left-hand side).

The broader black lines represent the inter-pseudo-tracheal plain areas of the disc.

If fed on a drop of moderate depth the proboscis does not seem to be so closely applied to the surface on which the drop is placed, though the disc is in an erected condition.

If a fly is allowed to feed on a large drop containing particles of various sizes it often sucks up all the fluid and leaves the larger particles in an irregular mass at one edge of the drop. When the area originally covered by the drop is examined with the aid of a lens it is found to be covered with numerous clear oval proboscis marks, indicated by fine lines of pigment at their peripheries. It is evident therefore that the fly at each application of its proboscis has sucked up and swallowed the fluid and smaller particles which are capable of passing through the inter-bifid spaces, and that the suction has caused the larger particles to adhere to the disc. After all the fluid has been swallowed the larger particles adhering to the proboscis are deposited either through the cessation of the suction, or by a small quantity of fluid being forced in a reverse direction to wash off the deposit.

A large number of experiments were carried out in order to ascertain the size of the largest bodies which could be swallowed. For this purpose flies were made to feed on drops of various fluids containing in suspension bodies of definite size and shape such as spores of moulds, pollen, etc. Immediately after feeding they were killed and dissected and the crop and intestinal contents examined for the presence of the suspended particles. It was found that the spores of *Nosema apis* and of various moulds measuring up to ·006 mm., in fact all bodies measuring in their smallest axis less than the diameter of the interbifid space, could be readily swallowed.

The case is however different with larger bodies such as pollen grains. Many feeding experiments were carried out with emulsions of the contents of bees' colons, containing many easily recognizable bodies of various sizes, including pollen grains in various stages of digestion. In most cases pollen grains, except of very small size, could not be detected in the crop or intestinal contents of the flies. On rare occasions however numerous pollen grains were found, both in the crop and in the intestine. On closer examination many of these were found to be empty flattened shells, readily distorted to a slight degree, but afterwards regaining their shape. Such bodies could be easily sucked through the interbifid spaces. Still more rarely one or two apparently undigested pollen grains were found. Also in some experiments with recently gathered pollen from the pollen baskets of the healthy bees the grains (·02 × ·04 mm.) could be detected in the crop or intestinal contents of a small proportion of the experimental flies. No object measuring more than ·02 mm. in its smallest diameter was ever swallowed.

It was found that objects of comparatively large size were more frequently ingested when suspended in viscid fluids, such as honey, or when flies were endeavouring to extract the fluid from semi-solid masses composed of large particles.

In experiments on the part played by flies on the dispersal of parasitic eggs Nicoll (1911, p. 18) found that flies could ingest such large objects as the eggs of tape-worms, measuring up to ·045 mm., which cannot pass into the pseudo-tracheæ[1].

[1] For an account of these experiments see Chapter XX.

These objects are extremely attractive to flies, which may suck at segments of tape-worms for several hours in order to extract their contents (Nicoll, 1911, p. 20). The flies appear to make great efforts to swallow the ova and probably the prestomal cavity is at times open so that the ova pass directly into the mouth without passing through the pseudo-tracheæ. This view is supported by the curiously uneven results obtained by Nicoll, who for example in one series of experiments fed seven flies on ruptured segments of *T. serrata* and found 400 ova in the intestines of two flies, two ova in one fly, and none in the other four flies. The most likely explanation seems to be that in the latter five flies the filter acted efficiently, whereas in the two former ova were allowed to pass into the mouth while the prestomal cavity was open. Possibly in their endeavours to swallow these ova the flies attempt to use their teeth to reduce their size. In order to do so the labellæ have to be so widely separated that the prestomal cavity is open, consequently if suction is made during the process of scraping large particles may pass into the mouth.

All the observations hitherto made indicate that under most conditions the filter acts very efficiently and prevents the entrance of particles larger than ·006 mm. in their smallest diameter into the mouth of the blow-fly. Exceptionally a few larger particles may be drawn forcibly through it, or pass directly through the prestomal cavity into the mouth.

SUMMARY.

All the non-biting flies examined, *C. erythrocephala*, *M. domestica*, *S. carnaria*, *F. canicularis*, *L. cæsar* and *O. anthrax*, possess a filtering apparatus situated in the pseudo-tracheæ of the suctorial disc. The anatomy and action of this filter have been most thoroughly studied in *C. erythrocephala*. The suctorial disc is grooved by pseudo-tracheæ which end near its centre in closed collecting channels. The latter open into furrows or gutters formed by the peculiar disposition of the prestomal teeth on the walls of the prestomal cavity. The opening of the mouth is situated at the base of the cavity. During natural feeding the lobes of the suctorial disc are pressed together so that the lumen of the prestomal cavity is obliterated, and no food can enter the mouth except through the collecting tubes. The pseudo-tracheæ are channels kept open by chitinous rings situated in their walls. Each ring has one bifid extremity, enclosing between the horns the 'interbifid space,' which forms an opening of definite size into the pseudo-trachea. A fold in the cuticle, the 'interbifid groove,' leads to each interbifid space.

The fluid food is sucked first along the interbifid grooves through the chitin-lined interbifid spaces into the pseudo-tracheæ. Particles of larger diameter than the interbifid spaces (·006 mm.) are usually prevented from entering the mouth and are rejected. The fluid and smaller particles are drawn along the pseudo-tracheæ, through the collecting channels and gutters between the prestomal teeth into the mouth. By means of strong suction two opposite interbifid grooves may be made to communicate with each other owing to the lateral fissures connecting with the longitudinal pseudo-tracheal fissure being forced open, and consequently a few larger particles, up to ·02 mm. in diameter, may be drawn into the pseudo-tracheæ.

Certain relatively large and very attractive objects, such as the ova of tape-worms, too large to pass through the filter, may occasionally be swallowed. Such objects probably pass directly into the mouth, when the prestomal cavity is open, during the prolonged sucking efforts made by the flies.

The large number of experiments which have been made leave little room for doubt that under natural conditions, especially when the fly is feeding on a thin film of moisture, the filtering apparatus works with a high degree of efficiency.

CHAPTER VI

THE FUNCTIONS OF THE CROP AND PROVENTRICULUS

"The structure and function of the crop and proventriculus are matters of considerable interest in considering the distribution of infectious material by flies. At the commencement of a meal the fluid is drawn up through the proboscis into the pharynx by the action of the dilator muscles of the pharynx and, as will be shown presently, the crop is first distended with liquid food. If the feeding is continued after the crop is fully distended, the food may pass directly into the ventriculus through the proventriculus. If, on the other hand, the fly is disturbed before any portion of the food has entered the intestine, the fluid which has been sucked into the crop is gradually passed into the ventriculus. In any case, after a variable period of time, the contents of the crop pass into the intestine. The proventriculus is capable, therefore, of being closed during the early part of a meal in order that the food may not enter the intestine but pass into the crop. On the complete distension of the crop, it opens in order to allow food to pass directly from the proboscis to the intestine. It also opens when it is necessary to allow material to pass from the crop into the intestine. After a meal flies usually regurgitate some of the fluid contents of their crops through the proboscis, and during this process the lumen of the proventriculus is closed in order to prevent the fluid from passing into the intestine. Lowne (p. 409) regards the proventriculus as a 'gizzard and nothing more,' and Gordon Hewitt (1907, p. 421) states that 'its structure suggests a pumping function and also that of a valve,' while Giles (1906) says that 'taking the structure as a whole, it is difficult to resist the idea that it must, in some way, have a valvular function, though it is difficult to say how.' The observations just quoted, of which some particulars are given later, seem to indicate that it acts as a valve, possibly controlled, at will, by the fly" (Graham-Smith, 1910, p. 4).

Since the paper quoted above was published, the writer has carried out a number of experiments on blow-flies to determine the function of the proventriculus by direct observation. Blow-flies were allowed to feed on syrup containing particles of Indian ink and immediately afterwards anæsthetized with chloroform. The insect was then fastened down on its side by means of hot sealing-wax at the bottom of a shallow tray, which was immediately filled with water. As rapidly as possible the upper side was dissected away so as to expose the thoracic œsophagus, crop-duct, proventriculus and ventriculus. Under these conditions it was seen that the crop contracted and relaxed at frequent but irregular intervals, causing the particles of the pigment to travel backwards and forwards in the crop-duct and its continuation, the œsophagus, below the opening of the proventriculus, which remained closed and prevented their passing into the ventriculus. At times the contractions of the crop follow each other in rapid succession. During some of these periods the proventriculus relaxes and allows large quantities of fluid containing particles of pigment to pass into the ventriculus, clearly showing that the proventriculus functions as a valve.

"Plate XV, fig. 1, shows a dissection of the proboscis, œsophagus, crop, proventriculus, and ventriculus of a fly which had been fed on milk and then starved for some time. The crop is nearly empty and the division of the œsophagus is well shown. Plate XV, fig. 2, illustrates a dissection of the same structures in a fly which had been fed just previously with liquid gelatin. The distension of the crop is well shown, though much greater degrees of distension have been often met with. In these photographs the organs have been arranged so as to show the several structures to their best advantage and are not in their natural relation to one another. The complete isolation of the structures as shown on Plate XV is a somewhat difficult dissection, since the œsophagus is very delicate and intimately attached to the chitin in the neck region. It was found, however, that if flies were kept in a cage in a warm incubator (37° C.) they soon gorged themselves on drops of liquid gelatin placed on the floor. On being removed from the incubator after 30—60 minutes, the whole intestinal canal, including the crop, was distended with gelatin and could be dissected out with ease, especially if coloured gelatin was used in feeding. If it was intended to subsequently cut sections, the flies were fixed with formalin.

"On several occasions flies which have been allowed to feed on syrup were killed and dissected. The fluid contained in the crop was collected in a capillary pipette and its volume measured. These experiments showed that the capacity of the crop varied between ·003 and ·002 c.c."

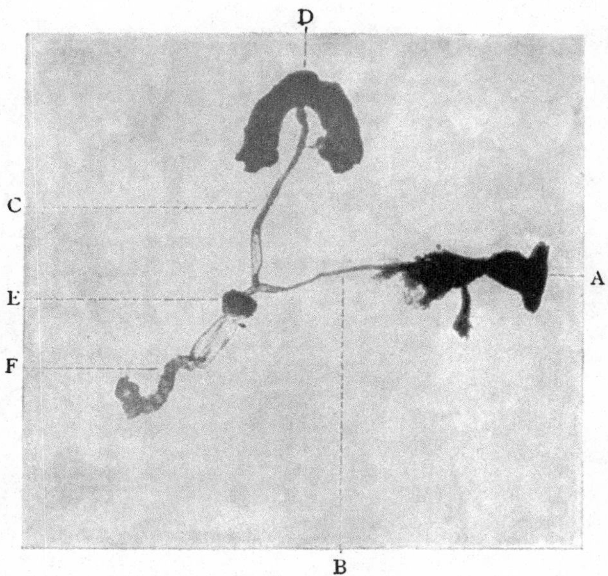

Fig. 1.

Photograph of a dissection (× 16) showing the proboscis (A), œsophagus (B), crop duct (C), crop, almost empty (D), proventriculus (E), and ventriculus (F) of a hungry fly.

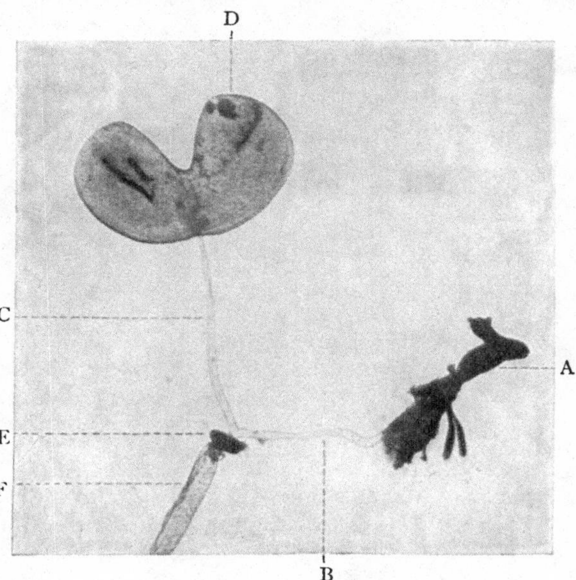

Fig. 2.

Photograph of a dissection showing the same structures in a fly recently fed on gelatin. Note distension of the crop.

(From Graham-Smith, *Reports to Local Government Board*, No. 40, 1910.)

FEEDING EXPERIMENTS.

Fluids.—Plain and coloured syrups.

"A series of feeding experiments with plain and coloured syrups was conducted in the following manner. Flies which had been kept for 24 hours or more without food were placed in clean cages and a few drops of syrup, made by dissolving brown sugar in water, placed on the glass floor plates. The flies began to feed almost immediately. It was noticed that the flies approached the drops and inserted their proboscides, but in many cases did not touch the drops with their legs. Occasionally the anterior legs were placed on the drops, but even then in many instances they did not appear to be soiled. If the drops were too close together, or were irregular, then the feet often became soiled. Occasionally a fly would fall into a drop and subsequently drag itself about the plate spreading the syrup and causing other flies which walked over the wet areas to soil their feet.

"If undisturbed a fly usually becomes gorged within a minute or less. Previous to feeding, the ventral surface of the abdomen of a hungry fly when viewed from the side is slightly concave. Immediately after feeding, the anterior half of the abdomen is greatly distended while the posterior half may still remain concave. This is due to the fact that the greater part of the food is first taken into the crop, which occupies the anterior portion of the abdomen, and greatly distends that organ. Plate XVI, fig. 1, represents the side view of an average unfed fly (× 7) and Plate XVI, fig. 2, the side view of a fly immediately after feeding on syrup. In the latter case the distention of the crop, which can be plainly seen, was so great that the lower portions of the tergal abdominal plates, which usually overlap each other, were forced some distance apart. Experiments with syrup coloured deep red with carmine or deep blue with nigrosin show very clearly the passage of the food material into the crop. As the fly feeds on carmine syrup a red area appears on the anterior portion of the ventral surface of the abdomen, and gradually enlarges till it occupies the whole of the anterior two-thirds of the surface of the abdomen, and usually shows a more or less well-defined convex posterior margin. (Pl. XVI, fig. 3.)

"On rare occasions the red area is situated near the posterior end of the abdomen, but is continued forwards to the thorax as a distinct median red line between colourless areas. In such cases dissection shows that the crop has been displaced by the distension of the large abdominal air sacs.

"Sometimes the flies continue to feed after the crop is full, and then the food passes directly into the intestine, and after a time the whole ventral surface becomes coloured.

"In order to check these observations a number of flies were killed and dissected (under a Zeiss binocular dissecting microscope) at various times after feeding on carmine syrup. The dissections showed that the crop was almost invariably distended with coloured material before any was found in the intestine. If feeding had continued beyond this point coloured material was found in the upper part of the intestine, and within a short time in the lower portion also. In one series of experiments, for example, hungry flies were fed on carmine syrup and killed and dissected at short intervals.

TABLE 3. *Showing the rate at which food passes from the crop into the intestine.*

Time after feeding	No. of flies dissected	Result
3 minutes	1	Crop full of red fluid, but none found in ventriculus or intestine.
6 ,, ...	1	Crop full of red fluid, but none found in ventriculus or intestine.
10 ,, ...	1	Crop full of red fluid, and some just beginning to pass into the ventriculus.
15 ,, ...	1	Crop full of red fluid, and upper third of intestine red.
20 ,, ...	1	Crop full of red fluid, and upper third of intestine red.
2 hours ...	3	Crop full of red fluid, and upper third of intestine red.
	4	Crop full of red fluid, and upper half of intestine red.
	1	Crop full of red fluid, and upper three-quarters of intestine red.

Plate XVI

Fig. 1.

Fig. 2.

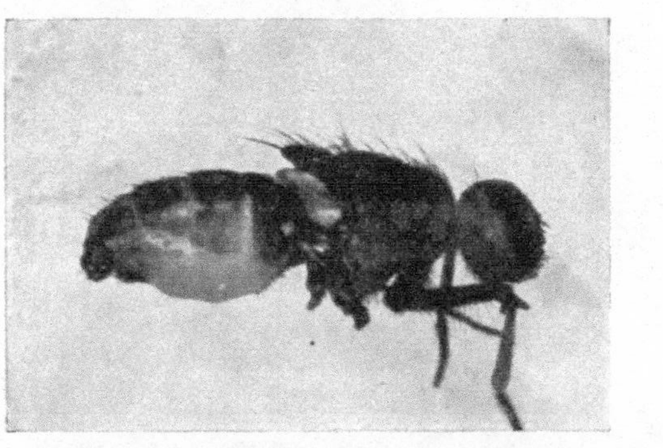

Fig. 3.

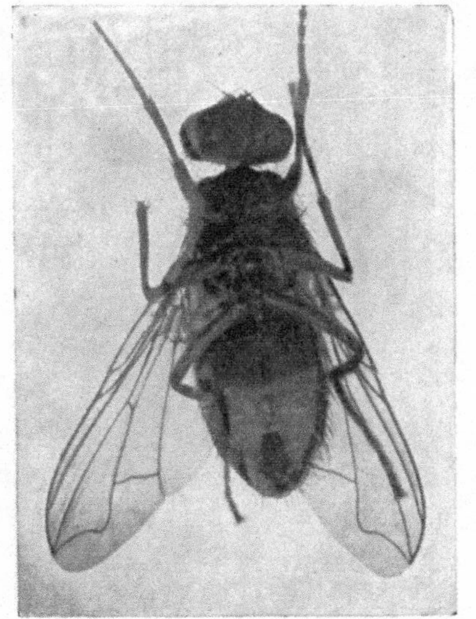

Fig. 1. Photograph (side view) of an unfed fly (×7).
Fig. 2. Photograph (side view) of a fly shortly after feeding on syrup. The distension of the anterior ventral portion of the abdomen in which the crop lies is well seen.
Fig. 3. Photograph (×7) of the ventral surface of a fly recently fed on syrup, coloured with carmine. The dark area in the anterior portion of the abdomen, which was coloured red, indicates the position of the crop.

(From Graham-Smith, *Report to Local Government Board*, No. 40, 1910.)

"The rate at which the food passes from the crop into the intestine appears to vary, depending to some extent on the temperature and the nature of the food. For example, if the flies are kept in the incubator at 37° C. and fed on carmine gelatin much of the food may reach the rectal valve within an hour.

"If the flies are disturbed before the crop is completely distended the contents of the crop are gradually passed into the intestine, but the organ is not completely emptied for many hours, or in some cases for days, even though no further food is given. In most examples which were dissected the crop was found nearly empty on the third day after feeding, but the intestine still contained large quantities of red material.

"Flies allowed to feed to their utmost capacity on carmine syrup showed a red colour all over the ventral surface of the abdomen within an hour or two, and dissections showed that the crop and intestine, down to the anus, were distended with coloured syrup. If such flies are subsequently fed on plain syrup it is found that most of the red material from the first meal is retained in the crop and only slowly passed into the intestine. Dissections show that a considerable quantity of the carmine, though diluted, is still present in the crop, under such conditions, after several days. For example a number of flies were fed once on carmine syrup, and were subsequently given plain syrup daily.

TABLE 4. *Showing the period during which coloured food may remain in the crop.*

Time after feeding	No. of flies dissected	Result
24 hours	2	Crop red and distended. Intestine red throughout.
48 "	3	Crop red and distended. Intestine red throughout.
3 days	3	Crop red and distended. Intestine red throughout.
4 "	2	Crop pink and distended. Intestine red throughout.

"From these experiments, of which a large number were performed at different times, it appears that in these insects the crop performs two important functions; (A) it acts, at the time of feeding, as a large receptacle, which can be filled with great rapidity, and which consequently enables a fly which is disturbed within a few seconds of commencing a meal to carry away sufficient food to live on for some days; (B) when food is abundant the crop seems to act as a reservoir in which material can be stored against a time when food may become scarce."

CHAPTER VII

THE HABITS OF ADULT FLIES

The habits of most of the species of flies which invade houses have up to the present been very insufficiently studied, only those of *M. domestica*, *F. canicularis* and *scalaris*, and of certain of the blue-bottles and green-bottles having received careful attention. The breeding habits of the various species have already been mentioned, and in dealing with the habits of the adults it may perhaps be most advantageous to consider them under the following headings:

A. Range of flight.

B. Outdoor habits.

C. Indoor habits.

D. Hibernation.

E. Habits after feeding.

F. Experiments on defæcation.

A. *Range of flight.*

Up to the present few observations have been made on the range of flight though the subject is obviously of considerable importance in relation to the whole question of the carriage of infection by these insects. The experimental investigations about to be quoted have all been carried out with house-flies.

The first series were undertaken by Arnold (1907, p. 262), who liberated from the window of the Administration Block of the Monsall Hospital, Manchester, a hundred flies marked with a spot of white enamel on the thorax, on three successive Sundays. This form of marking did not affect the energy of the fly, and the mark did not readily wear off. The fly traps in the wards were then watched for the marked flies. "Of the 300, five were recovered at distances varying from 30 to 190 yards. The liberations were always in fine weather, and the recoveries were within five days. In this experiment 190 yards was the greatest distance available, so that the experiments cannot be taken as giving any hint of the limit of range."

In the case of the biting fly, *Glossina morsitans*, the investigations of Bagshawe (1908) show that marked flies may be retaken up to 900 yards from the point of liberation.

A more extended series of observations were carried out by Copeman, Howlett and Merriman (1911) in 1910 at Postwick, a small village, situated about five miles east of Norwich, the inhabitants of which "were experiencing a plague of flies, so unprecedented in extent as to constitute a serious annoyance, and possible danger to health." More than 99 per cent. of the flies caught on the village fly papers were *M. domestica* and the remainder mostly *F. canicularis*. "As the result of careful investigations in the village itself, in which there existed no unusual accumulation of manure or other fermenting refuse, we came to the conclusion that no special opportunity was afforded there for the breeding of the house-fly in such quantities as had been present. It became obvious, therefore, that special conditions must be in operation, affording a reservoir of flies at some situation outside the village boundaries. Such conditions were afforded by the presence of enormous accumulations of dust-bin and other refuse deposited by the Norwich corporation on the Whitlingham Marshes, at a distance of a little over half-a-mile from the village church." In this mass of refuse fermentation was actively going on, the fresher portions steaming vigorously when the top layer was disturbed; it was in fact an almost ideal breeding ground for flies. Near this place was a workmen's shelter, which was warm but ill-lit. "On cold days it was often not easy to catch flies on the tip itself, but they could be caught in any numbers in the shelter, when some sacking, which covered the wall, and a bench near the stove, was sometimes literally black with them. Though the flies caught in the workmen's shelter, like those caught in the village, were practically all *M. domestica*, this must be due rather to the habits of this fly than to the failure of other species to breed on the tip, since the collection of 200 larvæ and pupæ from fresh tip refuse gave the following results.

M. domestica	143
M. stabulans	34
C. erythrocephala	18
P. rudis	3
F. canicularis	2

"A considerable number of undetermined *Phoridæ* were also bred out from samples of the refuse, which were kept as likely to be good for some of these larvæ.

"We see, therefore, that there was a considerable variety among the flies breeding in the refuse; just as on the sewage farm (near by) *Sepsis* and *Scatophaga* were the dominant species, so *M. domestica* predominated on the refuse heap."

These observers came to the conclusion that the tip did not attract flies for several reasons: marked flies did not return to it, eggs and young larvæ were not found on it, female flies did not predominate, and an examination of the fresh refuse showed that it already contained many larvæ and also pupæ. The tip was therefore a distributing centre of flies. On general grounds there is every reason to believe that the flies which infested the village were bred in the refuse heap and migrated from it, and further the investigators proved this experimentally. Flies were marked by shaking in a stout paper bag containing a small quantity of coloured chalk (using, as a rule, a different colour for each day) and liberated at the refuse heap. Some of these were subsequently found at the village. Other similar experiments showed that some of the flies occasionally travelled as far as 1700 yards, and that distances of 800 to 1000 yards were often traversed. Two marked flies were caught 800 yards from the refuse heap 35 and 45 minutes respectively after liberation.

Howard (1911, p. 54) says that in the summer of 1910 Hine made an effort to determine the distance flies can travel by liberating 350 flies, each marked with a spot of gold enamel on the thorax and on each wing. The marked flies were only found about dwellings a short distance off up to the third day. Howard also quotes Forbes who states that his experiments show that flies can spread naturally for at least a quarter of a mile.

Hewitt (1912, p. 2) carried out experiments on this subject at Ottawa, the flies being liberated from a small island in the Rideau River, which runs through a part of the city. The flies were obtained from pupæ and "were marked by spraying with rosolic acid in 10 per cent. alcohol, applied by means of a fine spray. This method is simple and harmless and reliable as a means of detection. The presence of a marked fly on a sticky fly-paper is indicated by its producing a scarlet colouration when the paper is dipped into water made slightly alkaline." "The papers were placed in as many as possible of the houses in the neighbouring districts on both sides of the river. The papers were placed chiefly in the kitchens of houses and were collected one or two days after being distributed. They were usually collected in that portion of the district towards which the wind had been blowing from the island, as it was found that the wind was the chief factor in determining the direction of distribution from day to day. The greatest range of flight obtained in these experiments, namely 700 yards, represents an actual flight of considerably greater distance than is represented by a straight line from the place of liberation to the point of capture."

The observations which have been quoted relate to the flight of house-flies in the open away from houses and show that under favourable conditions and assisted by the wind they can fly about a mile and frequently travel half-a-mile. It is not impossible, however, that they may travel still greater distances. As Hine says: "It appears most likely that the distance flies travel to reach dwellings is controlled by circumstances. Almost any reasonable distance may be covered by a fly under compulsion to reach food or shelter. When these are at hand the insect is not impelled to go far, and consequently does not do so."

The only observations hitherto published on the flight of flies in cities lend support to the last statement of Hine. Cox, Lewis and Glynn (1912, p. 309), working in Liverpool, came to the conclusion that "in cities where food is plentiful flies rarely migrate from the localities in which they are bred" (see Chapter X).

The larger species of house-frequenting flies can probably travel much further than the house-fly and other smaller species, if we may judge from the extraordinary powers of flight of some of the gad-flies of the family *Tabanidæ*, which can circle round fast trotting horses only alighting occasionally.

B. *Outdoor habits.*

In Chapter II it has been shown that most of the flies commonly found in houses breed in various decaying substances and excreta, and consequently the adults, especially the females, seek these substances for the purpose of depositing eggs, and at the same time walk over them and not infrequently feed on them. Though *M. domestica*, *M. stabulans*, and *Drosophilidæ* prefer to lay their eggs on fermenting vegetable matter, they also deposit them on horse manure and other excreta. *F. canicularis*, *F. scalaris*, *P. rudis*, *A. radicum*, *Sepsidæ* and the *Psychodidæ* prefer the latter. The larvæ of the larger flies, *Lucilia*, *Calliphora* and *Sarcophaga* feed on carrion, and the flies are attracted to such materials.

In fact most of these species are attracted to filth of all kinds. They are also frequently found feeding on over ripe fruit, both on trees and when exposed for sale in shops, and certainly contaminate it with fæcal and putrefactive bacteria. Many of them are also attracted to meat, both cooked and raw, milk, butter, sweets and other food materials exposed in shops and on stalls.

"In order to determine the distribution of the sexes" Hermes (1911, p. 521) made observations "under two different conditions, viz. first, six sweepings with an insect net were made over a horse manure pile on which many flies had gathered; second, flies were collected in one house, giving a fairly representative lot for indoors."

TABLE 5. *Showing results in regard to sexes and species in six sweepings from a horse manure pile on May 18 and 19, 1909.*

	First M.	First F.	Second M.	Second F.	Third M.	Third F.	Fourth M.	Fourth F.	Fifth M.	Fifth F.	Sixth M.	Sixth F.	Total M.	Total F.
House-fly (*M. domestica*)	7	153	4	81	3	64	9	77	4	210	5	112	32	697
Muscina stabulans	2	6	0	7	0	5	2	5	3	10	1	4	8	37
Blow-fly (*C. vomitoria*)	2	2	0	1	1	0	0	0	0	0	1	0	4	3
L. cæsar	0	1	0	1	0	1	0	1	0	0	0	0	0	4
Other species*	1	4	0	4	2	1	4	2	4	2	2	0	13	13
	12	166	4	94	6	71	15	85	11	222	9	116	57	754

* Excluding very small diptera.

TABLE 6. *Showing number of individuals collected in a screened dwelling, June 1, 1909.*

	M.	F.
House-fly (*M. domestica*)	86	116
Muscina sp.	3	
Homalomyia sp.	5	0
Calliphora	1	2
	95	119

"Table 5 shows that of those flies which frequent both the manure pile and the home, the house-flies compose 90 %, and that of the total collected, over 95 % were females. Thus, it is clear that it is the 'instinct' to oviposit that has mainly attracted these insects to this situation. In fact, fresher parts of the manure pile are often literally white with house-fly eggs in countless numbers. Observations made in the near vicinity of the manure pile proved that certainly the same percentage (over 95 %) of the flies clinging to the walls of the stable, boxes, and so on, were males."

"That the sexes in the house-fly are normally about equal in numbers is apparent, inasmuch as of a total of 264 pupæ collected indiscriminately and allowed to emerge in the laboratory, 129 were males and 135 were females."

In smaller villages the flies have many opportunities of frequenting especially filthy substances, and in larger towns, more particularly in some of the great cities, many courts and alleys are to be found in the poorer quarters, where decaying substances and excrement lie exposed and covered with flies.

The common house-fly and the raven fly (*M. corvina*) and other species annoy animals by settling on the more exposed portions of skin, and sucking the secretions from the skin and mucous surfaces. Human beings working or resting out-of-doors are annoyed in the same way. Flies are particularly attracted to open wounds and ulcers and to pus or other pathological secretions on dressings. Even in temperate climates disease-producing bacteria may be carried occasionally from one individual to another in this way. Whatever may be the significance of this mode of conveyance in temperate climates, it is obviously of far greater importance in the tropics, where insects are present in greater profusion throughout all seasons of the year. In Egypt and the Sudan, according to Sandwith (1904), flies "often alight on food, when coming direct from filth. They also crawl about the face and mouth of human beings and are most persistent in this, evidently in search of moisture." The natives, both adults and children, exhibit remarkable indifference to flies walking over their faces and eyes and there are good reasons for believing that many cases of ophthalmia are produced in this way in Egypt and other countries. Nicholls (1912, p. 85) believes "that the majority of cases of yaws in the West Indies are caused by the inoculation of surface injuries" by a small fly known as *Oscinis pallipes* (Pl. XVII, fig. 4).

In tropical countries where the lower classes are often unacquainted with the use of latrines, swarms of flies are bred in the fæcal deposits; some of these are found upon food, and in dry weather numbers will be found flying around pools and water supplies, and can be observed alighting at the edge of the water to drink. Some of these species for filthy associations far surpass the house-fly, and seem to have become adapted to breeding in human fæcal deposits, not being found elsewhere. Nicholls (1912, p. 81), in St Lucia, conducted experiments "by exposing human stools in various places on different days for about ten hours, after which it would be found that numerous ova and larvæ of flies had been deposited upon them. In all, twenty-five masses were used and approximately 18,000 flies hatched out; this gives an average of 720 for each stool." These flies belonged to six species, *Drosophila melanogaster* Mg., *Limosina punctipennis* Wied., *Sepsis* sp., *Sarcophaga aurifinis* Walk., *Sarcophaga* sp., and *Sarcophagula* sp. The undetermined *Sarcophaga* and the *Drosophila* are frequently found upon food, and the others, with the exception of the *Sepsis*, have occasionally been found upon provisions in houses. They are all liable to infect water supplies especially in dry weather. Reference to Chapter XXVI will show that the number of species that visit or breed in human excrement is very large.

Particular attention may, however, be directed to one of the species just mentioned, *L. punctipennis*, which occurs throughout the tropics, and to flies of the genus *Pycnosoma*.

In regard to *L. punctipennis*, Nicholls (p. 86) makes the following interesting statement:

"*Limosina punctipennis* lives and breeds almost exclusively upon human excrement, and in exposed places swarms of these little flies will be found. The only other situations in which I have caught it have been water pools, rivers and ravines in very dry weather, when it will fly a considerable distance in search of water. After a long period of dry weather I placed a small pan of water in a patch of 'bush' to which labourers were accustomed to resort, and in which these flies were consequently plentiful. Soon numbers of them were seen alighting on the vessel at the edge of the water and drinking; the next nearest water was 100 yards away and here also the flies were seen. The pan of water was left here for several hours; it was then removed and examined for fæcal contamination by means of cultures, and *Bacillus coli communis* was obtained. This experiment was repeated upon two other occasions, and in one of these the same organism was grown. Needless to say that both the vessel and the water were sterilised, and control samples were kept in sterilised bottles."

Especially in Africa and the East, flies of the genus *Pycnosoma*, which have habits similar to those of the house-fly, may carry disease organisms, especially *B. typhosus*. They swarm about filth trenches, and seem to breed in fæcal matter and offal of all kinds (see Chapter XIII).

Of this genus three species are common.

Pycnosoma marginale Wied. is a "thick-set, stoutly built fly, about 9 to 13 millimetres in length, with an average wing expanse of 22½ millimetres, with orange-buff-coloured face and shining, metallic plum-purple and metallic green body, recognisable at once by the dark brown front border to the wings. (Pl. XVII, fig. 1.)

"*Eyes* in male meeting together in the middle line above, in female separated by a cadmium-orange-coloured space (the front), practically equal to one-third of the head in width; male with an area on the upper half of each eye consisting of larger facets than the remainder; *antennæ* orange, the arista and hairs clothing it brown; ground colour of *thorax* and abdomen varying as indicated above; *thorax* with a shimmering, pollinose, transverse band of pearl-grey on its anterior and posterior third, making these areas duller than the remainder which appears in certain lights as a brown transverse band; *abdomen* with a shimmering, pollinose band on the basal portion of the second segment, and similar lateral patches on the third and fourth segments; first segment and hind borders of second and third segments usually darker than remainder of abdomen; *wings* hyaline, with a dark brown patch at the base, which is continued as a stripe along the fore border to the end of the second vein; *legs* metallic purplish-brown or black."

This species "has a very wide distribution in Africa and even ranges eastwards as far as Quetta" (Austen, 1904, p. 664).

Pycnosoma chloropyga Wied. is a smaller species, from 6½ to 10 millimetres in length, with an average wing expanse of 18 millimetres. "Metallic bluish-green, or metallic plum-purple, last two segments of abdomen brassy-green; wings hyaline, with a dark blotch near the base. (Pl. XVII, fig. 2.)

"*Head* in the male with the eyes almost meeting in the middle line above, in the female with eyes widely separated; lower part of head, including anterior portion of orbital margins, yellowish-grey, clothed with short silvery white hair; upper part of front in female shining purplish-black; *antennæ* black, arista and hair clothing it brown. *Thorax* marked as shown in Pl. XVII, fig. 2, the dark areas deep black, the lighter portions metallic

Plate XVII

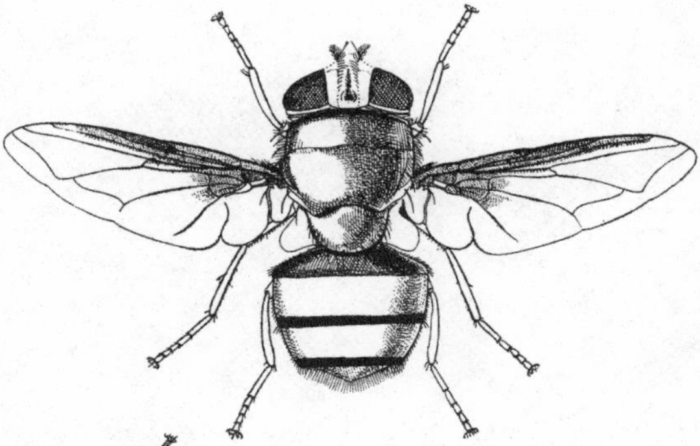

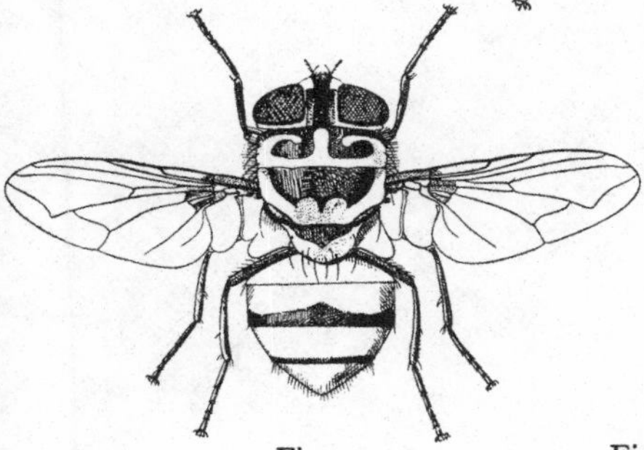

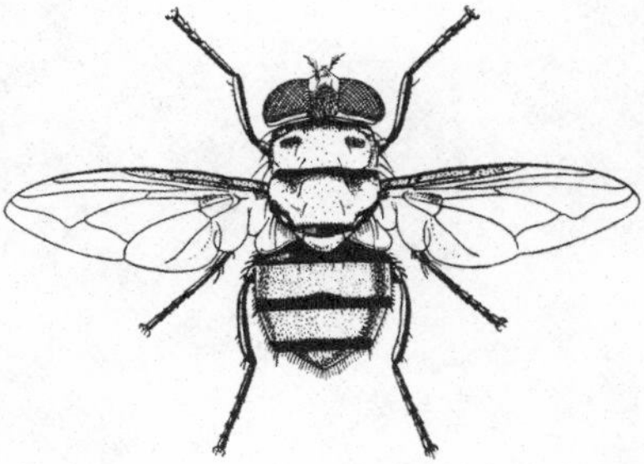

Fig. 2. Fig. 1. Fig. 3.

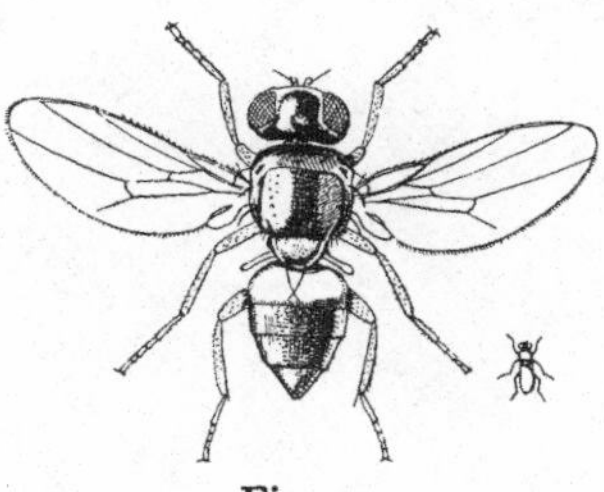

Fig. 4.

Fig. 1. *Pycnosoma marginale* Wied (× 4). Fig. 2. *Pycnosoma chloropyga* Wied (× 4).
Fig. 3. *Pycnosoma putorium* Wied (× 4). Fig. 4. *Oscinis pallipes* Lw. (× 8). Nat. size.

plum-purple or bluish-green, clothed with shimmering pearl-grey pollen, which is more conspicuous in front; *scutellum* generally more or less dull-black at the base, the distal two-thirds shining; *abdomen* with the first segment blackish, and the hind margins of the second and third segments dull-black, the dull margin of the second segment often double the depth of that of the third; shining portion of the second segment clothed with shimmering pearl-grey pollen; *legs* black."

This species "is widely distributed in South Africa, and ranges at least as far north as British East Africa."

Other species of this genus, very similar in size and general appearance to *P. chloropyga*, "are found in West Africa and elsewhere in the same continent, while yet other species occur in India, China and the East generally." (Austen, 1904.)

In some parts of India *M. domestica* and *M. determinata*, commonly breed in filth trenches, but, according to Patton, *M. nebulo* is the common species in Madras.

C. *Indoor habits.*

The species of flies found in the rooms of houses vary according to the time of year (see p. 17). Some flies apparently enter mainly for warmth and shelter, others are attracted by food, others seem to enter by accident, and some, which hibernate in houses, no doubt come in for the sake of shelter from the winter's cold. The bright and sunny rooms are usually the most attractive to all kinds of flies.

The lesser house-fly, *F. canicularis*, is most common in the earlier part of summer. It does not seem to be much attracted to food. Later, common house-flies (*M. domestica*) enter in greater numbers and apparently cause the lesser house-flies to retreat from the kitchens and dining-rooms to the bed-rooms.

The house-fly is a great feeder; it explores every part of the room, and to judge from the industrious way in which it travels over every article of furniture, constantly stopping to dab down its proboscis, it appears to extract some sort of nutriment from almost every household object. The vexatious persistency with which it repeatedly settles on any exposed skin surface, especially on warm days, is no doubt due to its anxiety to feed on the skin secretions.

Flies deposit vomit and fæces on almost every object on which they alight, whether food or not. In feeding, as has been shown already they frequently moisten soluble substances, and often attempt to dissolve insoluble materials with vomit and saliva, and even during feeding have been noticed to deposit fæces. Recently 1102 vomit marks, and 9 fæcal deposits were counted on an area six inches square of a cupboard window. Plate XVIII, fig. 1, is a photograph of part of this window showing a row of fæcal masses, probably deposited by one fly, and several vomit marks.

"One does not like to think that the fly now walking round the edge of the cream jug was a short time ago regaling its impartial palate on the choicest morsels in the dust-bin, ash-pit or garbage-can, or on more indescribable filth."

The house-fly is a diurnal species, resting during the night. It loves shady places, and is not specially attracted to bright windows.

The activity of flies is much influenced by temperature, a fall in the temperature often changing activity into stupor.

At midsummer flies probably do not often live more than two or three weeks, but accurate information on this point is difficult to obtain apart from experimental conditions. In the autumn they may be kept in captivity for several weeks. Under natural conditions, however, in the autumn the majority succumb to the attack of the fly fungus (*Empusa muscæ*, see Chapter XXIII), but some linger on until the early winter months. They do not disappear, however, altogether during the winter months as popularly thought, but may be found in such places as kitchens or bake-houses, where the temperature conditions are favourable. Possibly some of them may remain dormant throughout the winter in sheltered but cold situations.

The blow-flies (*C. erythrocephala* and *C. vomitoria*) and flesh flies (*S. carnaria*) often enter rooms apparently attracted by the presence of cold meat and similar substances, with the object of depositing eggs. Like the house-fly, however, they attempt to feed on every article of diet. The green-bottles

(*L. cæsar*) seem to be greatly influenced by light (p. 25), but are nevertheless frequently found in rooms, and then behave like blow-flies.

The cheese fly (*P. casei*) is attracted to cheese and fatty substances in which it lay its eggs, and the fruit flies (*Drosophila*) are frequently found about dishes containing fruit and jam.

D. *Hibernation.*

As has been stated in the last section, small numbers of house-flies probably hibernate. "In the first warm days of spring, they reappear in our houses invariably in those portions of our dwellings which are kept at a relatively high temperature; thus we get a marked domiciliary distribution or a preponderance of flies in those parts where both heat and food are available" (Newstead, 1909, p. 6).

Several other species occasionally hibernate in houses. The best known of these are the blow-flies, which remain hidden in various situations and come out on warm and sunny days; the raven fly (*M. corvina*), which frequently hibernates in country houses, and the cluster fly (*P. rudis*). A plague of the latter insects has been well described by Howard (1911, p. 237). "They were at once a terror to good house-keepers and a constant surprise, since they were found in beds, in pillow slips, under table covers, behind pictures, in wardrobes, and in all sorts of places. In clean, dark bed-rooms seldom used, they would form in large clusters about the ceilings....They were stated to be very sluggish—to crawl rather than to fly away when disturbed. They were said to be found often in incredible numbers under buildings, between the earth and floor."

E. *Habits after feeding.*

Observations on the functions of the proboscis, crop and proventriculus, and the ways in which flies feed have been quoted in previous chapters. Here it is only necessary to consider the habits of flies after feeding on various materials.

(1) *The habits of flies after feeding on fluids.*

"A number of observations were made on the habits of flies after feeding on various fluids. After gorging themselves the insects usually climb up the sides of the cage and move from place to place, frequently stopping to rub one leg against another or to clean their heads and wings by passing their legs over them. At intervals, however, they sit still and large drops of fluid, coloured red or blue, if the food has consisted of carmine or nigrosin syrup, or opaque and white if it has consisted of milk, exude from the tips of their proboscides. These drops gradually enlarge until they are about equal in size to the insect's head. After a longer or shorter period the drop is slowly withdrawn or deposited on the glass. Flies are frequently observed to exude and withdraw such drops several times. If disturbed they either deposit them or withdraw them

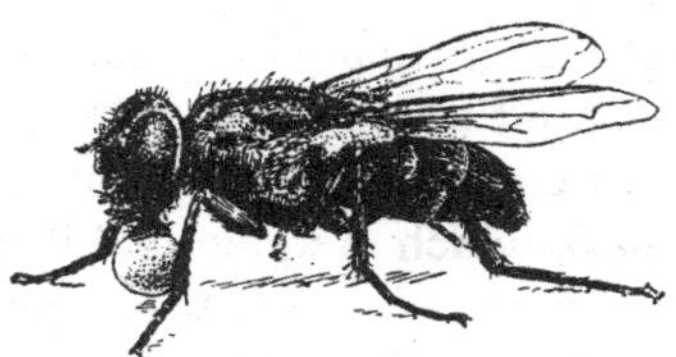

Fig. 23. House-fly in the act of regurgitating liquid food. Such a drop when deposited forms a 'vomit' spot. (From Hewitt, 1912, p. 30.)

with great rapidity. When deposited on the glass, as frequently happens, the drops gradually dry and each gives rise to a round stain with an opaque centre, surrounded by a clearer zone bounded by a distinct thin, more opaque marginal ring (see Plate XVIII, fig. 2). On watching these flies the impression conveyed is that the insects have distended their crops to an uncomfortable degree and that some of the food is regurgitated in order to relieve the distension.

"Flies have often been seen to suck up the drops deposited by their companions.

"Whatever may be the cause of the procedure the habit is very common after feeding on all kinds of fluids, such as milk, syrup and sputum, and the stains or 'spots' left by these drops can be recognised on all surfaces on which flies naturally settle.

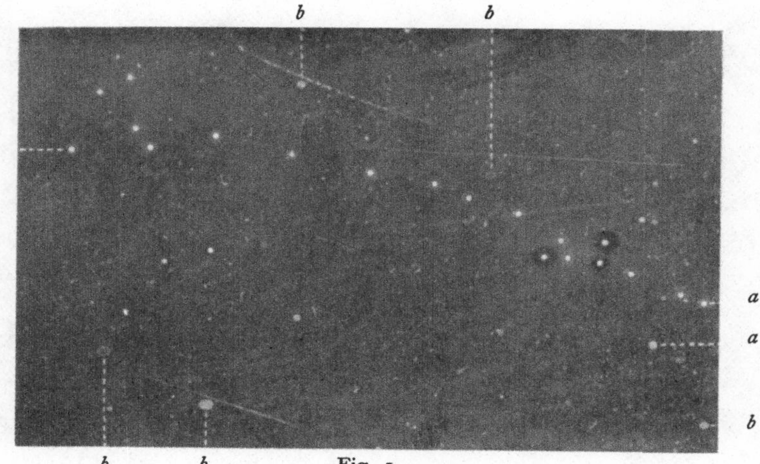

Fig. 1.

Photograph of part of a window pane soiled by flies. Natural size. (*a*...*a* fæcal deposits. *b*...*b* 'vomit' marks.)

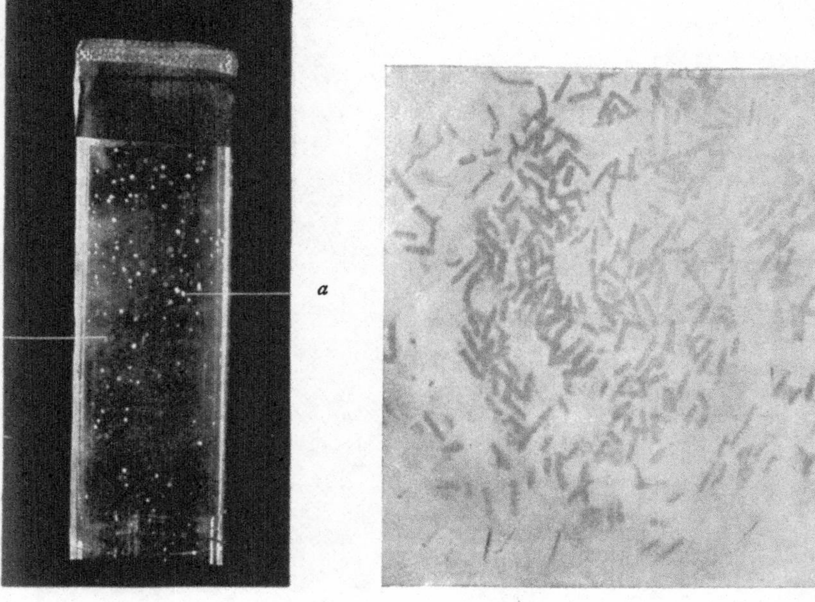

Fig. 2.

Fig. 3.

Fig. 2. Photograph of a cage ($\frac{1}{2}$ nat. size) in which well fed flies had been kept. Its surface is covered by numerous 'spots.' The white ones (*a*) are fæcal deposits and the lighter ones (*b*) with dark centres 'vomit' marks.

Fig. 3. Photograph of a film preparation made from the crop contents of a fly three days after feeding on the blood of a mouse just dead of anthrax. The preparation consists of a nearly pure culture of non-spore bearing anthrax bacilli.

(Figs. 2 and 3 from Graham-Smith, *Report to Local Government Board*, No. 40, 1910.)

"Flies fed on coloured syrup often regurgitate coloured fluid 24 or more hours later, though fed in the interval on plain syrup. When infected food has been given the infecting organisms are usually found in great numbers in these 'spots,' and moreover, as will be shown later, fluid regurgitated from the crop is used to dissolve or moisten sugar and other similar dry food materials. The importance of the habit cannot therefore be overestimated.

"The term 'vomit' will be used to differentiate the stains left by these drops from fæcal deposits and proboscis-marks made in half dried material.

"If a fly, which has been fed on coloured syrup, is killed with chloroform and pressure made with the forceps on the thorax some of the syrup may exude from the proboscis. Further pressure on the thorax or abdomen causes the proboscis to be protruded, and occasionally a large quantity of fluid may be exuded from it. Usually, however, though the proboscis appears to be distended with fluid, very little is exuded.

"Possibly some mechanism exists, near the tip of the proboscis, for preventing the expression of the fluid. If, however, the tip of the proboscis is cut off, or the head removed, the contents of the crop can easily be expressed from the cut end of the proboscis or the œsophagus, even up to five or six hours after feeding[1]."

(2) *Semi-fluid material.*

"At various times flies were allowed to feed on milk which had been spread on glass in a thin layer and allowed to partially dry, and on other materials of similar consistency. The flies walked over the areas covered by the dry milk and frequently applied their proboscides to them. In all cases the application was of some duration and fluid was often deposited by the fly on the area it was sucking. After each application an oval depression was made in the surface, in many cases showing most beautifully an imprint of the end of the proboscis, or an oval area was completely denuded. Plate XIV, fig. 2, shows

[1] Severe pressure on the sides of the head may cause turbid red-coloured fluid to be exuded. This seems to be derived from the eyes.

numerous imprints of flies' proboscides on a layer of Indian ink, and Fig. 3 one of the imprints more highly magnified, on which the tracings of the pseudo-tracheæ at the end of the proboscis can be clearly seen. If the flies had been fed previously on carmine syrup, red patches were frequently observed at the margins of these proboscis marks, either due to the deposition of carmine which had remained on the proboscis or to the regurgitation of carmine stained material to moisten the dried milk. The latter explanation is probably the correct one in most cases, for a single fly will leave many (100 or more) carmine-stained proboscis marks, and moreover carmine stains are more common when the layer of milk is rather dry, and requires more fluid to moisten it, than when it is less dry. In one experiment, made two hours after feeding on carmine syrup, half the proboscis marks showed carmine stains, and in another made 22 hours after feeding several of them showed carmine stains.

"It was also frequently noticed that flies which had the opportunity of feeding on either fluid or partially dried milk often chose the drier portions. Under natural conditions they can often be seen sucking the dried remains near the top of a milk jug.

"If flies are carefully observed under natural conditions, or in captivity in a cage, it is seen that they are constantly applying their proboscides to the surfaces over which they are walking, apparently attempting to suck up nutritive material. Under suitable conditions the imprints of their proboscides can often be made out."

(3) *Soluble solids.*

"Flies will feed readily on crystals of brown sugar. The mode of feeding can be very accurately watched by placing one or two flies in a small cage with a crystal of brown sugar on the bottom. The cage may be easily so arranged that the lens of a Zeiss binocular microscope can be focused on the sugar. The oral lobes of the proboscis are very widely opened and closely applied to the sugar. Fluid seems to be first deposited on the sugar and then strong sucking movements take place. When the proboscis is moved from one spot a depression in the sugar is observed, and, if the fly has been previously fed on carmine, red stains round its margin are often seen. In a number of experiments carmine stains were noticed on sugar 60, 80 and 90 minutes and even five hours after feeding on carmine.

"Infection experiments described later seem to prove that in the case of flies recently fed on syrup the fluid is mainly liquid regurgitated from the crop. When the crop is empty saliva alone is probably made use of.

"A fly was very carefully watched sucking an apparently quite dry layer of sputum. It put out large quantities of fluid from its proboscis and seemed to suck the fluid in and out alternately until a fairly large area was quite moist. Then as much as possible was sucked up and the fly moved on to another place." (Graham-Smith, 1910.)

F. *Experiments on defæcation.*

"Flies which have access to abundant food defæcate frequently. The fæces, consisting of thick brownish or yellowish semi-fluid material, are deposited in single masses and quickly dry, forming opaque raised rounded stains. Occasionally the stains are pear-shaped. At ordinary temperatures flies fed on coloured syrup do not deposit coloured fæces within two hours. The fæcal stains can be usually distinguished without difficulty from 'vomit' stains.

"Three different types of marks or 'spots' have therefore to be distinguished: (1) fæcal deposits, round, opaque, often raised and yellowish, brownish or whitish in colour; (2) 'vomit' stains, round, with a small opaque centre and clear peripheral portion, bounded by a darker zone, and (3) proboscis-marks left on half dried material.

"The extraordinary number of deposits, both fæcal and vomit, left by well-fed flies, can be judged from a small number of experiments which were made with the object of ascertaining the number of deposits (fæcal and vomit) produced. (Plate XVIII, fig. 2.)

"In the first series (A) 10 flies were given a single feed of milk. When all had fed they were transferred to a fresh cage. At intervals the flies were again transferred to other fresh cages and the deposits in the old cages counted. In the second series (B) the deposits of 11 flies were counted in the same way, but milk was always present in the cage so that the flies could feed as often as they wished.

TABLE 7. *To illustrate the number of deposits left by flies.*

	Series A			Series B		
Time after feeding	Vomit	Fæces	Total	Vomit	Fæces	Total
1st hour	30	11	41	22	10	32
2nd and 3rd hours ...	13	3	16	31	9	40
4th hour	18	6	24	6	4	10
5th hour	15	9	24	12	6	18
6th–22nd hour ...	49	10	59	108	16	124
	125	39	164	179	45	224

"Each fly in series (A) produced an average of 16·4 'spots,' and in series (B) of 20·4. In another experiment 10 flies which had been given one feed of milk, produced in nine hours 209 (191 vomit and 18 fæces) deposits, and in the complete 24 hours 307 (282 vomit and 25 fæces) deposits or an average of 30·7 'spots' per fly.

"No doubt the rate at which flies produce deposits depends on several factors, such as the temperature and the form of food, etc., but only a few experiments on this subject were made. Flies are more lively in hot weather or when placed in a warm incubator. That the kind of food exerts a considerable influence is shown by the following experiment. Three lots of flies were fed on syrup, milk and sputum respectively for several days. Those fed on syrup produced an average of 4·7 deposits per fly per day, those fed on milk 8·3 and those fed on sputum 27·0. In the latter case the fæces were much more voluminous and liquid than usual and in fact the flies seemed to suffer from diarrhœa." (Graham-Smith, 1910.)

Summary of feeding experiments, given in Chapters V, VI and VII.

Musca domestica feeds readily on various liquids such as syrup, milk and sputum. Provided the food is supplied in the form of well separated, discrete drops the flies do not usually appear to soil their legs. When undisturbed the flies gorge themselves in half a minute or less. The fluid first passes into the crop, which becomes distended, and if the food is coloured its contour can be seen through the ventral surface of the abdomen. Under ordinary conditions the fluid begins to pass into the ventriculus within 10 minutes and in two or three hours coloured material can be found throughout the intestine. At high temperatures it passes more rapidly. The crop, however, is not completely emptied for many hours. Sometimes flies go on feeding after the crop is full and then the food passes directly into the ventriculus and intestine. If flies are allowed constant access to food coloured material from the first meal remains in the crop for many days.

The crop therefore seems to act as a large receptacle which can be filled with great rapidity so that flies can obtain within a few seconds sufficient nourishment to keep them alive for several days. When food is abundant the crop acts as a reservoir in which surplus food is stored for use if necessity arises.

After feeding on liquid food flies habitually exude drops of fluid from their proboscides. Sometimes these drops are sucked up again and sometimes deposited on the surface on which the flies are walking. These deposits, which have been spoken of as 'vomit,' dry and produce round marks with an opaque centre and rim and an intervening less opaque area.

If allowed to feed on half dried materials the flies first moisten with vomit or saliva a small area and then suck it dry. In so doing they usually leave oval depressions, often exhibiting most beautifully the markings on the proboscis, or clear areas. If the flies have previously fed on coloured syrup these proboscis marks often show traces of pigment.

When feeding on sugar small areas are moistened, either with saliva or, in the case of flies fed on fluids, with vomit. Traces of pigment are often found on the sucked areas when the flies have previously been fed on coloured syrup.

Flies which have access to abundant food leave numerous 'spots' (vomit and fæces). The rate of deposition seems to vary with the kind of food and the temperature.

CHAPTER VIII

METHODS OF OBSERVING FLIES IN CAPTIVITY

Various workers have kept flies in large, specially constructed cages for some days, but very few seem to have been able to keep them alive in small, easily handled cages for more than a day or two. The methods adopted by the writer (Graham-Smith, 1910, p. 2), which gave excellent results, are therefore given in detail.

"Flies were captured in balloon traps baited with sugar moistened with stale beer or treacle and kept until required in a large gauze bag, about 12 inches in diameter and two and a half feet in length, suspended by a string. The sides of the bag were supported by wire hoops and the bottom was composed of a wooden disc. In the latter a square hole was cut the sides of which were fitted with grooves so that in place of the card-board panel which usually filled the space, a tray, containing watch-glasses of syrup and water, could be inserted, in order to supply the flies with food. A sleeve sufficiently large to admit the arm and communicating with the interior of the bag was attached about half way up. When it was not in use the sleeve was closed by a string tied round it near its junction with the bag (Plate XIX, fig. 3). The flies, when required, were captured by means of a large test-tube about 12 inches long, which was inserted through the sleeve. The mouth was placed over flies as they walked on the inside of the bag. Once in the tube the flies fell to the bottom and occasional shaking prevented them from getting out. In this way a considerable number of flies could

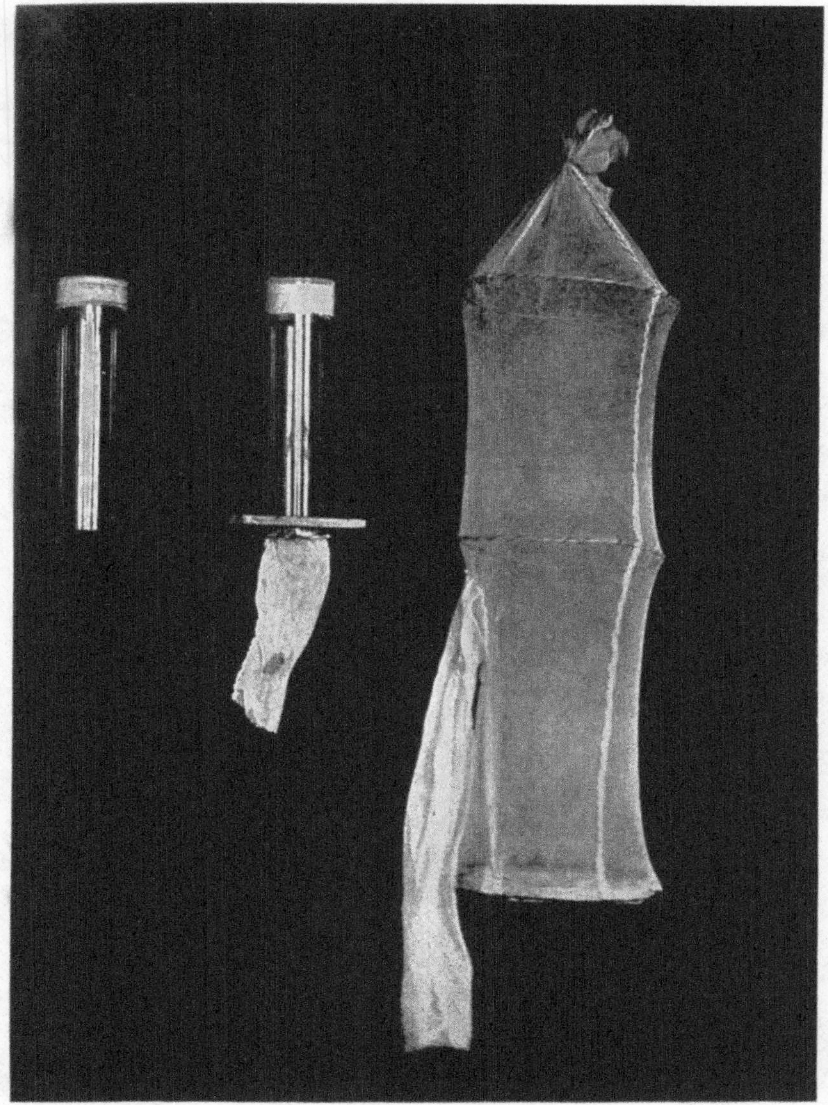

Fig. 1. Fig. 2. Fig. 3.

Fig. 1. Glass cage in which infected flies were kept, consisting of a glass cylinder 9 × 3 inches, covered with gauze at one end and open at the other. ($\frac{1}{8}$ nat. size.)

Fig. 2. Glass cage with apparatus, through which to extract flies, in place. The latter consists of a board in which a round hole slightly larger than the diameter of the cage had been cut and lined with cloth so as to grip the sides of the cage. On to the cloth gauze was sewn to form a conical bag open at the free end. ($\frac{1}{8}$ nat. size.)

Fig. 3. Gauze bag in which normal stock flies were kept. Note the sleeve at the side through which the flies were extracted. ($\frac{1}{8}$ nat. size.)

(From Graham-Smith, *Report to Local Government Board*, No. 40, 1910.)

be caught in a few minutes. After a sufficient number of flies had been captured they were placed in one of the experimental cages. These consisted of cylindrical glass chimneys about three inches in diameter and nine inches in length. One end of the chimney was closed by gauze kept in place by a piece of thin paper gummed round the chimney over the gauze. The other end was open and when in use rested on a clean quarter-plate negative glass (Plate XIX, fig. 1). Other cages of the same kind but smaller (one and a half by six inches) were also made use of. The transference of the flies from one such cage to another can be very easily accomplished. The fresh cage is placed on the bench with its open end upwards and the full cage with the negative glass still in place is placed on top of it. The negative glass is then slowly withdrawn leaving the two cages in free communication. By taking up the two cages in this position and holding the fresh one in the direction of the light most of the flies can be induced to pass into it. If any difficulty occurs they can be blown from the old cage into the other. A fresh glass plate is then inserted between the cages.

"Flies have been kept alive in such cages, with daily transfers to fresh cages, for more than three weeks. It was very rare for a fly to escape or to be injured during the process of transference from cage to cage.

"The flies were usually fed once daily. The liquid food (syrup, milk, sputum, etc.) was deposited in separate drops on a clean negative glass, which was placed in contact with the one on which the cage stood. The cage was then slightly tilted and slipped into position over the food on the new glass. Infected food was given in the same way.

"In order to obtain a few flies from a cage for cultural purposes the following plan was adopted. A piece of wood about six inches square, in which a round hole, slightly larger than the diameter of a cage, had been cut, was lined with cloth so as to closely grip the sides of the cage when the latter was placed in the hole. To one edge of the cloth gauze was sewn to form a conical bag about six inches in length and about two inches in diameter at its free end which was open (Plate XIX, fig. 2). When in use the cage is slipped from the negative glass over the wooden frame, and is made to fit into the hole in it. A long test-tube is then inserted into the cage through the gauze bag and the required number of flies caught in it. This apparatus worked extremely well for no flies escaped or were injured, in a large number of experiments, during the manipulations."

CHAPTER IX

THE WAYS IN WHICH FLIES CARRY AND DISTRIBUTE BACTERIA

There are several ways in which insects which play a part in the dissemination of disease serve as intermediaries. The organisms producing most of the diseases carried by biting flies of various kinds, mosquitoes, gnats, tse-tse flies, etc., are protozoa, and undergo certain of the necessary developmental changes in their life-cycles within the flies. In many cases a more or less prolonged period elapses between the time the fly sucks the blood of the patient and the time when it becomes infective to other individuals. Non-biting flies seldom have the opportunity of feeding on blood, and only occasionally feed on morbid secretions, and so far as we know none of the disease producing organisms they are capable of distributing undergo developmental changes within them. Moreover, since they cannot pierce the skin none of the organisms they carry can reach the circulatory system.

Micro-organisms are transferred either externally or internally by the fly from the source of infection. These organisms are mainly bacteria, some of which, the non-spore producing varieties, only survive drying for a few hours, while others, the spore-producing varieties, can survive drying for prolonged periods.

"As a means of transference the body of the fly is most excellently adapted, being thickly clothed with hairs or setæ of varying degrees of length (Plate I, fig. 1). Its legs, which chiefly come into contact with infected materials upon which it walks, resemble miniature brushes (Plate I, fig. 2), from which no cleansing can remove the organisms once these appendages have been defiled, with the result that they contaminate whatever substance they subsequently visit *within a certain length of time.*" (Hewitt, 1912, p. 72.)

These facts have been well recognized for years, and many writers during the latter part of the nineteenth century either attributed infection in certain cases to contamination by flies, or uttered warnings on the subject. From time to time the fact that a house-fly can carry micro-organisms on its legs, etc., was demonstrated experimentally by allowing a fly to walk over the surface of a culture and then causing it to walk over sterile culture media, on which the bacterium employed could be cultivated subsequently. By simple experiments of this nature, which closely resemble the ordinary methods adopted in transferring bacteria from one culture medium to another by means of a platinum needle, it was shown that flies can transfer a number of well-known disease producing bacteria, but very few attempts were made to ascertain how long the flies remained infective or whether they could carry the bacteria in any other way. The small number of more elaborate, usually isolated experiments which were made, are quoted in the chapters dealing with the specific diseases.

During 1909 and 1910 the writer (Graham-Smith, 1909, 1910) carried out for the Local Government Board Enquiry a large number of experiments on flies with *B. prodigiosus*, and several disease producing bacilli, including *B. anthracis* (see Chapters XIII—XVIII).

For the preliminary experiments *B. prodigiosus* was selected because it is an organism which is easily cultivated and identified on plate cultures. Moreover it seemed likely that the results would give some information as to the length of life of other non-spore-bearing and less easily recognizable bacteria under similar conditions, and afford some indications of the best methods of procedure in making investigations on them.

For the same reasons the spores of *B. anthracis* were employed to demonstrate the persistence of spores.

Methods.

Small numbers of flies were used and kept in the glass cages which have been alluded to (Chapter VIII). Infected material (usually an emulsion of *B. prodigiosus* in syrup) was only supplied to them for 15 minutes or less, and the cages were changed daily. In prolonged experiments they were fed, every day, with plain syrup or other food. For cultural purposes two or three flies were caught in a large test-tube and killed by chloroform vapour. The legs, wings, and heads were cut off and separately inoculated on different parts of an agar plate. In many cases fluid was also expressed from the proboscis by means of pressure on the head and separately cultivated. The body, after being placed in alcohol, or singed in the flame, was dissected, under a Zeiss binocular microscope, and the contents of the crop and intestines separately inoculated. The mounted Hagedorn needles and other instruments used for dissection were sterilized in the flame. After a little experience it is not difficult to dissect out the entire crop and sow its contents, and to subsequently remove the intestine without contamination with the crop contents. The agar plates on which the cultures were generally made were prepared and dried for a few minutes in the incubator at 37° C., and the legs, wings, head, and crop, and intestinal contents, etc. from one fly inoculated at different places. The spots where the crop and intestinal contents had been placed were marked by blue rings made with a glass pencil on the back of the plate, and when, as was often found possible, the organs of several flies were inoculated on one plate, those belonging to each fly were surrounded by a blue line and numbered.

Plate XX, fig. 1, illustrates a plate, before cultivation, inoculated with the organs of four flies infected with anthrax. Figure 2 shows the same plate after 24 hours' incubation.

(*a*) *Experiments on the duration of life of B. prodigiosus on the exterior, and in the alimentary canal of flies.*

The following table summarizes the results of four series of experiments, done at different times, on the length of life of *B. prodigiosus* on the feet and wings, and in the alimentary canal. In each case syrup infected with *B. prodigiosus* was placed for a few minutes in a cage containing hungry flies. After feeding, the flies were transferred to fresh cages, where, if the experiment was prolonged, they were fed daily with plain syrup. At intervals, specimens were caught and dissected, and their legs, wings, heads, and the contents of their crops and intestines inoculated on to agar plates.

TABLE 8. *Showing the length of life of B. prodigiosus on the exterior, and in the alimentary canal of flies.*

Time after infection	Flies used	Cultures from: Legs 1	Legs 2	Legs 3	Legs 4	Legs 5	Legs 6	Wings 1	Wings 2	Head	Crop	Intestine
1 minute	...	–	–	–	–	–	–	–	–	+ +	+ + +	+
30 ,,	(1)	+	+	+	+	–	–	–	–	+ +	o	o
	(2)	o	o	o	o	o	o	o	o	+ +	+ + +	+ + +
	(3)	o	+	+	o	o	o	o	o	+	+ + +	+ + +
	(4)	o	o	o	o	o	o	o	o	+ +	+ + +	+ + +
	(5)	+	+	+	o	o	o	+	o	+ +	+ + +	+ + +
60 ,,	...	+	+	–	–	–	–	+	+	+ +	+ + +	+ + +
90 ,,	(1)	+	+	+	+	o	o	+	+	+ +	+ +	+ +
	(2)	o	o	o	o	o	o	o	o	+	+ + +	+ + +
2 hours	...	+	+	+	o	o	o	o	o	o	o	o
2·5 ,,	...	o	o	o	o	o	o	o	o	o	+ +	+ +
3 ,,	...	o	o	o	o	o	o	o	o	+	+ + +	+ + +
3·5 ,,	...	+	o	o	o	o	o	o	o	+	+ + +	+ + +
4 ,,	...	o	o	o	o	o	o	o	o	–	–	–
5 ,,	...	o	o	o	o	o	o	o	o	–	–	–
5·5 ,,	...	+	+	+	o	o	o	+	+	+ +	+ + +	+ + +
12 ,,	(1)	+	+	+	+	+	o	+	+	+	+ + +	+
	(2)	+	+	+	+	+	o	+	o	+	+ +	–
	(3)	+	+	o	o	o	o	o	o	+	+ + +	–
	(4)	o	o	o	o	o	o	o	o	+	+ + +	+
	(5)	o	o	o	o	o	o	o	o	+	+ + +	+ +
	(6)	o	o	o	o	o	o	o	o	+	+ + +	+ +
18 ,,	(1)	+	+	+	+	o	o	o	o	+ +	+ + +	+ + +
	(2)	+	o	o	o	o	o	o	o	+ +	+ + +	+ + +
	(3)	o	o	o	o	o	o	o	o	+ +	+ + +	+ + +
	(4)	o	o	o	o	o	o	o	o	+	+ + +	+ +
24 ,,	(1)	o	o	o	o	o	o	o	o	+ +	+ + +	+ +
	(2)	o	o	o	o	o	o	o	o	+	–	–
	(3)	+	o	o	o	o	o	o	o	+	+ + +	+ +
	(4)	o	o	o	o	o	o	o	o	+	+ +	+ +
	(5)	+	+	o	o	o	o	o	o	+	+ + +	+ +
	(6)	o	o	o	o	o	o	o	o	–	+ + +	+
	(7)	o	o	o	o	o	o	o	o	+	+ +	+
29 ,,	(1)	+	o	o	o	o	o	o	o	+	+ + +	+ +
	(2)	o	o	o	o	o	o	o	o	+	+ + +	+ +
30 ,,	(1)	o	o	o	o	o	o	o	o	+	+ + +	+ +
	(2)	o	o	o	o	o	o	o	o	+	+ +	+ +
52 ,,	(1)	o	o	o	o	o	o	o	o	+	+	+ + +
	(2)	o	o	o	o	o	o	o	o	o	o	o
60 ,,	(1)	o	o	o	o	o	o	o	o	+	+ +	+ + +
	(2)	o	o	o	o	o	o	o	o	+	+ +	+ + +
3 days	(1)	o	o	o	o	o	o	o	o	o	o	o
	(2)	o	o	o	o	o	o	o	o	+	+ +	+
	(3)	o	o	o	o	o	o	o	o	o	+ + +	+
	(4)	o	o	o	o	o	o	o	o	+	+ + +	o
	(5)	o	o	o	o	o	o	o	o	+	+ +	+
	(6)	o	o	o	o	o	o	o	o	o	+ +	+
	(7)	o	o	o	o	o	o	o	o	+	+ +	+

+ indicates a few colonies of *B. prodigiosus*, + + several colonies, and + + + numerous colonies. The numbers in brackets after the later results indicate the number of colonies found. o = no colonies appeared, – = no cultures made, ... = one fly used.

TABLE 8 (*continued*).

Time after infection	Flies used	Cultures from: Legs 1	2	3	4	5	6	Wings 1	2	Head	Crop	Intestine
4 days	(1)	o	o	o	o	o	o	o	o	+	+ + +	+ +
	(2)	o	o	o	o	o	o	o	o	o	+ +	+ + +
5 ,,	(1)	o	o	o	o	o	o	o	o	o	+	+ (3)
	(2)	o	o	o	o	o	o	o	o	+	+ + +	+ +
	(3)	o	o	o	o	o	o	o	o	o	o	+ (1)
8 ,,	(1)	o	o	o	o	o	o	o	o	+ (1)	+ + (40)	+ + (31)
	(2)	o	o	o	o	o	o	o	o	+	o	+ (3)
	(3)	o	o	o	o	o	o	o	o	o	o	+
9 ,,	...	o	o	o	o	o	+ (1)	o	o	o	o	o
11 ,,	...	o	o	o	o	o	o	o	o	+ (1)	–	+ (4)
12 ,,	(1)	o	o	o	o	o	o	o	o	o	–	o
	(2)	o	o	o	o	o	o	o	o	o	o	+ (2)
14 ,,	...	o	o	o	o	o	o	o	o	o	–	+ (5)
15 ,,	...	o	o	o	o	o	o	o	o	o	–	+ (5)
16 ,,	...	o	o	o	o	o	o	o	o	o	–	o
17 ,,	...	o	o	o	o	o	o	o	o	o	–	+ (13)
18 ,,	...	o	o	o	o	o	o	o	o	o	o	o
19 ,,	...	o	o	o	o	o	o	o	o	o	o	o
20 ,,	...	o	o	o	o	o	o	o	o	o	o	o
21 ,,	...	o	o	o	o	o	o	o	o	o	o	o

+ indicates a few colonies of *B. prodigiosus*, + + several colonies, and + + + numerous colonies. The numbers in brackets after the later results indicate the number of colonies found. o = no colonies appeared, – = no cultures made, ... = one fly used.

It is evident from the above table that *B. prodigiosus* may remain alive on the legs and wings for at least 18 hours after feeding. Exceptionally it may remain alive longer. It is present, in large numbers, in the contents of the crop and intestine and on the proboscis for four or five days. After this time its numbers gradually diminish, cultures after 17 days yielding negative results.

(*b*) *Experiments to determine whether B. prodigiosus multiplies in the crop.*

A fine capillary was drawn out of thermometer tubing and marks scratched on it with a file, one about half an inch and the other about two inches from the end. Flies were fed on a dilute emulsion of *B. prodigiosus*. Some of this emulsion was drawn up to the first mark, and water to the second mark to dilute it. The fluids were mixed and the mixture sown on an agar plate.

At intervals flies were killed and their crops dissected out. Some of the fluid from the crop was drawn up to the first mark, diluted and sown. Between each culture the pipette was sterilized with alcohol and washed and dried. Approximately the same number of colonies grew in cultures made from the emulsion and from the crop contents of flies dissected one, four, five and a half and eight hours after feeding. About half the number of colonies grew in cultures made from the crop contents of flies dissected 24 and 31 hours later, which had been allowed to feed once in the interval on plain syrup.

In another similar experiment the colonies were counted.

A fly was dissected 45 minutes after feeding and 4500 colonies were counted.

A fly was dissected 75 minutes after feeding and 5490 colonies were counted.

A fly was dissected 2·75 hours after feeding and 4900 colonies were counted.

A fly was dissected 5·5 hours after feeding and 4098 colonies were counted.

A fly was dissected 24 hours after feeding and 247 colonies were counted.

A fly was dissected 3 days after feeding and 10 colonies were counted.

These experiments seem to indicate that in the case of *B. prodigiosus* multiplication does not take place in the crop.

(*c*) *The infection of agar plates by living flies.*

In each of the following experiments two or more flies which had previously fed on syrup infected with *B. prodigiosus* were allowed to walk for 30 minutes over the surface of agar plates. For the first few minutes the flies generally walked rapidly over the surface, but subsequently they frequently stopped, and applying their proboscides apparently sucked the agar. In some cases, especially if the agar was not too dry, oval marks were left where the proboscides were applied, and it was round these marks that the prodigiosus colonies grew. The following table shows the result of these experiments.

TABLE 9. *Showing the results of experiments with living flies allowed to walk over the surface of agar plates.*

Time after feeding on infected syrup	No. of flies allowed to walk on plate	Result
1 day	2	About 600 colonies of *B. prodigiosus*
3 days	2	Numerous colonies of *B. prodigiosus*
4 "	3	" " "
5 "	3	" " "
6 "	6	Several " "
7 "	3	" " "

(*d*) *Experiments on the infection of sugar.*

Flies were allowed to feed on syrup infected with *B. prodigiosus* for 15 minutes, and were then removed to fresh cages. At various times one or two crystals of brown sugar were placed in the cage and the flies allowed to suck them for some time. The crystals were then taken out and dissolved in a drop of water, and the solution sown on agar. The results of three series of experiments of this kind are incorporated in the following table:

TABLE 10. *Showing results of allowing infected flies to feed on sugar.*

Time after infection when sugar given	Results		
3 hours ...	*B. prodigiosus*	cultivated.	Numerous colonies
3·5 " ...	"	"	100 colonies
4 " ...	"	"	few "
4·5 " ...	"	"	22 "
5 " ...	"	"	30 "
5·25 " ...	"	"	1 colony
5·5 " ...	"	"	many colonies
7·75 " ...	"	"	50 "
20 " ...	"	"	2 "
32 " ...	"	"	6 "
42 " ...	"	"	8 "
46 " ...	"	"	1 colony
56 " ...	"	not cultivated	
66 " ...	"	cultivated.	3 colonies
3 days ...	"	not cultivated	
4 " ...	"	"	
5 " ...	"	"	
6 " ...	"	"	
7 " ...	"	"	
8 " ...	"	"	

From these experiments it appears that flies are able to infect sugar for at least two days after feeding on an emulsion of *B. prodigiosus* in syrup.

(*e*) *The period during which infected fæcal material is deposited.*

Several experiments to ascertain the period during which infected fæcal material may be deposited were conducted in the following way. Flies were allowed to feed on syrup infected with *B. prodigiosus* for 30 minutes, and then transferred to fresh cages. At various intervals they were again transferred to fresh cages, and the fæces left in the old cages emulsified in water, and the emulsions sown on agar.

TABLE 11. *Showing the period during which infected fæces are deposited.*

Time after infection when fæces collected		Result
2 hours	...	*B. prodigiosus* cultivated from 3 out of 4 deposits
3 ,,	...	,, ,,
4 ,,	...	,, ,, from 3 out of 5 deposits
6 ,,	...	,, ,,
8 ,,	...	,, ,,
10 ,,	...	,, ,, from 3 out of 5 deposits
18 ,,	...	,, ,, from 6 out of 8 deposits
26 ,,	...	,, ,,
36 ,,	...	,, not cultivated from 5 deposits
48 ,,	...	,, cultivated from 3 out of 6 deposits
3 days	...	,, not cultivated from 5 deposits
4 ,,	...	,, cultivated from 3 out of 7 deposits
5 ,,	...	,, not cultivated
6 ,,	...	,, cultivated. One colony in cultures from 8 deposits
7 ,,	...	,, not cultivated
8 ,,	...	,, ,,
9 ,,	...	,, ,,

These experiments show that heavily infected fæcal material may be deposited for at least two days after infection.

(*f*) *The influence of various kinds of food on the period during which infected fæcal material is passed.*

As it had previously been found that the rate of deposition of fæces depended to some extent on the kind of food, an experiment was made in order to ascertain whether the period during which the fæces continued infective was influenced by the food. Different batches of flies were allowed to feed for 15 minutes on syrup, milk and sputum infected with *B. prodigiosus* and then transferred to fresh cages. Every day the cages were changed and the flies fed on non-infected syrup, milk and sputum respectively. The fæcal material present in the old cages was emulsified in water and the emulsion was sown on agar. The following table gives the results of these experiments.

TABLE 12. *Showing the influence of the food on the infectivity of the fæces.*

Time after infection when fæces collected	Cultures from the fæces of flies fed on		
	Milk	Syrup	Sputum
1 day	+	+	+
2 days	+	+	+
3 ,, ...	+	+	o
4 ,, ...	+	+	o
5 ,, ...	+	o	o
7 ,, ...	+	o	o
8 ,, ...	o	o	o
9 ,, ...	o	o	o
13 ,, ...	o	–	–

This table shows that *B. prodigiosus* cannot be cultivated from the fæces of flies fed on sputum after 48 hours. It was noticed that the fæces of these flies were much more voluminous than those of the flies fed on milk or syrup. The fæces of the flies fed on milk were infective for 7 days and those of the flies fed on syrup for only 4 days.

To ascertain how long *B. prodigiosus* is capable of surviving in various fluids dried on glass, small drops (about the size of the fæcal deposits) of the syrup, milk and sputum used to infect the flies and of an emulsion in water were placed on glass and cultures made from them at intervals. It was found that *B. prodigiosus* could no longer be recovered from the dried watery emulsions after 18 hours. They were still present in small numbers in the milk and syrup drops after 28 hours. In the sputum emulsions similarly treated they were present after 3 days in considerable numbers.

(*g*) *The infection of fresh flies from the deposits of infected flies.*

Several experiments were made to ascertain whether clean flies became infected if placed in cages lately occupied by infected flies. For example flies were fed on syrup infected with *B. prodigiosus*. One hour after feeding they were transferred to a fresh cage, and allowed to remain there for two hours, and then transferred to a third fresh cage. In the second cage numerous deposits of fæces and vomit were left. Eight clean hungry flies were then put into the second cage, and immediately sucked at the deposits left by the infected flies. After being allowed to remain in the cage for various times these eight flies were dissected and cultures made from their organs, with the following results.

TABLE 13. *Showing the infection of clean flies from the deposits of infected flies.*

In infected cage for	No. of fly	Cultures from: Legs 1	Legs 2	Legs 3	Legs 4	Legs 5	Legs 6	Wings 1	Wings 2	Head	Intestine
1·5 hours	1	o	o	o	o	o	o	o	o	+	+++
	2	o	o	o	o	o	o	o	o	o	o
	3	o	o	o	o	o	o	o	o	o	+ (1 colony)
	4	o	o	o	o	o	o	o	o	o	+
3·5 "	5	o	o	o	o	o	o	o	o	+	+ (3 colonies)
	6	o	o	o	o	o	o	o	o	o	o
5 "	7	o	o	o	o	o	o	o	o	o	+ (3 colonies)
	8	o	o	o	o	o	o	o	o	+	+ (1 colony)

Several experiments of this type were carried out which seem to indicate that clean flies may sometimes infect themselves from the vomit and fæces deposited by infected flies even up to several days after infection.

(*h*) *Experiments designed to ascertain whether flies can infect fluids on which they feed.*

In 1909 the writer carried out some experiments on this subject but they were few in number and inconclusive, so in 1910 he (Graham-Smith, 1911) re-investigated the subject using both *M. domestica* and *C. erythrocephala*, the latter having been bred in captivity from eggs. The fluids used for the experiments were syrup and sterilized milk. Two out of several experiments are quoted.

Experiments with house-flies (*M. domestica*).

Six flies were carefully fed on an emulsion of *B. prodigiosus* which was placed on the floor of their cage in single drops. During the process of feeding the flies did not fall into the syrup or soil their wings. Their proboscides and legs were the only organs which could become infected by direct contact with contaminated syrup. They were then transferred to a clean cage. Sterile milk was poured into a sterile watch-glass and the latter was placed in the incubator until some of the milk had evaporated and a rim of partially dried milk was left round the fluid portion. Three hours after the flies had fed on the infected emulsion, a watch-glass of sterile milk was placed in the cage, and left there for some hours. It was noticed that the flies fed on the dried parts as well as on the fluid milk. On examination of the watch-glass after it had been removed from the cage, there was noticed on the areas covered with partially dried milk, not only numerous proboscis marks, but also several red marks produced by vomit composed of an emulsion of *B. prodigiosus*. Cultures were made from (*a*) the fluid milk, (*b*) the dried parts (not obviously contaminated with vomit) and (*c*) vomit marks. Similar experiments were carried out 24, 26 and 28 hours after the infection of the flies with positive results as shown in Table 14.

TABLE 14. *Showing the results of cultures made from fluid and partially dried milk on which flies infected with B. prodigiosus had been allowed to feed.*

Time after flies were infected	Fluid milk	Partially dried milk	Vomit
3 hours	+ +	+ + +	+ + +
24 ,,	+ + +	+ + +	–
26 ,,	+ + +	+ +	–
28 ,,	+ + +	+ + +	–

In other series of experiments with large numbers of flies infection of the milk was obtained in the case of *B. prodigiosus* and the spores of *B. anthracis* up to the 11th day.

All the experiments done show that artificially infected flies (*M. domestica*), kept in captivity, may contaminate milk on which they feed for several days.

Experiments with blow-flies (*C. erythrocephala*).

Several experiments were also carried out with blow-flies (*C. erythrocephala*), of which one is quoted.

About 20 blow-flies were confined in each of four cages, the flies in two of the cages being infected by feeding on an emulsion of *B. prodigiosus* in syrup, and those in the other two cages being similarly infected by feeding on an emulsion of *B. pyocyaneus*.

In each instance the emulsion was placed in a watch-glass, and a short distance above it was fixed a piece of zinc pierced with round perforations about three-sixteenths of an inch in diameter. Through these perforations the flies put their proboscides and drank the fluid, and occasionally, though rarely, soiled their legs by putting them through. It was, however, impossible for them to fall into the fluid. It was noticed that, after feeding, they not infrequently deposited vomit on the zinc, and no doubt sometimes infected their feet and wings by walking and falling into it. They also infected their limbs by contact with their proboscides by cleaning them (p. 107). The two sets of flies infected with *B. prodigiosus* and the two sets infected with *B. pyocyaneus* were fed daily through sterilized perforated zinc trays on syrup and sterilized milk respectively, and cultures were made from the remains of these fluids. The results of these experiments are given in Table 15.

TABLE 15. *Showing the results of cultures made from the remains of syrup and milk on which blow-flies infected with B. pyocyaneus and B. prodigiosus had been allowed to feed through perforated zinc trays.*

Time after flies were infected	Infection with *B. pyocyaneus*		Infection with *B. prodigiosus*	
	Syrup	Milk	Syrup	Milk
1 day	–	+ + +	–	+ + +
2 days	+ + +	+ + +	+ + +	+ + +
3 ,,	+ + +	+ + +	+ + +	+ + +
4 ,,	+ + +	+ + +	+ + +	+ + +
5 ,,	+ + +	+	+ +	+ +
7 ,,	+ + +	+	+ +	+
8 ,,	+ +	+	+ +	o
9 ,,	+ +	+	+ +	+
10 ,,	+	+	+ +	+
11 ,,	+ (2 colonies)	+	+ +	+
13 ,,	o	+	+ +	+
14 ,,	+	+	+	o
15 ,,	+ (1 colony)	+	+	o
16 ,,	+	+	+ (1 colony)	o
17 ,,	o	+	+	+ (1 colony)
18 ,,	+	o	+	o
20 ,,	o	o	+	+ (1 colony)
21 ,,	o	o	+	+ (2 colonies)
22 ,,	o	o	+	o
23 ,,	o	o	+	o
24 ,,	+	o	+ (1 colony)	o
25 ,,	o	o	+	o
26 ,,	o	+ (1 colony)	+	+ (2 colonies)
27 ,,	o	o	+ (1 colony)	o
28 ,,	+ (1 colony)	o	+	o
29 ,,	o	o	+	o
30 ,,	o	o	o	o
31 ,,	o	o	+ (1 colony)	o
33 ,,	o	o	o	o

These experiments show that blow-flies infected with non-spore bearing micro-organisms are capable of seriously contaminating both syrup and milk for at least a week by feeding on them. Blow-flies originally fed on an emulsion of *B. pyocyaneus* constantly produced some degree of infection in both syrup and milk for 16 days, and at even later periods occasional colonies of *B. pyocyaneus* could be cultivated from their food. Milk was apparently not infected after the 26th day, or syrup after the 28th day. Blow-flies which had been fed on *B. prodigiosus* constantly produced infection in syrup up to the 29th day, though the degree of infection was small after the 14th day. Milk was infected to a smaller extent, and only occasional colonies were cultivated from it after the 8th day.

It is of course likely that the table shows a smaller degree of infection than really existed since only a small proportion of the milk was cultivated on each occasion.

Observations on the habits of blow-flies and their bearing on feeding experiments[1].

Blow-flies spend a large proportion of their time, when in captivity, in cleaning their limbs and proboscides in the following manner:

The wings are usually cleaned with the posterior pair of legs, which are passed over and under each wing. Often two legs are simultaneously applied to a wing which is drawn between them. Subsequently the legs which have been used are rubbed together. The posterior legs are also used for cleaning the abdomen, and, in so doing, are passed over the anus. Probably they are frequently infected in this way and, later, infect the wings. For cleaning the proboscis and head the anterior pair of legs is made use of. During this process the proboscis is usually extended to its fullest extent, and the legs are passed along it from its proximal to its distal extremity. Occasionally the oral discs are applied to some part of the leg, probably in order to remove some irritating material. Flies have been seen to clean their proboscides immediately after feeding, and to leave infected material on their legs.

The efforts made to cleanse their limbs are often very prolonged when flies have been allowed to feed upon very sticky materials, such as concentrated syrup, and some observations which have been made appear to indicate that, under such circumstances, gross re-infection of the limbs may occur. On one occasion a fly sucked at some semi-solid syrup mixed with carmine for a long time and moved away from the food with a large mass adhering to its proboscis. This mass was

[1] See also Chapter XX.

deliberately removed with the anterior pair of legs. The same thing was frequently noticed in subsequent similar experiments.

From all the observations which have been made it seems highly probable that blow-flies frequently re-infect their limbs when cleaning themselves. It is, however, almost impossible to determine by actual experiments how frequently or to what extent this occurs. Probably both the frequency and the extent vary with the consistency of the food.

Measurements which were made of the contents of the crops of recently fed blow-flies showed that more than 0·02 c.c. of fluid might be contained in them. On one occasion a blow-fly which had recently fed on coloured syrup was held by the wing and the material which it vomited collected and measured. It was found that 0·01 c.c. of coloured syrup had been deposited. Subsequently the fly was killed and dissected and 0·01 c.c. of fluid obtained from its crop.

All the experiments which have been made on this subject show that blow-flies take up large quantities of fluid in feeding, and are capable of vomiting at least half of the contents of their crops.

If flies are allowed to feed on fairly large volumes of milk contained in watch-glasses they often fall into the milk. After emerging they leave long trails as they crawl up the sides of the watch-glasses. Frequently also they soil their limbs while feeding, and in walking away leave trails like those just mentioned. On several occasions these trails have been proved to be infected. Other flies approaching the milk usually stop and suck at the half dried trails and drops left by previous flies, and probably infect their feet and take up micro-organisms into their crops.

The experiments and observations on the feeding habits of blow-flies all show that the individual blow-fly (*C. erythrocephala*) is capable of distributing greater numbers of bacteria, and over a longer period of time, than the individual house-fly (*M. domestica*). House-flies, however, are probably a greater source of danger owing to their greater prevalence and to their more frequent occurrence where food can be easily contaminated.

Summary of experiments with B. prodigiosus.

The experiments which have been carried out in relation to the period during which *B. prodigiosus* remains alive on the legs and wings and in the crops and intestinal contents of infected flies, on the infection of sugar and agar plates by living flies, and on the time during which infected material may be deposited, are sufficiently numerous and conclusive to allow of definite statements being made on these points.

B. prodigiosus may be cultivated from the legs and wings of infected flies for 18 hours (and occasionally longer) after infection. It can be cultivated from the contents of the crop and intestine in large numbers up to 4 or 5 days, and has been found surviving in the intestine up to 18 days. There is no evidence to show that *B. prodigiosus* multiplies in the crop. Flies allowed to walk over agar plates are capable of infecting them (probably by means of material regurgitated through their proboscides) for at least 7 days. They are capable of infecting sugar for at least 2 days. Contaminated fæces may be deposited during several days after infection, the periods varying with the kind of food. Flies fed on milk deposited infected fæces during 7 days, those fed on syrup during 4 days, and those fed on sputum for 2 days. Clean flies may infect themselves by feeding on the deposits left by infected flies, especially if the latter have been freshly passed shortly after infection. Milk seems to be frequently contaminated by infected flies whether they merely drink it or fall into it. In the single experiment which was tried, flies which walked and fed on meat did not infect it. Possibly *B. prodigiosus* is not a suitable organism for the last experiment.

CHAPTER X

THE BACTERIOLOGY OF CITY FLIES

Two important contributions to the *general* bacteriology of city flies have been published recently, one by Torrey (1912) working in New York and the other by Cox, Lewis and Glynn (1912) working in Liverpool.

Torrey (1912) investigated in detail the bacterial content of a considerable number of flies caught entering the windows of the Loomis Laboratory, Cornell University Medical School, New York. The flies caught were amongst those continually circulating in and out of the open windows of a row of tenements of the poorer grade 75 ft. distant. The flies caught in large sterile test-tubes were examined in lots of ten.

"They were shaken for 5 minutes in 10 c.c. of sterile normal salt solution, and the wash was set aside and labelled I. The flies were then rinsed thoroughly in 20 c.c. of salt solution, which was drained off and discarded. The washed flies were next placed in 10 c.c. of the salt solution and the abdomens were so squeezed with a sterile platinum spatula that the contents of the intestine exuded into the fluid. The thoroughly emulsified intestinal matter of 10 flies was labelled II. Platings were made from I and II, suitably diluted, in agar, litmus lactose agar and Conradi-Drigalski medium. These plates were incubated 24 hours at 37° C. The number of colonies on the nutrient agar plates was taken as the total count.... The types of colonies, which appeared to be dominant, were isolated and identified, and in addition a special search was always made for colonies of the dysentery bacillus type."

He found that up to the latter part of June the flies were free from fæcal bacteria, showing mainly cocci. "During July and August there occurred periods in which the flies examined carried several millions of bacteria, alternating with periods in which the number of bacteria was reduced to hundreds." He thinks "the scanty flora probably indicated the advent of swarms of recently hatched flies." "The bacteria in the intestines of the flies were 8·6 times as numerous as on the surface of the insects." Bacilli belonging to the colon group were three times as numerous in the intestine as on the surface. The figures given in his table show "that the surface contamination of these 'wild' flies may vary from 570 to 4,400,000 bacteria per insect, and the intestinal bacterial content from 16,000 to 28,000,000."

The most extensive and important investigation was carried out by Cox, Lewis and Glynn (1912) in Liverpool. They caught flies in sterilized balloon traps; owing to the bait being protected by sterilized gauze the flies were unable to touch it. By making the flies swim in sterile water they were able to simulate as closely as possible the way in which flies naturally pollute liquids if they fall into them, and to estimate the rate at which bacteria are given off. They also determined the gross numbers carried in and on flies, and isolated some of the varieties obtained. Their experiments show that:

(1) "The number of bacteria derived from house-flies whilst struggling in a fluid, and which are taken as a measure of their capacity to pollute food by vomiting, defæcation, etc., may be very large, and increases with the time they remain in the fluid" from 2000 in five minutes to 350,000 in thirty minutes, "but that the number of bacteria carried inside the fly is much greater."

(2) "Flies caught in congested areas always carried and contained more ærobic bacteria (800,000 to 500,000,000), including those of the intestinal group, than flies from cleaner areas (21,000 to 100,000)."

(3) Flies caught in a 'sanitary oasis' in the midst of a slum area carried and contained less bacteria of all kinds than those from the dwelling rooms of a street with insanitary court property on either side.

(4) Flies caught in the office of a refuse destructor, situated in the Offensive Trades Area, and in a slaughtering room of a knacker's yard contained enormous numbers.

(5) "Flies caught in milk shops apparently carry and contain more bacteria than those from other shops with exposed food in a similar neighbourhood. The reason of this is probably because milk (when accessible), especially in summer months, is a suitable culture medium for bacteria, and the flies first inoculate the milk and later re-inoculate themselves, so establishing a vicious circle."

(6) "The fact that flies from congested and relatively insanitary areas of the city carry more bacteria than those from

cleaner areas, may be explained by the lower standard of general cleanliness in the house, the yard, the street, and the alley; human excrement is frequently found in the courts of the slums." "It might have been imagined that flies move constantly from one street or locality of the city to another, and consequently the number of bacteria carried by them would be approximately the same, and bear no relation to the amount of street refuse and the habits of the people.

"Our observations, however, prove that such migrations from one area to another do not occur to any great extent."

(7) "We have shown that the amount of dirt carried by flies measured in terms of bacteria bears a definite relation to the habits of the people and the state of the streets."

Esten and Mason (1908) have also published some observations on flies mainly caught in cow-stables and 'swill barrels.' Estimations of the numbers carried on their bodies appear to have been made by washing the bodies of the flies. These observers found that "the numbers of bacteria on a single fly may range all the way from 550 to 6,600,000." "The average for 414 flies was about 1,250,000 bacteria for each," but the flies from dirty areas carried a far greater number than those from clean areas.

A few investigations have also been made in regard to the *fæcal bacteria* of the colon and non-lactose fermenting types carried by flies.

Jackson (1907) found as many as 100,000 fæcal bacteria in a single fly, and recognized that these bacteria might survive the passage through the intestinal canal. Graham-Smith (1909) examined 148 flies caught in various parts of London and Cambridge. Of these 35 (23·6 %) were infected externally or internally or in both situations with bacilli belonging to the colon group.

Nicoll (1911, p. 381) examined the intestines of flies from dwelling rooms of houses in London for fæcal bacteria.

"The flies were first well washed in sterile broth, then in 2 % lysol or absolute alcohol for 10—20 minutes. They were then thoroughly washed in sterile water, dried over the flame, and the whole alimentary canal was placed in broth. After incubation at 37° C. overnight the broth cultures were plated in MacConkey's bile-salt medium, and from each plate about a dozen colonies were picked off and their characters determined. Altogether 145 specimens of *Musca domestica* were examined, 25 of these were examined individually, the rest in 23 lots of 5 to 7 each."

About 75 per cent. of these flies showed colon bacilli representing 27 different varieties. From his investigations he concludes that "it is apparent that a considerable similarity in respect of the colon bacilli exists between the bacterial flora of flies and the bacteria met with in the fæces of man and other animals. The most striking feature is the marked predominance of the characteristic fæcal organism *B. coli communis* and MacConkey's bacillus No. 71."

Graham-Smith (1912) examined 642 flies from diarrhœa infected houses in Birmingham and Cambridge and 600 from non-diarrhœa infected houses. Of the former 283 (44 %) and of the latter 212 (35 %) contained bacilli of the colon type. Further analysis of the results shows that during the whole period (July 10th to October 14th) covered by these examinations at least 20 per cent. of flies from all sources were infected with colon bacilli. The degree of infection was greatest during August and the first three weeks of September. It is of interest and importance to note that the percentage of infection in flies of different batches, obtained from one place on different occasions, varied greatly. For example, from one diarrhœa infected house eleven batches of flies were obtained. The infection with colon bacilli varied from 25 per cent. to 78 per cent. (mean 44 per cent.). The infection in flies from a farm house varied from 50 per cent. to 93 per cent. Similar variations were seen in batches from different diarrhœa infected houses in Birmingham, the infection varying from 0 per cent. to 87 per cent.

Conclusions.

It is evident from the investigations which have been made on city flies that these insects carry both on and in their bodies very large numbers of bacteria, many of which are derived from fæcal material. In the chapters dealing with the specific diseases it will be shown that in the few special examinations that have been made disease-producing types, or varieties closely allied to them, have been found occasionally.

CHAPTER XI

THE SURVIVAL IN THE ADULT FLY OF MICRO-ORGANISMS INGESTED BY THE LARVA

Faichnie (1909, p. 580) seems to have been the first to suggest that bacteria ingested by the larva might survive the pupal stage and be present in the intestine of the adult. He put forward this hypothesis because, during the investigation of a small outbreak of typhoid at Kamptee, India, he realized that "infection by the excrement of flies bred in an infected material" might explain "many conclusions previously difficult to accept." Shortly afterwards he carried out the following interesting experiments (p. 672).

"On August 12th, 1909, three ounces of fæces, containing *B. typhosus*, were thrown into a box of earth and covered with a wire cage, and about 30 flies were let loose inside. These flies all died in a day or two, but on August 26th, 14 days later, one fly hatched; on August 27th, 12 flies were hatched; on this same day, after the flies were hatched, the box of earth was replaced by an earthenware plate which had been previously washed in a solution of 1 in 500 perchloride of mercury; sugar and water as food in separate porcelain saucers were also introduced, and the wire cover was changed for a bell-shaped mosquito net. On August 26th, one fly, one day old, was transfixed with a red hot needle after chloroforming it, flamed and put into a bottle of sterile salt solution. It was shaken up and 1 c.c. of the solution put into McConkey broth, which remained unchanged for 48 hours. After this the fly was crushed with a sterile glass rod and a drop plated; *B. typhosus* was found." Four other flies one day old gave the same results, and two flies 6 days old and two flies 9 days old also gave the same results. "On September 10th two flies 13 days old were put into a dry sterile bottle and left for 24 hours; they were then removed, and some salt solution was poured into the bottle, and from this solution of excrement *B. typhosus* was obtained." The two flies were treated as the previous ones had been and *B. typhosus* was obtained. From one fly 16 days old and from its excrement *B. typhosus* was also obtained, but not from another.

From the foregoing experiment it will be seen that out of the 13 flies bred from a typhoid stool at least 6 contained *B. typhosus* in their intestines; and the bacillus was recovered from the intestines and excrement of a fly 16 days old.

"A second series of experiments was carried out with the fæces of a man suffering from paratyphoid fever (*B. paratyphosus* A) the diagnosis having been made by a blood culture.

"On August 22nd two ounces of liquid fæces, containing *B. paratyphosus* A, were put into a box of earth and about 30 flies allowed to feed on it; as the flies had no water given to them they died in a day or two. On September 1st one fly hatched out; on September 3rd 12 flies were seen. On the same date the earth was replaced by a plate as before. On September 1st one fly, one day old, was examined; the McConkey control was negative; and after being flamed and crushed *B. paratyphosus* A was obtained. On September 3rd four flies, each one day old, were examined; the McConkey control was negative; and from the crushed flies *B. paratyphosus* A was separated. On September 10th 3 flies, each seven days old, were put through the sterile bottle test, the excrement was examined, and from it *B. paratyphosus* A was obtained." It was also obtained from the crushed flies. "On September 13th one fly, 10 days old, was examined, but the bacillus was not recovered. Two other flies, also 10 days old, were examined and *B. paratyphosus* A was recovered.'

These very suggestive experiments have influenced several workers to make observations on the same lines, and their experiments are recorded in the order of publication.

Bacot (III. 1911) experimented with *Musca domestica* and *B. pyocyaneus.*

"About an inch of dry silver sand was placed in a one-pint card cream jar. A mixture consisting of cooked meat, baked rice, rice pudding, custard, boiled potato, gristle of meat, was chopped up, and, together with the contents of several agar tubes of pure cultures of *B. pyocyaneus*, was placed on the sand, ova of *Musca domestica* being added. By the time the larvæ were from half to two-thirds grown, the food was exhausted, so a small quantity of lean uncooked beef was minced, wetted with distilled water, mixed with the contents of a tube of pure *B. pyocyaneus* and allowed to remain at 29° C. for three or four hours. It was then given to the larvæ. When the larvæ were full fed, all remnants of the food were removed and some clean sand added at the bottom of the jar."

Twelve of the pupæ obtained were placed in lysol (5—10 %) for 5 to 7 minutes. Then transferred to a tube of broth and shaken up. The time of immersion in this medium varied between five minutes and 13 hours. Afterwards they were removed to a second tube of broth and broken up with sterile needles. In all cases the second broth tube gave a copious growth of *B. pyocyaneus*, showing that this organism was present within the pupæ and in several cases the first broth tube gave a slow growth of the organisms, probably indicating that some communication exists through the air passages.

Ten flies which emerged from pupæ were also examined. Four were placed in 5 % lysol, and then washed in a tube of broth and then transferred to a second tube and broken up. On incubation the second tube gave a marked growth and the first tube a slow growth. Five flies were treated with 5 % lysol, and after being washed in two successive broth tubes broken up in a third. Only the latter gave growths on incubation. Lastly a fly was seen to emerge, and removed to 5 % lysol before it had any opportunity of infecting itself. Thence it was passed through a broth tube and broken up in a second. Only the latter gave a growth of *B. pyocyaneus.*

From his experiments the author comes to the following conclusions:—"(1) Pupæ and imagines of *Musca domestica* bred from larvæ infected with *B. pyocyaneus* under conditions which exclude the chance of re-infection in the pupal or imaginal period undoubtedly remain infected with the bacillus; (2) in the imago the infection is maximal at emergence and then diminishes suddenly; (3) the possibility of a dangerously pathogenic organism being taken up by the larva and subsequently distributed by the fly is one which deserves serious consideration."

Ledingham (III. 1911) made some experiments with pupæ sent to him by Bacot, employing another method of disinfection.

"After washing the pupæ in successive tubes of broth and saline solution, they were transferred to a Petri dish containing a small quantity of absolute alcohol, where they remained for three or four minutes. The alcohol was then ignited and allowed to burn out almost completely. Some of the pupæ, as the result of the process, seemed to be slightly desiccated externally. They were then placed in 10 % formalin for four to five minutes. Thereafter they were removed one by one to a tube of sterile broth and shaken up. From this tube they were removed to a second broth tube and shaken. Finally from this second tube each pupa was removed to an agar slope and mashed up with a strong platinum loop. The two broth tubes and the series of agar slopes were incubated at 37° C. Next day both the broth tubes were sterile but *all the agar slopes showed abundant growth in which B. pyocyaneus was present.*"

Graham-Smith (V. 1911) carried out several series of experiments with blow-fly larvæ.

In one series the larvæ when seven days old were placed in several tin boxes containing moist earth and allowed to feed on meat infected with (*a*) a spore-bearing culture of *B. anthracis*, (*b*) *B. typhosus*, (*c*) *B. enteritidis* (Gaertner), (*d*) *B. prodigiosus* and (*e*) *V. choleræ* derived from cultures respectively. After seven days the remains of the meat were removed, and the larvæ fed on fresh meat. At intervals specimens of the larvæ were placed in alcohol for 15 minutes and then passed through the flame and dissected. Cultures from their organs yielded *B. anthracis*, but none of the other organisms. The flies emerged from the 18th to the 25th days after infection. Each morning the cages in which the pupæ had been placed were examined, and the flies which had emerged removed. Some were killed and dissected within a few hours, and others were placed in glass cages and kept alive for various periods of time on syrup.

"Altogether about 70 flies emerged from larvæ fed on meat infected with *B. anthracis*. Of these, 17 were dissected and cultures made from their organs within a few hours of emerging. From four specimens *B. anthracis* was not cultivated, but from the other 13 cultures were obtained. It was present in the intestinal contents of 10; on one or both wings of 8; on one or more legs of 12; and on the heads of 8."

Three specimens were dissected after living two days in a cage. From the legs, wings and intestinal contents of all *B. anthracis* was obtained. One or more colonies were obtained from the organs of some of the flies up to the 19th day, but not after that time though some of the flies survived up to the 33rd day. Several of the cultures obtained were proved to be virulent.

"A few other experiments were carried out with these flies. Four flies were allowed to walk over agar plates a few hours after emerging. Numerous colonies of *B. anthracis* developed on these plates.

"Twelve flies a few hours old were kept in a glass cage and fed on syrup. Shortly after their first meal some of the remains of the syrup on which they had been feeding was smeared on the surface of agar plates. Numerous colonies of *B. anthracis* developed on these plates. Nearly every fly very shortly after emerging deposited a large quantity of whitish, semi-fluid material. Cultures made from this material were negative. The fæces deposited by flies two days old contained *B. anthracis* in considerable numbers, as also did the remains of syrup on which they had fed.

"*B. anthracis* was not found in cultures made from the fæces of flies 22 and 23 days old, nor in those made from the remains of syrup on which they had been feeding, but a single colony of *B. anthracis* was obtained from the remains of syrup on which flies 21 days old had fed."

The experiments with the flies bred from larvæ fed on *B. typhosus* (45 flies), *B. enteritidis* (14 flies), *B. prodigiosus* (25 flies) and *V. choleræ* (20 flies) were entirely negative.

Two other series of experiments with these organisms were also negative, and the writer came to the conclusion that "these experiments seem to indicate that, under the conditions described, none of the non-spore-bearing organisms mentioned commonly survive sufficiently long to be found in the blow-flies which emerge from infected larvæ."

Ledingham (X. 1911) in several series of experiments found that "although typhoid bacilli were liberally supplied to larvæ of *Musca domestica*, all attempts to demonstrate *B. typhosus* in the pupæ or imagines were unsuccessful until recourse was had to disinfection of the ova."

In one of his experiments the eggs were thoroughly disinfected by a short sojourn in lysol. The young larvæ were placed on a sterile agar slope, which remained sterile. "Human blood mixed with typhoid bacilli was spread on the agar and this process was repeated, the larvæ being transferred to a fresh agar slope with blood every day." Under these highly artificial conditions *B. typhosus* was isolated from the larvæ and from one pupa. No imago was obtained.

"In the experiments with unsterilized ova great difficulty was experienced in determining whether *B. typhosus* was present in MacConkey plates owing to the almost invariable occurrence of the colourless typhoid-like colonies of *Bacillus* '*A*[1]' which was evidently an organism thoroughly adapted to the conditions prevailing in the interior of the larvæ, pupæ and imagines."

[1] This organism appears to be identical with one, Ca. 8, commonly found in adult flies (see Chap. XIV).

"From the practical point of view the main conclusions to be drawn from the experiments detailed in this communication is that the typhoid bacillus can lead only a very precarious existence in the interior of larvæ or pupæ which possess, at least in so far as these investigations warrant, a well-defined bacterial flora of their own."

Nicholls (1912), working with the larvæ of *Sarcophagula* and *Sarcophaga*, came to the conclusion that "during development the fly possesses very great powers of destroying micro-organisms" and that "a freshly hatched fly may be considered probably sterile." When breeding larvæ of *Sarcophagula* in fæces infected with *B. typhosus* he found that these bacilli rapidly disappeared from the larvæ if they were removed from their infected surroundings.

Graham-Smith (1912) carried out a further series of experiments, using blow-flies, green-bottles and house-flies. In his previous paper it was pointed out that "possibly they (the bacteria) might be found in flies which emerge from larvæ which had fed on the flesh of infected animals."

Series I.

"In one series therefore half-grown larvæ of *C. erythrocephala* and *L. cæsar* were allowed to feed on the bodies of guinea-pigs which had died from infection with *B. enteritidis* and *B. anthracis*. The larvæ pupated in 10—15 days and the flies began to emerge in 20 days. In order to avoid the possibility of the flies re-infecting themselves after emerging the pupæ were removed to clean cages and placed on clean sand. In some cases before the preparation of cultures the flies were sterilized in various ways, while in other cases no sterilization of the exterior was attempted. Sometimes the flies were killed shortly after emerging, while on other occasions they were kept for some hours or days. In the latter case they were fed on syrup.

"*B. anthracis.*—Cultures on agar were prepared in the way previously described (1910) from the intestinal contents of 511 flies, 170 *C. erythrocephala* and 341 *L. cæsar*, which emerged from larvæ which fed on the body of a guinea-pig dead of anthrax. Only three colonies were met with which resembled in any way those produced by *B. anthracis*. By subcultures they were proved not to be those of *B. anthracis*.

"*B. enteritidis.*—Cultures on MacConkey's lactose neutral-red agar were made from the intestinal contents of 27 flies, all *C. erythrocephala*, which emerged from larvæ which had fed on the body of a guinea-pig dead of infection with *B. enteritidis*. A large number of colonies of non-lactose fermenting organisms developed on the plates; but although subcultures were made from many no example of *B. enteritidis* was isolated."

These experiments confirm the results previously obtained and indicate that non-spore-bearing organisms, not accustomed to the conditions prevailing in the intestine of the larva, do not commonly survive even when the larvæ feed on the bodies of animals which have died as the result of infection from such organisms. The results obtained from the spore-free forms of *B. anthracis* are in remarkable contrast with the previous experiments with spore-bearing forms (see p. 116).

In two other series of experiments the larvæ of *M. domestica* were used.

SERIES II.

"In this series house-flies, *M. domestica*, were allowed to deposit eggs on food consisting of a mixture of boiled meat, potato, and rice. The larvæ which emerged were kept in clean card cream boxes containing clean sterile sand. About three days after hatching, batches of the larvæ were transferred to six fresh boxes and fed on similar food infected with pure cultures of various organisms. The food in one box was not infected. That in the second box was infected with *B. prodigiosus*, that in the third with a *coccus* producing pink colonies, that in the fourth with Morgan's bacillus, that in the fifth with *B. enteritidis* and that in the sixth with *B. anthracis*.

"After a day or two the surface of the food became dry, but the larvæ lived and fed on the moist part below, as they do under natural conditions. The boxes were inspected daily and as pupæ developed they were transferred to fresh boxes, so that the flies on emerging should not become contaminated by crawling over the infected materials. Some of the pupæ were examined by cultures. The end of the pupa was sterilized by the application of a cautery, and the contents were removed by means of a fine pipette through the sterilized surface. After emulsification in salt solution, agar and MacConkey plates were sown. The former usually showed large numbers of colonies of cocci and other organisms, and the latter colonies of lactose fermenting and non-fermenting bacilli. Nineteen pupæ from the non-infected box were examined. In four non-lactose fermenting bacilli were met with. Of these a large number were isolated and examined and one turned out to be an example of Morgan's bacillus. In cultures made from fifteen pupæ which had developed from larvæ infected with the coccus one colony of the coccus occurred. Cultures made from eleven pupæ which developed from larvæ infected with *B. prodigiosus* yielded no colonies of that organism.

"From each box a large number of flies emerged. Cultures were made from the intestinal contents of these, usually within a few hours after hatching. In some cases the exterior of the fly was sterilized, and in others no sterilization of the exterior was attempted. Cultures from 40 flies which emerged from the control box yielded no organisms of special interest, though on the MacConkey plates a number of non-lactose fermenting organisms developed whose characters will be discussed later. Cultures from 194 flies which emerged from larvæ infected with the *coccus* producing pink colonies, and from 117 flies which emerged from larvæ infected with *B. prodigiosus*, yielded negative results. Cultures from 21 flies which emerged from *B. enteritidis* infected larvæ also yielded negative results.

"Cultures from 37 flies which emerged from Morgan infected larvæ gave numerous colonies of non-lactose fermenting bacilli. Three out of the many isolated proved to be examples of Morgan's bacillus. Cultures were made on agar from 95 of the flies which emerged from larvæ infected with the spores of *B. anthracis*.

"Cultures from 11 out of 14 newly hatched flies showed *B. anthracis* (78 %).

"Cultures from 48 out of 62 flies one day old showed *B. anthracis* (78 %).

"Cultures from 2 out of 8 flies 3 days old showed *B. anthracis* (25 %).

" " 1 " 6 " 4 " " " (16 %).

" " 1 " 5 " 6 " " " (20 %).

"Positive results were obtained from 63 (66 %) out of the 95 flies examined. A few of the flies which emerged were kept in a clean cage without food and died in a few days. After they had been dead some weeks cultures were made from three of them. *B. anthracis* was found in cultures from two."

These experiments appear to indicate that non-spore producing organisms such as *B. prodigiosus*, *B. enteritidis* and certain *cocci*, which are not adapted to the conditions prevailing in the interior of the larva and pupa, seldom survive long enough to appear in the adult. Morgan's bacillus, however, which is sometimes found in the intestine of the fly under natural conditions, appears to be capable of surviving. Colonies of various non-lactose fermenting organisms were frequently found, a fact which seems to show that many organisms of this class are specially adapted to the conditions which prevail in the intestine of the larva and of the adult fly. Many cocci and other organisms are also capable of surviving during the metamorphosis.

The spores of *B. anthracis* persist, and are present in a large proportion of the adults which develop. The spores of other bacilli can probably behave in the same way.

SERIES III.

The third series of experiments was undertaken in order to compare the results obtained by breeding larvæ in different artificially infected foods.

"Sets of card cream boxes containing sterile sand were prepared. In one set was placed food consisting of cooked meat and potato sterilized in the autoclave, in the second human fæces sterilized in the autoclave, and in the third unsterilized human fæces. In the first and second sets the organisms originally present had been destroyed. One box of each set was infected with *B. typhosus*, one with *B. enteritidis*, one with Morgan's bacillus, one with *B. prodigiosus*, and one was kept as a control. Flies were placed in a cage containing sterile food and the eggs and young larvæ removed and placed in the boxes described. The flies infected the food in the cage to some extent.

"The larvæ developed rapidly in each box and the pupæ when formed were transferred to fresh boxes containing clean sterile sand. The flies began to emerge in about a month.

"Cultures from the control flies showed no organisms similar to those which had been used for infecting purposes. At first cultures were made from single flies, but as these yielded negative results, batches of 10 flies were later emulsified and the emulsion plated on MacConkey plates. No colonies of *B. prodigiosus* developed on any of the plates although cultures were made from a large number of flies. In searching for *B. typhosus*, *B. enteritidis*, and Morgan's bacillus, MacConkey's medium was used. Numbers of colonies of non-lactose fermenting bacilli developed and from each plate several colonies were picked off and put through various tests in order to establish their identity. Neither *B. typhosus* nor *B. enteritidis* was ever isolated. Eight colonies of Morgan's bacillus were, however, obtained, three from flies which emerged from larvæ fed on sterilized fæces, four from flies which emerged from larvæ fed on unsterilized fæces, and one from flies which emerged from larvæ fed on sterile food."

"The foods used seemed to exercise little effect. These experiments again indicate that Morgan's bacillus and certain other non-lactose fermenters can survive the metamorphosis. On the other hand, it cannot be claimed that they conclusively prove that other organisms, such as *B. typhosus* and *B. enteritidis*, are entirely incapable of surviving, since all the colonies were not tested and some undetected examples of these organisms may have been present on the plates. Nevertheless sufficient colonies were isolated and tested to show that these organisms very rarely survive sufficiently long to appear in adult flies under the experimental conditions. Under natural conditions it is certain that if such organisms happen to be present in the material in which the larvæ feed they have to compete with many varieties of organisms better adapted to the conditions prevailing in the intestine of the larvæ, and their persistence in large numbers is improbable."

The varieties of non-lactose fermenting bacilli found in flies from different sources are fully discussed in Chapter XIV.

From his experiments the writer came to the following conclusions:

(1) "The blow-flies which develop from larvæ allowed to feed on the bodies of animals dead of infection due to *B. enteritidis* or *B. anthracis* are not infected with these organisms.

(2) "A large proportion of the house-flies (*M. domestica*)

which develop from larvæ infected with the spores of *B. anthracis* are infected.

(3) "Of non-spore producing organisms only those which are adapted to the conditions prevailing in the intestine of the larva, such as Morgan's bacillus and certain non-lactose fermenting bacilli, survive through the metamorphosis and are present in the flies. Organisms such as *B. typhosus*, *B. enteritidis*, and *B. prodigiosus* rarely survive."

Tebbutt (1913) carried out experiments in the following way.

"Ova of *M. domestica* were placed upon agar slopes to which a little fresh human blood was added together with the organisms with which the young larvæ were to be infected. Sometimes the ova were sterilized by washing in 3 % lysol for two or three minutes. Larvæ when full-grown were placed on sterile sand to pupate and the pupæ were stored in sterile test-tubes till they were examined or till imagines emerged. The method of examining the pupæ was that described by Ledingham (1911), the blunt end being seared with a hot iron, a capillary pipette inserted and the contents sucked out and plated on MacConkey's neutral red lactose agar.

"The imagines were examined either as soon as they were first noticed or after feeding on sterile sugar-cane solution. The method used was to wash them separately in 2 % lysol for seven to ten minutes, then in two or three successive tubes of broth, after which each was crushed in a small amount of broth and the latter plated out on several MacConkey lactose plates, so that the whole of each imago was bacteriologically examined. The broths used to wash the fly were also incubated in order to detect bacteria on the external surface, and subcultures were made from the last broth in which the fly was washed before being crushed and plated.

"The ova, larvæ, pupæ and imagines were kept throughout at a temperature of 25° C."

With regard to the bacteria met with and employed in this research a few comments are necessary. The principal pathogenic organism on which larvæ were fed was one of the mannite types of the dysentery bacillus, viz. Bac. 'Y' of Hiss and Russell.

Tebbutt (p. 525) came to the following conclusions:

(1) "Pathogenic organisms such as *B. dysenteriæ* (type 'Y') cannot be recovered from pupæ or imagines reared from larvæ to which these organisms have been administered.

(2) "When the larvæ have been bred from disinfected ova and are subsequently fed on *B. dysenteriæ* (type 'Y'), this organism may be successfully recovered from the pupæ and imagines in a small number of cases.

(3) "Under similar conditions *B. typhosus* was not recovered in a single case from pupæ or imagines.

(4) "In those cases in which *B. dysenteriæ* ('Y') was successfully recovered from pupæ, the colonies on the plate were invariably fewer than those obtained from pupæ and imagines after administration to the larvæ of more adaptable organisms such as '*Bac. A*' (Ledingham).

(5) "A certain proportion of the pupæ remained sterile, so that the process of metamorphosis is undoubtedly accompanied by a considerable destruction of the bacteria present in the larval stage.

(6) "The possibility of flies becoming infected from the presence of pathogenic organisms in the breeding grounds of the larvæ may be considered as very remote."

GENERAL SUMMARY.

The evidence hitherto published relating to the possibility of the micro-organisms ingested by the larvæ surviving in the adult fly has been fully quoted because the subject is one of great importance. Though it seems to have been proved that the spores of *B. anthracis* may survive, most observers agree that such non-spore bearing pathogenic organisms as *B. typhosus*, *B. enteritidis* and *B. dysenteriæ derived from cultures* and added to the food of the larvæ are not present in the flies which emerge, except under very special and highly artificial conditions. Most of these observers conclude from their experiments that the possibility of flies becoming infected from the presence of pathogenic organisms in the breeding ground of the larvæ may be considered as remote. On the other hand Faichnie working with *uncultivated B. typhosus* and *B. paratyphosus* A stated that he was able to isolate these organisms from the flies which emerged. All the other investigators have failed to take into account the possibility of *cultivated bacilli* behaving in a different manner to *uncultivated bacilli*. Faichnie's experiments are not altogether conclusive since the experimental conditions were such that the newly emerged flies might have re-infected themselves by feeding on the contaminated material. There is no evidence in his paper that he separated the larvæ which had fed on infected material and examined the pupæ and imagines under conditions which would exclude the possibility of re-infection.

Before forming a final judgment his experiments ought to be repeated with suitable precautions against re-infection.

It must be remembered, however, that under natural conditions flies which emerge from infected larvæ may be able to re-infect themselves if the contaminating organism still survives in the material surrounding the pupæ.

One point, however, has been clearly demonstrated. Both the larva and adult fly have a peculiar flora, consisting, so far as is at present known, of non-lactose fermenting organisms, adapted to life within their alimentary canals, and capable of surviving the pupal stage. These bacilli are of considerable practical importance since they are often present in large numbers and render the search for pathogenic bacilli of the typhoid-enteritidis group one of great labour, since they resemble them in many cultural characters and can only be certainly distinguished from them by means of elaborate cultural and serological tests.

CHAPTER XII

FLIES AND 'SPECIFIC' DISEASES

Though there is at the present time a widespread tendency to believe that under special conditions non-biting flies are often partly responsible for the spread of certain diseases, few undoubted instances of infection by flies have yet been recorded. This is partly due to the fact that sufficient attention has not been devoted to the enquiries; partly to the difficulty of excluding other possible sources of infection and partly to the difficulty of obtaining direct proof of infection by flies alone.

In dealing with each specific disease the evidence relating to the possibility of the virus being distributed by flies will be summarized under the following headings:

(1) Experiments showing to what extent and in what manner flies can carry and distribute the causative organisms.

(2) The discovery of the specific organism or related types in 'wild' flies.

(3) General observations on the relationship of flies to outbreaks of the disease.

In considering the bearing of experimental work on natural transmission of the disease organisms, it must be borne in mind that most experiments have been conducted with cultures. Much grosser infection of the fly is, therefore, produced than can usually occur under natural conditions, and moreover 'cultivated' as opposed to 'uncultivated' bacteria are used. The latter fact introduces a factor about which we have at present little accurate knowledge. We know that 'cultivated' bacteria usually grow better under artificial laboratory conditions, but we have little information as to how they behave, as compared with 'uncultivated' bacteria direct from the body, in competition with the different organisms present under varying conditions in the alimentary canal of the fly. While it is probable that the 'uncultivated' strains persist longer in the fly, it is certain that their powers of producing infection in the human subject or in experimental animals are greater.

In judging of the value of the records relating to the finding of 'specific' pathogenic bacteria in 'wild' flies, it must be remembered that many of the records were published several years ago, when the means of differentiating allied organisms were not so complete as at present, and further, that comparatively little was then known of the numerous species, which very closely resemble the specific pathogenic forms, both in appearance and in culture. The greatest caution must therefore be observed in accepting statements unaccompanied by full descriptions of the methods employed.

The general observations which have been published on the relationship of flies to outbreaks of disease are obviously of very unequal value. Many are mere surmises unaccompanied by evidence; in many cases other possible sources of infection have not been excluded and the evidence brought forward is of very doubtful value; in some statistical evidence requiring very careful interpretation and often covering an insufficient period is mainly relied on, but in a few instances the evidence appears to be conclusive.

It is evident, therefore, that the greatest care has to be exercised in criticizing and sifting the mass of evidence of various kinds, which has been brought forward in favour of the transmission of disease by non-biting flies, and that prolonged and accurate investigations in all departments are necessary before we can hope to have an accurate knowledge of the precise part played by flies in disseminating various diseases.

Flies do not seem to be affected in any way by bacteria pathogenic to man.

In the following chapters an endeavour has been made to place before the reader an account of all the bacteriological investigations which have been made in relation to each disease. The more recent work has been quoted at sufficient length to enable a judgment to be formed as to its merits. Selections from the more important papers dealing with general observations have also been quoted very fully.

CHAPTER XIII

TYPHOID OR ENTERIC FEVER AND DISEASE CAUSED BY ALLIED ORGANISMS

Though the possibility of the spread of typhoid fever infection by flies has been generally acknowledged for some years, but few records are to be found of instances in which *B. typhosus* has been recovered from infected flies in connection with outbreaks of the disease. In spite of this fact much evidence has accumulated to show that *under certain favourable conditions* flies are important agents in spreading the disease. Howard (1911, p. xvi) has even gone so far as to propose the name 'typhoid-fly' as a substitute for the name 'house-fly' now in general use, though he admits that "strictly speaking the term 'typhoid-fly' is open to some objection as conveying the erroneous idea that the fly is solely responsible for the spread of typhoid." For many reasons exact bacteriological proof of the conveyance of this infection by flies is difficult in the majority of outbreaks and consequently we have to rely on indirect evidence as is done in water analyses. If on bacteriological examination a sample of water is found to contain fæcal bacteria, and it can be shown that the source of supply is liable to contamination with human sewage, the water is considered to be dangerous, not because the ordinary fæcal bacteria are themselves the cause of specific disease, but because the organisms causing typhoid fever and other intestinal diseases may find their way into the water in the same way as the fæcal bacteria. Typhoid bacilli have only rarely been isolated from infected waters, though numerous undoubted water-borne epidemics have been recorded. Flies we know constantly carry and distribute fæcal bacteria and no doubt carry the bacteria of intestinal diseases, when suitable opportunities occur.

The difficulties in the way of producing definite bacteriological proof of infection through flies are due to several different causes. The typhoid bacillus does not originate in the fly; the latter must obtain infection from some pre-existing case of the disease in the human subject either by contact with some article soiled by the patient or more usually by visiting infected excreta.

Modern research has shown that many patients continue to excrete *B. typhosus* in the urine or fæces long after the symptoms of the disease have disappeared. Such persons, who often have the disease in a mild and almost unrecognizable form, and subsequently remain in perfect health, are termed 'carriers.' Some of these carriers constantly excrete the bacilli, while others only do so at intervals, but the majority continue to excrete them for prolonged periods, often many years. Numerous outbreaks have been traced to unrecognized carriers, and it is now universally recognized that many of them, especially those who have to do with the preparation of food, constitute a serious danger to the health of the community in which they live.

Flies cannot obtain *B. typhosus* from the excreta of normal individuals, but can do so from the fæces of apparently healthy 'carriers,' and of unrecognized, incipiently mild, atypical and typical cases of typhoid. Morgan and Harvey (1909) made some very interesting observations on the persistence of *B. typhosus* in the urine and fæces of a typhoid carrier. The bacilli could be cultivated from a patch of ground exposed to bright sun six hours after a typhoid carrier had voided urine on it. In the corner of a dark hut the bacilli were present in large numbers for five hours and in smaller numbers up to thirty hours. Fæces were passed into a 'gumlah' half filled with dry earth and then covered with dry earth. *B. typhosus* was isolated from the surface of the fæcal deposit on the seventh day and could be recovered from the interior up to eighteen days. From a sample of blanketing soiled with liquid fæces *B. typhosus* was isolated up to the fortieth day, but not later.

In properly sewered towns these discharges are disposed of without flies being able to gain access to them, except in dirty and ill-kept courts and alleys, and consequently in such towns flies probably play an insignificant part in the spread of the disease. In towns and villages with privies and privy-middens the flies have greater opportunities of infecting themselves, and further research will probably show that under these conditions they may be factors in the spread of the disease. In towns and military camps where the night-soil is buried in inefficiently constructed trenches, they appear to play a most important part in the spread of the disease as will be shown later.

Even when infected flies are found it is difficult to state definitely the exact means by which infection has been carried to the individual. The probability is that food is the medium through which the specific organisms reach the person infected; and the article of food which offers the best medium for the growth and multiplication of the bacilli is milk. The chief difficulty in tracing the exact channel of infection in a series of cases of this disease is that the incubation period is long, i.e. in most cases over ten days, so that investigations cannot be commenced for at least a fortnight after actual infection has taken place. After this time there will be no remains of the food which has been the actual means of infection, and unless the contamination of food continues to take place it is improbable that infected food will be found. It is therefore difficult to prove the connection between infected flies and cases of the disease.

Finally it is by no means an easy task to isolate and identify *B. typhosus* from the fly. In the fly's intestine there are very frequently present many non-lactose fermenting bacilli (see Table 21), apparently well adapted to life in this situation, closely resembling *B. typhosus.* Not only do the colonies which many of them produce on the original plate cultures resemble those of *B. typhosus,* but some of these bacilli cannot be distinguished with certainty from *B. typhosus* even when isolated and cultivated in suitable media. Such species can only be distinguished by means of agglutination and absorption tests with known immune sera. The occurrence of these non-lactose fermenting bacilli probably often leads to failure in isolating *B. typhosus* even when it is present, and in any case renders its detection a long and laborious undertaking.

Experimental evidence.

Celli (1888) was apparently the first observer to make experiments on flies with *B. typhosus.* He fed flies with pure cultures and examined their fæces and contents and came to the conclusion that these bacilli could be found in the excreta. His experiments are of doubtful value owing to the inadequate means of differential diagnosis at that time.

Firth and Horrocks (1902) carried out experiments in

"a large box measuring 4 ft. by 3 ft. by 3 ft. One side of it was occupied by a pane of glass and at one end was a large circular aperture closed by means of a muslin funnel. This muslin had an opening through it, which was readily closed either by a tape or by a clamp. Through this muslin-closed opening flies were introduced, and also a bottle containing larvæ and chrysalids of flies; these gradually developing, maintained a steady supply of flies within the box. When a sufficient number of flies were in the box, a small dish containing a rich emulsion in sugar made from a twenty-four hour agar slope of Bacillus typhosus recently obtained from an enteric stool, and rubbed up with some fine soil, was introduced; also a small pot containing some honey, the margin of which was smeared with honey and scrapings from a fresh agar slope of Bacillus typhosus.

"At the same time some sterile litmus agar plates and also some dishes containing sterile broth were exposed and placed at a spot some distance away from the infected soil and infected honey. A sheet of clean paper was also placed in the box. The flies were seen through the glass pane to settle on the infected matter and also on the agar plates, the broth and the paper. After a few days the agar plates and the broth were removed, incubated at 37° C. for 20 hours and respectively examined and subcultured for the presence of the enteric bacillus. No difficulty was experienced in finding colonies of the Bacillus typhosus on the agar plates and also in recovering it from the exposed broth, in which the flies were seen to walk."

The paper was covered with fly-specks, but *B. typhosus* was not obtained from them. Several somewhat similar experiments were carried out and the writers came to the conclusion that the bacilli adhered to the external parts and did not pass through the alimentary canal. This is probably due to the fact that the 'specks' were left for several days before examination, and in consequence the bacilli in them died owing to drying.

Ficker (1903) carried out a more elaborate series of experiments, keeping various numbers of flies in 10 litre flasks, and allowing them to feed on pure cultures of *B. typhosus*. After 18 to 24 hours the flies were transferred to clean flasks, and were subsequently transferred to clean flasks every two or three days. Cultures were made from crushed flies at frequent intervals. In his series of experiments *B. typhosus* was recovered from flies 5 to 23 days after they had been infected. Agglutination tests were made use of to prove the identity of the bacilli isolated. Graham-Smith (1910) carried out experiments with large numbers of flies kept in gauze cages and fed for eight hours on emulsions of *B. typhosus* in syrup. After that time the infected syrup was removed and the flies were fed on plain syrup. *B. typhosus* was isolated up to 48 hours (but not later) from emulsions of their fæces and from plates over which they walked. In the latter case infection was largely due to inoculation by the flies' proboscides. The bacillus was isolated up to the sixth day from intestinal contents.

The isolation of B. typhosus from 'wild' flies.

Hamilton (1903) seems to have been the first to isolate *B. typhosus* from five out of eighteen 'wild' flies in Chicago, caught in two undrained privies, on the walls of houses and in the room of a typhoid patient. She thought that the outbreak, which was confined to a certain ward of Chicago, was in large measure due to flies acting as carriers of the specific bacilli. In the same year Ficker (1903) briefly stated that he had isolated *B. typhosus* from flies caught in a house in Leipzig in which eight cases of typhoid had occurred. Klein (1908, p. 1150, footnote) examined 12 living flies caught by Wilshaw in a row of houses in which typhoid had occurred. The flies "were minced in a sterile dish with $\frac{1}{2}$ cm. of sterile salt solution. The whole of the resulting turbid fluid was used for cultures." In each plate he found two or three typhoid-like colonies. "These agreed in all respects culturally with the stock *B. typhosus*, including distinct agglutination in 10 minutes with a 1 : 50 dilution of anti-typhoid serum, but in litmus glucose bile salt peptone water produced acid and 'very slight gas after three days.'" Odlum (1908) briefly states that he isolated *B. typhosus* from two flies out of several hundreds at Nasirabad (see p. 139). Bertarelli (1910) made a more extensive investigation on 120 flies caught in an Italian house in which several cases of typhoid had occurred. He isolated *B. typhosus* from the bodies of eight flies, proving their identity by cultural and agglutination tests.

On this subject the most interesting investigations are those of Faichnie (1909) and Cochrane (1912), whose observations are fully quoted.

Faichnie (1909) investigated a small outbreak of typhoid at Kamptee, and, after excluding all other sources, was obliged to suspect the flies. They were not very numerous. About 40 were collected, 20 each from the verandahs of the artillery and infantry kitchens.

"Twelve flies from the artillery lines were mashed up in sterile normal salt solution and a drop plated, with the result that *B. typhosus* was separated. This bacillus was agglutinated by a solution of 1—10,000 of a specific *B. typhosus* serum" and gave the usual reactions on various media. "Also 12 flies from the infantry kitchen were treated as follows: Each was transfixed with a sterile needle, and passed two or three times through a flame, until the legs and wings were scorched; they were then put into normal salt solution and stirred without breaking with a glass rod. One c.c. of this solution was seeded into MacConkey broth which remained unchanged thereby showing the absence of *B. typhosus* on the legs and wings after burning. After this the flies were mashed up and a drop of the fluid plated. *B. typhosus*, as above, was again found, thereby demonstrating that the bacillus was present in the intestine, but not on the legs."

Summing up he says:—"Experience seems to show that infection conveyed by flies' legs, natural though it may appear to all from experiments carried out to prove its possibility, is not a common nor even a considerable cause of enteric fever. On the other hand infection by the excrement of flies bred in an infected material explains many conclusions previously difficult to accept. In a word, it is the breeding ground that constitutes the danger, not the ground where the flies feed."

The cultures which have just been described were sent to Lieutenant-Colonel Semple, Director of the Central Research Institute, Kasauli, who stated that they were undoubtedly *B. typhosus*. Amongst other tests he immunized rabbits with these cultures and found that their serum agglutinated stock cultures of *B. typhosus* in high dilutions.

In a later paper (p. 675) Faichnie says:—"Since writing my first paper on this subject, I have found *B. typhosus* in flies from Sehore, once; from Kamptee, twice; from Nasirabad, once in flies from the bungalow of an officer who had enteric fever, and once from flies in the Officers' Mess there; from Nowgong, twice, once in the flies from the Royal Artillery Coffee Shop, and again in flies from the trenching ground, making a total of nine in three months. Except those from Nasirabad, the flies were always flamed before examination, and a control of the washed flies was taken before crushing, so there is no doubt the bacillus was actually in the interior of the fly, probably in the intestine." He does not state whether agglutination tests were applied or not to these organisms.

Cochrane (1912) gives an interesting account of a small outbreak of eight cases which occurred in April and May 1911 at St George's, Bermuda. The first patient became ill on April 15th, the second on the 21st, the third on the 23rd, the fourth on the 24th, the fifth and sixth on May 1st, the seventh on May 7th and the eighth on May 8th.

Well-marked agglutination reactions with *B. typhosus* were obtained in cases 1, 5, 6, 7 and 8, and the bacillus was isolated by blood cultures from cases 2, 3 and 4.

"Investigations made at St George's on April 30th suggested no definite source of infection for the first four cases, but it was found that there had been a fatal case of enteric in a coloured woman's house (Mrs P.) near Alexandra Battery in September, 1910, and that in December, 1910, Gunner O., who lived as caretaker in the Battery, contracted the disease. The occurrence of further cases amongst the coloured people in the vicinity of the Cut Road since that date could not be ascertained."

On May 3rd, 1911, five or six flies (*M. domestica*) were caught at each of the following places and placed in a sterile test-tube and numbered: No. 1, kitchen of case 3. No. 2, kitchen of case 1. No. 3, kitchen of case 3. No. 4, Mrs P.'s washhouse, which is close to a dry earth latrine used by her household.

"The flies from each place were put into 5 c.c. of sterile salt solution in a test-tube, the contents of the test-tube were well shaken for a minute, and bile salt broth or 'Fawcus medium' plates inoculated from the fluid. These tubes or plates were labelled 'external washing' and numbered 1, 2, 3 and 4 respectively. The flies were now emulsified with a glass rod in sterile salt solution, and another series of tubes or plates made and similarly numbered. The growth of the liquid medium was plated out on the following day. The inoculated plates were examined after incubation in the usual manner. The final result was that from Nos. 1 and 2 no suspicious organisms were isolated. From No. 3 'fly emulsion' a non-Gram staining motile bacillus was recovered which resembled *B. typhosus* in cultural reactions on sugars, milk, gelatine and peptone solutions; morphologically, it was very short, no filaments could be seen and it was more motile than a typical *B. typhosus*, gave a thicker and whiter growth on agar, and did not agglutinate with an anti-typhoid serum. From No. 4 'external washing' a non-Gram staining motile bacillus was recovered which gave the following reactions:

Lactose litmus broth	No acidity.
Saccharose	" "
Glucose	Acid, no gas.
Mannite	" "
Peptone solution	No indol after six days.
Gelatine	No liquefaction in ten days.
Neutral red agar	No fluorescence.
Litmus milk	Acid, no clot in ten days.

"Agglutination tests:—

"As no immunized animals or specific typhoid serum was available the specific serum was obtained from the patients. The sera of cases 6 and 8 were found to give the most complete agglutination with the stock *B. typhosus*.

"The bacillus under investigation was clumped completely in half-an-hour in 1 in 30 dilution of these sera as seen under the microscope, and completely sedimented in twenty-four hours in dilutions up to 1 in 180 in capillary tubes. Similar control results were obtained at the same time with the stock *B. typhosus*."

"These reactions proved that a true *B. typhosus* had been recovered from the 'external washing' of flies caught at Mrs P.'s house on May 3, 1911. From this it may be concluded that flies at this house had access to some specially infected matter, and that the organisms were probably carried on their feet or proboscis. Having definitely ascertained that a focus of infection existed at Mrs P.'s house on May 3, 1911, it is reasonable to assume that this had existed previous to this date, and that infected flies were the probable carriers of infection to case 1." The distance "is less than 300 yards. It is possible that cases 2, 3, 4 and 5 were infected in a similar way from this house, but the infection in cases 6, 7 and 8 was probably directly from other cases."

"It is interesting to note that the prevailing direction of the wind during April, 1911, was north-east." An east wind would blow directly from Mrs P.'s house to the house of case 1. Unfortunately "Mrs P. refused to allow any investigation of excreta or blood examination to be made."

General Observations.

Temperate climates.

The general evidence relating to the spread of typhoid fever by flies in cities in temperate climates is at present far from conclusive. The majority of the cases of the disease are discovered early and are removed to hospital before the excreta contain large numbers of the bacilli, and under any circumstances the opportunities for flies to pick up infection, even from unrecognized typhoid carriers, in well-sewered cities and towns are small, since the bulk of the excreta is immediately passed into the drains. It must be remembered, however, that even in reasonably clean and well-sewered cities flies have some opportunities of infecting themselves. "The city of Washington has the reputation of being perhaps the cleanest and best-sewered city in the United States and yet it is possible any summer morning to find human dejecta in alleyways and vacant lots deposited there overnight by irresponsible persons, and in the light of day swarming with flies. In the poor quarters of the city uncared-for children of the indigent ease themselves almost wherever they happen to be" (Howard, 1911, p. 141). Newstead (1907, p. 16) in his Liverpool report writes to the same effect. "In the course of my investigations, more especially on hot days, numbers of flies were seen hovering over or feeding on 'human dejecta.' The fæces were generally those of children, and were lying, as a rule, a few feet from the doorways, in the courts or in passages behind the houses. In one instance no less than five patches of human excreta were lying in one court, and all of them were attended by house-flies." It is not improbable that a small proportion of these dejecta are deposited by 'typhoid carriers.' Moreover the possibility of fly infection has received little attention hitherto, even in those towns in which suitable conditions occur.

In certain cities data have been obtained which are sufficient to afford information as to the general time relationship between fly prevalence and the incidence of typhoid fever. Niven (1910) has carried out investigations of this nature since 1904 in Manchester, Rosenau, Lunsden, Kartle and Howard made similar investigations in Washington in 1909 and Hamer (1909) in London. As a whole these observations seem to indicate that there is little relationship in these cities between the prevalence of flies and the incidence of typhoid fever. It must be remembered, however, in considering this question, that in large cities many factors are in operation and that it is not impossible as Niven believes that increased fly prevalence determines the increased incidence of typhoid fever in London and Manchester at the end of summer.

More detailed observations were made in Washington by Lumsden and Anderson (1911) who found that the incidence of typhoid fever upon the population using privies or yard closets was greatest during the fly season.

Howard (1911, p. 148) quotes the opinions of several observers living in rural districts in the United States, who believe that flies are chiefly responsible for the spread of the disease in country places. Reliable information on this subject is still lacking.

Tropical climates.

Numerous workers have recorded their belief that flies play an important part in the dissemination of typhoid fever in stations in the tropics. The observations of Faichnie (1909) and of Cochrane (1912) have already been quoted, and a few extracts from other interesting reports will be sufficient to indicate the observations on which this very general belief is founded. Reports concerning Poona and Nasirabad in India, and Bermuda have been chosen because they cover a series of years.

Writing of Poona, Ainsworth (1909) says:

"We find then, year by year, that in Poona and Kirkee enteric fever begins in July, reaches its maximum in August, maintains a high level in September, dies down in October, and nearly disappears in November and December. The admissions for the two months, August and September, are considerably higher than those for all the other ten months put together, and for the four months, July, August, September and October, rather more than two and a half times greater than the sum of the other eight months. This is a very striking fact, and points unmistakably to a regularly recurrent cause. Now these four months are the monsoon months, and at first it would seem to afford proof positive that the germs are water-borne; but, apart from the fact that there is a pipe supply from a distant catchment area, not very liable to contamination, and that analyses, both chemical and bacteriological, exonerate the water, it is practically certain that if water were the agent the first outburst would follow the break of the monsoon in the average incubation period, say fourteen days, and the maximum intensity would be reached within the month, as the accumulated filth of the antecedent dry days would be washed down by the first floods. But this is not so, as reference to the annexed charts will show; on the contrary the monsoon breaks invariably in the middle of June, and enteric does not become epidemic until August. But heat and moisture, combined with suitable breeding media, will for certainty produce flies. Unfortunately, I can only speak of this one season, which local residents did not consider to be a bad year for flies, yet in July, 1908, the flies were simply appalling, and one medical officer, who is most particular in regard to the sanitation of his bungalow and compound, told me that in two days with six large glass traps he filled a stable bucket with dead flies caught in his own kitchen and back verandah. This will give some idea of their prevalence."

The two following charts from Ainsworth's paper sufficiently explain themselves.

The fly prevalence was estimated in the following manner. "A half-sheet of 'tangle foot' was placed in three different kitchens and changed every twenty-four hours; a count was

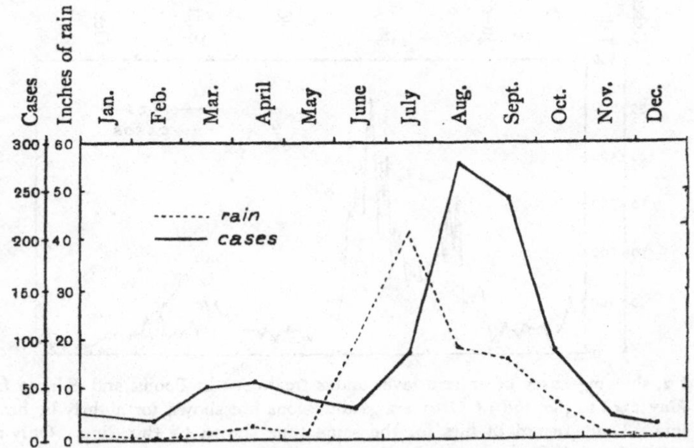

Chart 1, showing the total number of admissions for enteric fever to the Station Hospitals, Poona and Kirkee, from Jan. 1st, 1894, to the end of October, 1908, and the total rainfall, from January 1st, 1905, to the end of October, 1908.

thereafter made and a daily average struck—a rough and ready method, no doubt, but sufficiently accurate for practical purposes, especially when I add that, at the height of the fly plague, over 700 were caught on a half-sheet of paper. Incidentally also, two facts may be quoted, first, that the kitchens used were supposed to be fly-proof, being elaborately protected by gauze; and, second, that the daily average of flies caught in the kitchen of the Station Hospital, Poona, during the period the observations were carried out (May to October) was thirty, whilst in the worst of the three experimental kitchens it was just 200." Ainsworth also makes the following interesting statement. "I would remark that there are a great many more cases of enteric fever amongst the natives than is usually conceded—for instance out of ninety-two cases of enteric fever collected by me in Poona during the first ten months of 1908, no less than forty were genuine attacks in natives, from whose blood in many instances I isolated pure cultures of the *Bacillus typhosus.* Now when the habits of the natives of India are considered the danger of these cases to the general community cannot be over-estimated."

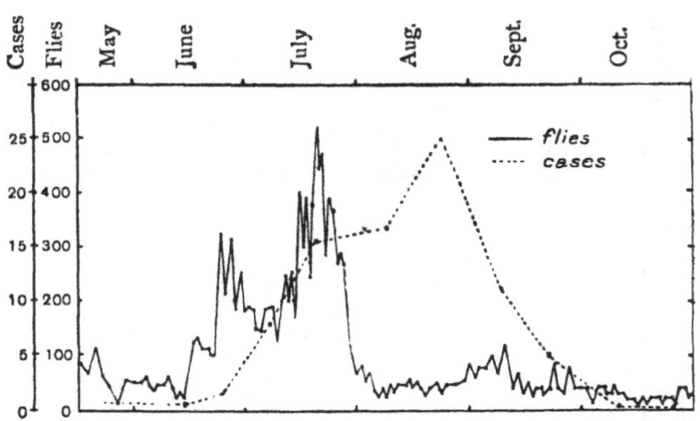

Chart 2, showing cases of enteric fever under treatment in Poona and Kirkee from May 23rd to the end of October. Admissions are shown fortnightly by broken line. Daily record of flies for the same time shown by thin line. Only nine cases of enteric fever were under treatment for the first four and a half months of the year, viz. Jan. 1st to May 15th, 1908.

Finally no better comment could be made on this paper than that of Ainsworth himself:—"I readily admit that the observations recorded and the arguments advanced are open to the objection that they afford but scanty data upon which to base so important a conclusion that the house-fly is frequently the intermediary and probably by far the most common intermediary, in the propagation of that *bête noire* of Indian sanitarians, enteric fever. Nevertheless, scanty though these data undoubtedly are, rough though the methods employed may be, and brief the period over which the observations extend, there is an isochronism shown in the appended charts between the advent of the house-fly in Poona and the seasonal prevalence of enteric fever, which is highly significant and at least suggests that a *primâ facie* case has been established for further investigation."

In connection with Ainsworth's observations Quills' (1905) experiences several years before are of interest. "I well remember an experience at Poona which will bear relating. Enteric fever, at the time I speak of, was very prevalent at that Station, and a close observation was being made in relation to the cause of the outbreak. Among other matters it was considered advisable to make an inspection of the place where the sewage of the city of Poona was deposited. This place was some two miles from the city, and about an equal distance from the barracks. When some half a mile from the odoriferous spot we were in search of a 'booming sound' was heard, the cause of which was a mystery. We continued our journey; the 'booming sound' steadily increased in intensity, and explained itself on the sewage ground being reached. There we found three large tanks, one full, the others partly full, of putrescent filth, giving out an overpowering stench; on the surface of these filth tanks was an incredible swarm of flies, all busily engaged in sucking in the foul, green corruption. The buzzing of these flies was the cause of the 'booming sound' which had so puzzled us when first heard over half a mile distant. The putrid contents of these tanks was eagerly bought by natives for agricultural purposes—a suggestive subject. But further, what of the poison-laden flies? Did they migrate? If so, where to, and with what result?"

Perhaps the station from which the most interesting series of reports is available is Nasirabad. Odlum (1908) records the conditions prevailing there about ten years ago. "In 1903, the Seaforth Highlanders, stationed at Nasirabad, suffered from a very bad epidemic of typhoid fever, and when all other means had failed, it was decided to try to exterminate the flies. This at first appeared to be a hopeless task, as we were not then conversant with the habits and methods of breeding of these insects. Finally the flies disappeared and enteric ceased. We had not a case of enteric fever in Nasirabad from July 1905 to August

1906, on which latter date flies reappeared. Although we searched diligently for their breeding ground, it could not be found, and as a result we daily expected an outbreak of enteric. In this we were not disappointed, as we got ten cases, each from a separate barrack room."

Jones (1907, p. 22), who instituted the measures, pointed out that since a raid on flies had been commenced in Nasirabad, in 1904, the enteric fever rate there had very much diminished, and that the results obtained were partly due to a better system of trenching the night soil, by which the breeding of flies was prevented.

Later Faichnie (1909, p. 580) gives an interesting account of his experiences in this neighbourhood.

"One of my first duties as sanitary officer of the division in which Nasirabad is situated was to report on its water supply. As a result of my inspection and analysis I was satisfied that the water was above suspicion, and probably had been so for many years. Meanwhile the improvement in the enteric rate, which had commenced in 1904, has been maintained up to August 1909.

"At my first visit to Nasirabad, in January of this year, flies were present both in the barracks and in the hospital, but only a few were then found at the trenching ground; at my second visit, at the end of May, none at all were found at that place. In my head-quarter station, Mhow, there was also a sudden diminution in enteric in 1907, which has been maintained ever since. This diminution coincides with the inspection of the station by Surgeon-General Trevor, who found the trenching grounds swarming with flies. Since then, owing to the skill and watchfulness of the Cantonment Magistrate, Major Hunts, a marked change in this respect has followed, and now for eighteen months scarcely a fly has been bred there.

"This drop in the enteric fever rate is very marked, but it cannot be put down solely to anti-typhoid inoculation, for although the majority of the people in the station have been inoculated, many have not, and of those who have been many were done in 1907, and are now showing only slight signs of protection, judging by their agglutinins. There are also in the station over 60 men who had enteric fever before the days when convalescents were examined to eliminate 'carriers.' An examination of these men has been recently begun, and already I have found two men who have been carriers since 1906, so that it cannot be said that anything more than usual has been done to prevent direct infection. The Mhow water supply is from a pure source, and does not require boiling, so there can be very little doubt that the essential cause of the improvement is the fact that flies do not breed in the trenching grounds.

"At the beginning of this year the only station in the division that was suffering from enteric fever was Jubbulpore, which has an unquestionable water supply, but which is swarming with flies, even in the cold weather. A visit to the trenching grounds always brings back numbers of them, conveyed by horse and trap.

"A consideration of the conditions of these three stations points clearly to the assumption that trenching grounds are very important factors in the causation of enteric fever....I venture to say that the evidence points strongly to the conclusion that... the chief and most common method is by excrement when the flies are bred in an enteric infected material. By this I mean that one station may swarm with flies, bred only from the excreta of cows and horses, and yet have no enteric; while another place, where there are very few flies, but where these are bred from human excreta either in or out of the station, may have an epidemic, the source of infection being the excrement of the flies, and the insects themselves being the carriers."

Woodhouse (1908) "believes flies to be the channel by which enteric fever is most frequently propagated in India" and Aldridge (1907) came to the following conclusions:

"There is a large mass of evidence pointing to the close connection of epidemics of enteric fever with a great prevalence of house-flies in dwellings, places where food is stored and latrines. As far as observations up to the present have been made, the seasonal prevalence of flies agrees very closely with that of enteric fever. Flies are bred at certain seasons of the year in enormous numbers in latrine trenches, and in excrement after it has been buried in comparatively shallow trenches. Statistics show that, in Indian cantonments with 500 British troops or over, the five having the lowest enteric fever admission rates have no filth trenches; and in the only remaining ones in which there are no trenches, or only at a considerable distance from barracks the rates are much below the average."

The observations just quoted, covering a number of years, were made in various parts of India by independent workers, and are so suggestive that it is to be hoped that more extended investigations will be carried out to confirm or disprove the hypotheses advanced by these writers.

One other record may be quoted. Wanhill (1907) investigated the cause of the prevalence of enteric fever among the troops stationed in Bermuda. "At Warwick camp cases of enteric began to appear among the men of this battalion in September, 1904, and continued till the end of the year, some seventeen cases in all being admitted." The water, milk and food supply was excellent but "the latrines were of a bad pattern...and the use of dry earth to cover fæcal matter was neglected. As a result, the pails were full to overflowing early in the morning and were exposed to flies for the rest of the day, since by the law of the Island they were only allowed to be emptied at night. The resultant condition of things will be imagined; and of the possibilities of food contamination there could be no doubt.... The precautionary measures necessary, therefore, resolved themselves into a campaign against flies."

"The result of these measures was the complete disappearance of enteric fever from the camps for the next two years."

In connection with Cochrane's experiences seven years later (see p. 132) in Bermuda, this account is particularly interesting.

Military camps in the Spanish-American and South African Wars.

The Commission appointed to investigate the cause of the epidemics of enteric fever in the volunteer camps in the United States during the Spanish-American War of 1898 found that "the water supply was in most places good, and was not responsible for the spread of the fever. This was effected, in the opinion of the members of the Commission, by the flies which swarmed in all the camps and devoted their attentions impartially and alternately to the fæcal matter in the open and not disinfected latrines 'and the food of the troops.'" "These pests had inflicted greater loss upon American soldiers than the arms of Spain." These remarks of the American Commissioners are supported by Veeder (1898, p. 429) who states with reference to standing camps in the same campaign that he "has seen fæcal matter in shallow trenches open to the air, with the merest apology for disinfection, and only lightly covered with earth at intervals of a day or two. In sultry weather this material, fresh from the bowel and in its most dangerous condition, was covered with myriads of flies, and at a short distance there was a tent, equally open to the air, for dining and cooking. To say that flies were busy travelling back and forth between these two places is putting it mildly." "There is no doubt that air and sunlight kill infection, if given time, but their very access gives opportunity for the flies to do serious mischief as conveyers of fresh infection wherever they put their feet. In a few minutes they may load themselves with the dejections of a dysenteric or typhoid patient, not as yet sick enough to be in hospital or under observation, and carry the poison so taken up into the very midst of the food and water ready for the next meal. There is no long roundabout process involved. It is very plain and direct, and yet when the thousands of lives are at stake in this way the danger passes unnoticed, and the consequences are disastrous and seem mysterious until attention is directed to the point; then it becomes simple enough in all conscience."

Vaughan states that during 1898, in some of the large military camps, where lime had been sprinkled recently over the contents of the latrines flies with their feet whitened with lime were seen walking over the food.

Munson (1901) remarked that "the typhoid epidemics of 1898 gradually decreased with the approach of cold weather and the disabling of the fly as a carrier of infection. Where a strong wind constantly blows from the same direction, a fly-borne infection will chiefly extend down wind, as this insect always rises and generally moves in the direction of air currents" (see p. 77).

During the South African War many observers made similar reports.

Tooth and Calverley (1901, p. 73) remarked that "in a tent full of men, all apparently equally ill, one may almost pick out the enteric cases by the masses of flies they attract. This was very noticeable at Modder River, for at that time there were in the tents men with severe sunstroke who resembled in some ways enteric patients, and it was remarkable to see how the flies passed over them to hover round and settle on the enterics. The moment an enteric patient put out his tongue one or more flies would settle on it....It was impossible not to regard them as most important factors in the dissemination of enteric fever. Our opinion is further strengthened by the fact that enteric fever in South Africa practically ceases every year with the cold weather, and this was the case at Bloemfontein.... It seemed to us that the cold weather reduced the number of the enteric cases by killing these pests."

Both Smith (1903) and Austen (1904, p. 656) make very similar remarks on the conditions of the latrine trenches during this campaign. The former states that a neglected trench "becomes an open privy with an infected surface soil around it; the flies browse on it in the day time, and occupy the men's tents at night. On visiting a deserted camp during the recent campaign it was common to find half-a-dozen or so open latrines containing a fetid mass of excreta and maggots. This because the responsible persons so often failed to comply with the regulations for encampments by filling in latrines on the departure of the troops." The latter vividly describes visiting a latrine in a certain standing camp. "On visiting this latrine after it had been left undisturbed for a short time, a buzzing swarm of flies would suddenly arise from it with a noise faintly suggestive of the bursting of a percussion shrapnel shell. The latrine was certainly not more than one hundred yards from the nearest tents, if so much, and at meal times men's mess tins, etc., were always invaded by flies. A tin of jam incautiously left open for a few minutes became a seething mass of flies (chiefly *Pycnosoma chloropyga* Wied.), completely covering the contents."

Enough has been said in regard to this question from the

point of view of practical experience and it is needless to multiply instances to prove that swarms of flies in camps with open latrines, used by incipient and ambulant cases of typhoid and typhoid carriers, constitute a very serious danger.

Austen (1904, p. 658) considers that many cases of intestinal myiasis at home are due to flies, belonging to the genus *Fannia*, ovipositing on the anus of the patient when using a country privy, and thinks that in camps flies may inoculate typhoid in a similar way.

Summary.

It has been shown experimentally that flies are capable of carrying and distributing *B. typhosus*, by means of infected feet, proboscides and fæces for several days, and on several occasions this organism has been isolated from 'wild' flies caught in places where outbreaks were in progress. In clean and well-sewered cities flies have few opportunities of infecting themselves, but under suitable conditions may act as carriers of the disease, mainly by infecting themselves with bacilli derived from mild unrecognized cases and 'carriers.' In smaller towns and in country districts their opportunities are greater, but up to the present sufficient evidence has not been obtained on which to found a final judgment. Sedgwick and Winslow (1902), after a careful study of the seasonal prevalence of typhoid fever, came to the following conclusions: "Of the three great intermediaries of typhoid transmission, fingers, food and flies, the last is even more significant than the others in relation to seasonal variation....There can be little doubt that many of the so-called 'sporadic' cases of typhoid fever, which are so difficult for the sanitarian to explain, are conditioned by the passage of a fly from an infected vault to an unprotected table or an open larder. The relation of this factor to the season is of course close and complete, and a certain amount of the autumnal excess of fever is undoubtedly traceable to the presence of large numbers of flies and to the opportunities of their pernicious activity."

Medical officers in India have published numerous articles placing on record their belief that flies, bred in the trenching grounds, are important agents in spreading the disease. In several instances campaigns undertaken to exterminate flies have met with marked success. The reports relating to military camps in war time show very conclusively that flies are under those conditions the principal agents in spreading the disease. Both in Indian stations and in military camps it is probable that 'carriers' and incipient cases are largely responsible for providing the necessary infected material.

Much investigation is still required before the part played by the fly in various circumstances is fully understood.

Diseases caused by allied organisms.

(i) *Dysentery.*

Though it is very probable that flies may occasionally distribute the bacilli of dysentery, little evidence directly bearing on the subject has yet been published. Orton (1910) in America investigated an outbreak of 136 cases of dysentery in the Worcester State Hospital for the insane, and came to the conclusions that flies, which were present in unusual numbers, were entirely responsible for the outbreak. *B. dysenteriæ* was not isolated from flies, but an interesting experiment was made with *B. prodigiosus.* Cultures of this organism were exposed in the laundry, where the bedding and clothing were cleaned, and from some of the flies subsequently caught in other rooms of the hospital this bacillus was isolated. Since many of the non-lactose fermenting bacilli found in the intestines of flies are indistinguishable culturally from *B. dysenteriæ*, agglutination and absorption tests would have to be employed in identifying any suspicious organisms that might be isolated from suspected flies.

(ii) *Paratyphoid and food poisoning.*

Graham-Smith (1910, p. 14) carried out the following experiments with *B. enteritidis* (Gaertner).

"An emulsion of an agar culture of *B. enteritidis* (Gaertner) in syrup was placed in a gauze cage containing a large number of flies. Eight hours later the emulsion was removed and plain syrup substituted. Each day a certain number of flies were caught in a large test-tube; some were allowed to walk over Drigalski-Conradi plates, and others were killed and their intestines dissected out and emulsified and sown on similar plates. The fæces deposited on the test-tube were also emulsified and sown on plates.

"The results of these experiments are given in the following table:

TABLE 16. *Showing the results of experiments with B. enteritidis (Gaertner).*

Time after infection	Plates from: Intestinal contents	Plates from: Fæces	Plates from: Flies allowed to walk over plates
24 hours	+ (11)	–	o (3)
48 ,, ...	o (17)	o	+ (7)
3 days	o (15)	o	+ (5)
4 ,, ...	+ (22)	o	+ (5)
5 ,, ...	+ (9)	–	+ (6)
6 ,, ...	+ (12)	–	+ (4)
7 ,, ...	+ (8)	–	+ (3)
8 ,, ...	o (7)	–	o (6)

+ indicates that *B. enteritidis* was isolated and proved by cultures on suitable media, including sugars; o that the suspicious colonies isolated did not turn out to be *B. enteritidis* and – that no cultures were made. Some of the plates were completely overgrown with colon-like organisms. The figures in brackets indicate the number of flies used in each experiment.

"On the 7th day six flies (I—VI, Table 17) were captured and killed. The legs and wings were removed with sterile forceps and plated separately. After flaming, the bodies were dissected and the crops and intestines isolated, separate cultures being made from the contents of each. The head was also removed and separately cultivated. On the 8th day five flies (VII—XI) were treated in the same way. The results of these experiments are given in the following table:

TABLE 17. *Showing the results of further experiments with B. enteritidis.*

No. of fly	Cultures from: Legs 1	Legs 2	Legs 3	Legs 4	Legs 5	Legs 6	Wings 1	Wings 2	Head	Crop	Intestines	
I	o	o	–	–	–	–	o	o	o	o	–	Flies dissected on the 7th day after infection
II	o	o	o	o	o	o	o	o	+	+ +	–	
III	o	o	o	o	o	o	o	o	+	+ +	+	
IV	o	o	o	o	o	o	o	o	+	+	+	
V	+	o	o	o	o	o	–	o	o	–	o	
VI	o	o	o	o	o	o	o	o	o	–	o	
VII	o	o	o	o	o	o	o	o	–	o	o	Flies dissected on the 8th day after infection
VIII	o	o	o	o	o	o	o	o	o	+	o	
IX	o	o	o	o	o	o	o	o	o	o	o	
X	o	o	o	o	o	o	o	o	o	o	o	
XI	o	o	o	o	o	o	o	o	o	o	o	

+ + indicates that numerous colonies of *B. enteritidis* were found.

"These experiments show that *B. enteritidis* may be present in the contents of the crops and intestines of flies for a least 7 days after infection. Flies can infect plates over which they walk for some days in spite of the fact that the organism can seldom be isolated from their legs (once in 32 cultures). When walking over plates flies constantly place their proboscides on the medium and in most cases leave imprints on its surface. The colonies develop round these marks. The infection of the plate is therefore probably due, in large measure, to inoculation by the fly's proboscis.

"It is not improbable that by means of more careful and extensive experiments *B. enteritidis* might be isolated for even longer periods, since several of the plates in this series gave negative results owing to being overgrown by *B. coli*-like organism."

Faichnie's (1909) experiments on breeding larvæ in the fæces of a man suffering from paratyphoid fever (*B. paratyphosus* A) and similar experiments with cultivated strains have already been quoted (p. 115).

Torrey (1912) isolated *B. paratyphosus* A from three cultures from 'wild' flies caught in New York. He employed agglutination and absorption tests with sera made from stock cultures in identifying these organisms. "Inoculations into guinea-pigs of these fly paratyphoid cultures disclosed approximately the same degree of toxicity as the stock paratyphoid cultures. Feeding experiments with white mice resulted negatively." Nicoll (1911, p. 383) isolated *B. paratyphosus* B from two flies, "from the external surface and intestine of one fly and from the intestine of the second. The identity of the bacillus was confirmed by Dr F. A. Bainbridge."

The observations which have been quoted show that flies, if suitable opportunities of visiting infected material occur, may carry and distribute organisms of this type for several days. No instances of infection by flies have yet been recorded. In the identification of these bacilli serological tests are necessary, since allied organisms frequently occur in the intestine of the fly.

CHAPTER XIV

EPIDEMIC OR SUMMER DIARRHŒA

Epidemic or summer diarrhœa is a term applied to an affection marked by a somewhat definite group of symptoms, in which vomiting, copious diarrhœa, rice-watery and green stools, and finally convulsions play a conspicuous part. From the studies of a large number of histories Ballard (1889) concluded that he was dealing with a definite disease, and observers since his time have been of the same opinion. Yet no doubt enteric fever and other diseases of infants are often mistaken for it. "Whether summer diarrhœa is produced by a definite micro-organism or is an illness conditioned by several allied bacilli, it is a clinical entity possessing a very definite course, and as such is susceptible of study" (Niven, 1910, p. 133). It is a disease, which occasions great mortality among infants under five years of age, but also produces symptoms, though of a less marked character in older persons. Between infancy and old age the fatality is so slight, that its widespread distribution escapes attention. "As a rule the sufferer is able to go out to the closet, a fact which may prove of considerable significance."

It is doubtful whether many people realize the full extent of the ravages of the disease. In the United States, and in Great Britain, and in many European countries the general death rate is largely dependent on the infant mortality, a very large proportion of which is due to epidemic diarrhœa. In the registration area, for example, of the United States 189,865 children under five years of age died in 1908, and of these 52,213 died of epidemic diarrhœa (Howard, 1911, p. 157).

From time to time various hypotheses, which need not be summarized, have been put forward connecting the disease with emanations from the soil, atmospheric conditions, etc. It is now generally admitted that the disease is infectious, but up to the present the infective agent has not been identified with certainty, and the mode of spread is uncertain. There can be little doubt that direct contact, infected food, especially milk, whether infected before reaching the house or within it, and carelessness in dealing with soiled articles, all tend to spread the disease, but in this chapter the influence of flies only will be considered.

In considering the relationship of flies to epidemic diarrhœa we have two sets of data on which to base an opinion: (*a*) epidemiological evidence and (*b*) bacteriological analyses.

(*a*) *Epidemiological evidence.*

Many papers have been published on the epidemiology of epidemic diarrhœa, but definite statistical evidence in regard to the relationship of flies to the disease is rare. Niven (1910) has however studied this subject with great care during a series of years, 1903—1909, in Manchester, and has described the results of his investigations in an admirable paper, which is extensively quoted in this chapter.

As Niven rightly remarks: "it is a great advantage, in forming conclusions as to the explanation of facts, to deal with areas all the characters of which are quite familiar to the reasoner. The atmosphere, the temperatures of the soil, and the rainfall are approximately the same throughout" (p. 132).

Though a few cases are recorded week by week throughout the year the disease is not much in evidence until the annual summer outbreak which never occurs before June. In winter, spring and early summer the mortality is low, and on investigation of a number of individual cases "infection from person to person becomes highly probable in a considerable proportion of the cases, the agency being left vague." During the summer outbreak, however, the mortality is often high.

"We may take it as proved that there is an intimate relation between the storage of excreta in privy-middens and a high diarrhœal mortality." The social condition of the population has also much influence on the diarrhœal death rate, owing chiefly to ignorance and carelessness on the part of many mothers.

"The essential problem in summer diarrhœa is the summer wave, ascending as it does steeply, and descending with but a little less abruptness. It is to this period that the fatality is due. Broadly speaking it corresponds to a similar upward movement and descent of the temperatures registered at a depth of 4 ft. in the soil. The readings of the air thermometer do not correspond closely to the course of the wave of deaths, being subject to considerable fluctuations."

It has been conjectured that under favourable conditions micro-organisms in the earth multiply and cause diarrhœa. After a full consideration of this subject Niven concludes that "one is driven to abandon the idea that the growth of bacteria, whether in or on the soil, has to do with the annual wave of diarrhœa."

Another hypothesis is that fruit may be responsible. "But, in the case of diarrhœa, the disease appears first in the infant in house after house, and it is certain that the infant has no fruit; the effect produced by fruit in the annual course of the disease can therefore only be partial."

"Another view is that heat may itself cause the disease, or if not the disease at any rate the fatality....Clearly, however, heat can in no way account for the rapid spread of the disease among particular classes of the population" (see also p. 158).

Transmission by dust is also an inadequate explanation.

"What we require for the explanation of the facts of summer diarrhœa is the presence of some transmitting agent rising and falling with the rise and fall of diarrhœa, the features pertaining to which must correspond to and explain the features of the annual wave of diarrhœa."

"None of the other factors of which we have cognizance do afford such an explanation, and we come by exclusion to consider the house-fly. The process of conveyance of infection is not striking and arresting as it is in military camps abroad; nor does the number of flies usually approach that observed in tropical and subtropical countries. We are therefore obliged to attack the question *de novo*, and examine such evidence as we possess to see whether we may rest reasonably confident that in flies we have found the transmitting agent sought for.

"If the house-fly is the transmitting agent in summer diarrhœa, the following conditions should be fulfilled:

(1) (*a*) "There should be evidence that the house-fly carries bacteria under the ordinary summer conditions; (*b*) house-flies should be present in sufficient numbers in houses invaded by fatal diarrhœa.

(2) "There should be a close correspondence between the aggregate number of house-flies in houses and the aggregate number of deaths from diarrhœa week by week.

(3) "The life-history of the house-fly should explain any discrepancy between the observed number of flies and the observed number of deaths.

(4) "The minority of breast-fed children not apparently accessible to infection should receive explanation.

(5) "There should be a closer correspondence of diarrhœal fatality with the number of flies than with any other varying seasonal fact.

(6) "Any other closely corresponding seasonal fact should be capable of interpretation in terms of the number of house-flies.

(7) "Any variation from district to district in the annual curve of deaths should be accompanied by a similar variation in the curve of flies.

(8) "No other available hypotheses must be capable of explaining the course of summer diarrhœa."

In regard to 1 (*a*) it has been shown in previous chapters that flies carry numerous bacteria under ordinary summer conditions.—1 (*b*) and 2.—In order to estimate the number of flies in houses from 1904 onwards, Niven provided certain reliable householders with bell-glass traps, which were baited with beer. Careful and continuous daily counts were made. At each station the numbers caught per week varied, and it was only when the numbers caught at all the stations were added together that coherent and graduated curves could be obtained. Niven records for five years the number of deaths week by week, the number of flies captured, the mean atmospheric temperature and the mean temperatures at depths of 1 ft. and 4 ft. Charts 3 and 4 giving the numbers of flies captured and the diarrhœa deaths in 1904

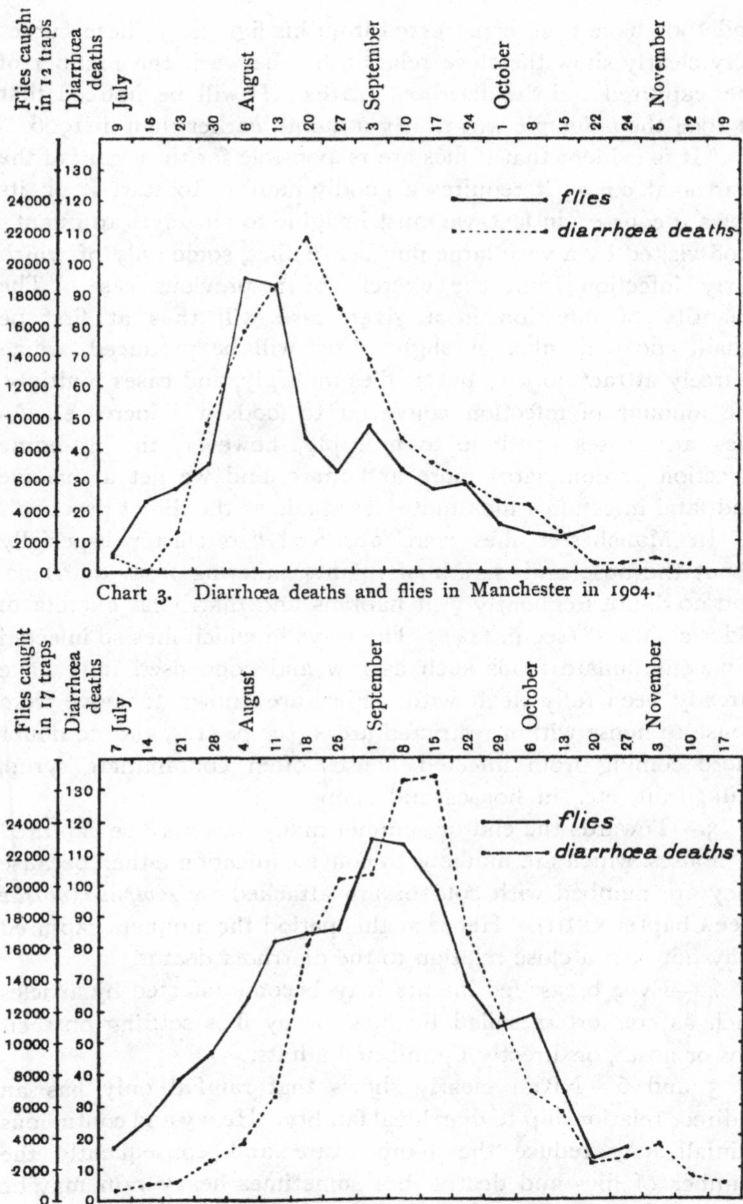

Chart 3. Diarrhœa deaths and flies in Manchester in 1904.

Chart 4. Diarrhœa deaths and flies in Manchester in 1906.

and 1906 have been constructed from his figures. These curves very clearly show the close relationship between the number of flies captured and the diarrhœa deaths. It will be noticed that in 1904 the epidemic was nearly a month earlier than in 1906.

"It is evident that if flies are responsible for the ascent of the diarrhœal curve, it requires a goodly number to start it on its upward course; in fact, we must imagine to ourselves an infant's food visited by a very large number of flies, some only of which carry infection from the excreta of a previous case. The quantity of infection in a given case will thus at first be small, and a number of slight cases will be produced, which scarcely attract notice; but as flies multiply, and cases multiply, the amount of infection conveyed to foods will increase....As flies and cases continue to multiply, however, the fly-borne infection predominates more and more, and we get a massive and fatal infection which quite overshadows the direct process."

In Manchester flies were observed "to cluster especially about the nose and mouth of infants suffering from diarrhœa, and no doubt frequently visit napkins and diarrhœal excreta of older children" (see p. 144). The ways in which flies so infected can contaminate foods such as raw and condensed milk have already been fully dealt with. Flies are known to move from house to house within restricted areas (see p. 112), and no doubt those coming from infected houses often contaminate syrup, milk, fruit, etc., in houses and shops.

3.—Towards the end of summer many flies may be captured in houses, which are unlikely to convey infection either because they are numbed with cold or are attacked by *Empusa muscæ* (see Chapter XXIII). Hence at this period the numbers captured may not bear a close relation to the diarrhœa deaths.

4.—Even breast-fed infants may become infected by articles such as comforters soiled by flies, or by flies settling on their lips or noses, or directly by infected adults.

5 and 6.—Niven clearly shows that rainfall only has an indirect relationship to diarrhœal fatality. Heavy and continuous rainfall may reduce the temperature and consequently the number of flies and deaths, but sometimes heavy rain may be accompanied by a rise in the atmospheric temperature, and then

there is no diminution in the number of flies or of deaths. Summing up his observations on rainfall for five years Niven (p. 162) comes to the following conclusions. "Thus heavy rainfalls tend to lower the temperature of the surface, but have less effect on the atmospheric temperature, which may rise in spite of them. They produce a greater effect on flies than they do on temperature, and this effect on flies is reflected on the number of fatal cases commencing, and on the number of deaths in the week but one following. This is not a quite accurate statement for the end of the curve....There can be no doubt that heavy rainfall exerts on the whole a disastrous influence on the production of flies. This does not occur in rainfalls of 0·8 inches or under, which appear to have the reverse effect, at all events so long as the atmospheric temperature is rising. In the nice balance more or less rainfall over the quarter cannot much matter. In fact, in Manchester no sustained correspondence can be made out between the main rainfall in the third quarter and the number of deaths from diarrhœa. The years of highest rainfall—viz., 1891, 1892, 1893, 1895 and 1903—have all been years of fairly high diarrhœal fatality; 1907, the year of lowest diarrhœal fatality, was not a year of exceptionally low rainfall. Even heavy rainfall, it will be seen, does not necessarily exert any unfavourable influence on the development of flies or the extension of diarrhœa. Its doing so will depend entirely whether it is able to lower the surface temperatures below those which are favourable to the development of the larvæ or the escape of the imago. If it will fail to effect this, its influence will probably be in the opposite direction, owing to the great need of moisture for the development of the larvæ, and, one may add, for the health of the flies."

The course of the 4 ft. thermometer corresponds more closely to the curve of diarrhœa deaths than any other 'varying seasonal fact.' Its course corresponds generally to the excess of heat entering over heat leaving the surface the week before. Many of the breeding grounds of the larvæ are greatly influenced by the temperature of the soil, and flies in their development and reproduction respond to all the influences which affect the 4 ft.

thermometer[1]. Flies stand, however, in a more intimate relation to deaths from diarrhœa than does the 4 ft. thermometer.

7.—Up to the present sufficient data have not been collected to establish or disprove this hypothesis, but the known facts from districts in Manchester lend a general support to it. The data could be collected without great difficulty by planting a sufficient number of traps in different districts of sufficient size.

8.—Up to the present no other available hypothesis seems capable of explaining the course of summer diarrhœa.

Niven (p. 174) sums up the analysis of his investigations as follows:

"Summer diarrhœa is an infectious disease. This is shown by the course of the annual wave, by the manner of its incidence on the different sanitary districts of Manchester, and by the history of individual cases. The summer wave is not due to dust, nor is it conditioned by any growth of bacteria in or on the soil. There is nothing to support the view that the infective organisms are of animal origin, and the connection between privy-middens goes far to prove the contrary. The disease becomes more fatal only after house-flies have been prevalent for some time, and its fatality rises as their numbers increase and falls as they fall. The correspondence of diarrhœal fatality is closer with the number of flies in circulation than with any other fact....Certain facts in the life-history of the fly throw light on discrepancies arising in the decline of flies and cases. The close correspondence between flies and cases of fatal diarrhœa receives general support from the diarrhœal history of sanitary subdivisions of the Manchester district. The few facts available for the study of the correspondence of flies and fatal cases in different subdivisions, in the course of the same year also lend support to this view. No other explanation even approximately fits the case."

Hamer made observations, somewhat similar to those of Niven, in various parts of London in 1907, 1908 and 1909, on a larger scale. He, however, caught the flies in the neighbourhood of refuse and manure dépôts, where flies are bred, and

[1] For a clear discussion of the 'varying seasonal facts,' see Niven, pp. 163—166.

consequently his figures do not necessarily represent the fly population in houses. Nevertheless his curves representing diarrhœa fatality and fly prevalence closely resemble those of Niven. Hamer, Peters (1910) and other critics have pointed out that if variations in the number of fly transmitters of an infective agent existing in the stools of infants were the sole factors concerned, the curve for diarrhœa cases should shoot up beyond and come down later than that representing the number of flies, because the opportunities afforded to flies to pick up the infective agent increase with the development of the epidemic. This, however, does not happen. On the contrary the epidemic is arrested while flies are numerous, and declines more quickly than the fly population. In this exhaustion of susceptible material probably plays some part. The decrease in the activity of the flies owing to Empusa disease in the autumn, and to colder weather also probably has a very important effect. Possibly the fall in the temperatures has a decided effect in checking the multiplication of the infecting agent as Martin (1913, p. 5) suggests.

Peters (1910, p. 717), who most carefully studied epidemic diarrhœa in the town of Mansfield, but who did not make accurate estimations of the numbers of flies in houses, gives the following summary of *the evidence specially favouring fly carriage.* "(1) The low level of the winter cases—in the absence of flies. (2) The facts suggesting that the house, and not the individual, is the centre of infection. (3) The sudden outbreak in a 'clump,' supervening upon solitary preceding cases, suggests that flies have suddenly gained access to infection. (4) The fact that within the 'clump,' infection appears to some extent to rain down equally upon all persons and houses included, suggests systematic dissemination by flies. (5) Variations of prevalence with variations of temperature. (6) The almost identical temperature limitations of fly and diarrhœa prevalences, as regards their rise and fall: the significant immobility of the diarrhœa curve till the first fortnight of favourable fly temperature has passed by. (7) The correlation of the fly and diarrhœa curves is such as to be quite compatible with a theory of causal connection between flies and diarrhœa. (8) The large amount of evidence for personal origin of infection is mostly also evidence for fly carriage. (9) No real evidence has been produced *against* the fly theory."

Peters also produces evidence to show that flies do not bring infection from the manure heaps in which they have been bred.

Several previous observers had expressed the opinion that flies spread summer diarrhœa, amongst others Fraser (1902), Nash (1903, 1904), Copeman (1906), Shell (1906) and Sandilands (1906), held strong views on the subject. Newsholme (1903, p. 21) thinks that food in the houses of the poor can scarcely escape fæcal infection. "The sugar used in sweetening milk is often black with flies, which may have come from a neighbouring dust-bin or manure heap, or from the liquid stools of a diarrhœal patient in a neighbouring house. Flies have to be picked out of the half empty can of condensed milk before its remaining contents can be used for the next meal." He considers that the greater prevalence of diarrhœa among infants fed on Nestlé's milk is due to the fact that flies are more attracted to it than to ordinary cow's milk on account of its sweetness. The investigations of Lewis (1912, p. 276) are specially interesting in this connection. Out of twenty-eight samples of milk bacteriologically examined seventeen showed non-lactose fermenting bacilli, and in six of these the bacilli were of the same variety as had been found in the fæces of the children for whom the supply was provided.

Several interesting observations have been made on this subject in other parts of the world. Ainsworth (1909), though dealing with very small numbers of cases, shows clearly by means of a chart the close correspondence between the numbers of flies and the cases of diarrhœa in Poona, India. Peters (1909) has pointed out that in Melbourne, Australia, the epidemic often declines notwithstanding the fact that the temperature may continue to rise for several weeks. This may be attributed in part to exhaustion of susceptible material, and in part to the effect of the extremely hot dry winds which are very fatal to flies both in the larval and imago stages.

Whatever part flies may play in the dissemination of the disease direct infection and carelessness must always be factors of great importance.

(*b*) *Bacteriological investigations.*

Up to the present the infective agent of summer diarrhœa has not been identified with certainty. Different organisms have been reported as being particularly prevalent in the fæces in different epidemics in various localities. In America *B. dysenteriæ* (Flexner type) has been encountered in the stools in some epidemics [Wollstein (1903), Park, Collins and Goodwin (1903), Duval and Schorer (1903), Cordes (1903) and Weaver, Tunnicliffe, Heineman and Michael (1905)], but not in others.

Various other organisms, including *B. enteritidis sporogenes*, *B. enteritidis* (Gaertner), *B. vulgaris*, have been regarded as the causative agents in certain outbreaks.

During the epidemics in London in the years 1905, 1906, 1907 and 1908 Morgan (1906, 1907), and Morgan and Ledingham (1909) carried out extensive investigations on the non-lactose fermenting and non-gelatin liquefying bacilli in the stools of infants. A very large number of such organisms were isolated and examined, but the only one whose prevalence was found to be related to infantile diarrhœa was a non-motile bacillus of this group, which fermented glucose with the production of gas, but failed to ferment any of the other 'sugars' on which it was tested. This is now generally known as "*Morgan's No.* 1" bacillus. This bacillus was frequently recovered from the organs of fatal cases, and produced diarrhœa when fed to monkeys and young rats. It was rarely met with in children not suffering from acute diarrhœa. In 1905 this bacillus was found in the fæces of 54 % of acute diarrhœa cases, in 1906 in 56 %, in 1907 in 16 % and in 1908 in 53 %.

Since 1910 several investigations[1], published in the 40th and 41st Annual Reports of the Medical Officer, have been carried out for the Local Government Board. In the summer of 1910, when epidemic diarrhœa was relatively uncommon, Lewis (1911) made observations in Birmingham, Ross (1911) in Manchester, Orr (1911) in Shrewsbury and O'Brien (1911) in London. Ross and Orr found that non-lactose fermenting bacilli, which do not

[1] The bacilli found in all these investigations are recorded in Table 23.

liquefy gelatin, were at least twice as numerous in the fæces of children suffering from diarrhœa as in those of healthy children, but neither they nor O'Brien detected any type which largely predominated. During the summer of 1911, when the disease was very common, Alexander (1912) carried out similar investigations in Liverpool, and Lewis (1912) continued his investigations in Birmingham. Alexander found non-lactose fermenting bacilli in the fæces of 56 % of children suffering from diarrhœa and in the fæces of 49 % of healthy children. Morgan's No. 1 bacillus occurred in 13·2 % of the former class and in 6·6 % of the latter.

On the other hand Lewis, as the result of two years' very careful and extensive work, came to the following conclusions: "(1) The frequency of non-liquefying and non-lactose fermenting ærobic bacilli in the fæces of children suffering from diarrhœa is greater than in the fæces of normal children; this fact is suggestive that one or more types of this wide group of organisms may have a causal relationship to the disease. (2) Absolute proof of this relationship is still defective. (3) The evidence adduced brings under such strong suspicion the possible causal relationship of one variety, viz., variety 8 of the subgroup (*a*) of the group G (i.e. Morgan's No. 1 bacillus) that further concentration of research upon this variety is desirable."

In 1910 Lewis found non-liquefying, non-lactose fermenting bacilli in the fæces of 21 (14 %) out of 146 normal children and in the fæces of 47 (77 %) out of 62 cases of diarrhœa in children, while in 1911 they occurred in the fæces of 38 (38 %) out of 100 normal children and in the fæces of 103 (95 %) out of 140 cases of diarrhœa. In 1910 Morgan's bacillus was isolated from the fæces of 30 % of diarrhœa cases, while in 1911 it was isolated from 78 %. In 1910 it was not encountered in any of the samples of fæces from 146 normal children, but in 1911 it was found in the fæces of 17 out of 100 normal children. The organism was also isolated from the heart's blood or spleen of 9 (64 %) out of 14 children who had died of the disease. Feeding experiments on rats, mice and rabbits showed that 23 (76 %) out of 31 strains of Morgan's bacillus, whether isolated from the fæces of normal children or of those suffering from diarrhœa, proved fatal to these animals, whereas of the other non-lactose fermenting bacilli tested only 35 % proved fatal.

From the investigations, which have been quoted, it seems evident that Morgan's bacillus is intimately associated with summer diarrhœa in certain epidemics, whilst its connection with other outbreaks has not been established.

During 1911 the writer (Graham-Smith, 1912, i.) carried out the only extensive series of investigations on non-lactose fermenting bacilli in flies which has yet been made.

These observations were carried out for the purpose of ascertaining the frequency and distribution in house-flies (*M. domestica*), obtained from different sources, of bacilli which neither ferment lactose nor liquefy gelatin, and more particularly for the purpose of determining whether the varieties which occur in districts where epidemic diarrhœa is prevalent differ from those which occur elsewhere. A record was kept also of the number of flies infected with lactose fermenting bacilli of the colon type, and of the non-lactose fermenting bacilli which liquefy gelatin.

From 14th July to 16th October, 1911, 1242 flies were examined, of which 624 were obtained in Cambridge and 618 came from Birmingham. The Cambridge flies were collected in several different localities; 97 (Series B) from seven houses in the town in which cases of epidemic diarrhœa had occurred, and 74 (Series C) from a farm house, situated on the outskirts of the town, in which all the inhabitants suffered severely from diarrhœa. The remaining flies were obtained from houses in which diarrhœa did not occur, 157 (Series F) from a bake-house, 51 (Series E) from a house in the centre of the town, 90 (Series H) from a house outside the town and 155 (Series G) from a farm house situated two miles out of the town.

Dr Robertson, the Medical Officer of Health, very kindly arranged for sending flies from Birmingham. Specimens were received from 53 houses in which cases of epidemic diarrhœa had occurred, and of these 471 (Series A) were examined. Specimens were also received from seven houses, in the neighbourhood of the others, in which no cases of epidemic diarrhœa had occurred, and of these 147 (Series D) were examined.

Altogether 642 flies from diarrhœa infected houses were examined and 600 from non-diarrhœa infected houses.

Methods.

"The flies were caught in balloon traps and examined as soon as possible. The whole trap was placed in a bell-jar and the flies killed by the addition of a few drops of chloroform. For examination each fly was placed on a sterile glass plate and the intestinal canal, including the crop, dissected out with sterile needles. The intestinal contents were emulsified in a small quantity of sterile salt solution. In many cases an emulsion was also made from the external parts of the fly. With the fluids thus obtained plate cultures were made. The medium used for the plates was MacConkey's bile-salt lactose neutral red agar with crystal violet (1—100,000). The plates were incubated at 37° C. for 48 hours. At the end of this period the plates were examined, and the red lactose fermenting colonies, resembling those produced by bacilli of the colon type, recorded. When non-lactose fermenting colonies were present, sub-cultures were made from three of them in different tubes of litmus lactose peptone water. These cultures were incubated for seven days. If at the end of that time acid had not been produced, cultures were made from these tubes on to agar slopes. After incubation the latter cultures were kept until the further cultural characters of the bacilli could be determined. Previous to testing the fermenting properties, plate cultures on MacConkey's medium were again made in order to test the purity of the cultures. From single colonies on these plates lactose litmus peptone water tubes were inoculated and from them cultures on agar prepared. Thus, every precaution was taken to procure pure cultures before the fluid media were inoculated.

"In order to test the fermenting properties, six litmus peptone water tubes (each provided with a Durham's tube) containing 0·5 per cent. of the following substances, glucose, mannite, dulcite, saccharose, salicin and sorbite, were inoculated. The reactions of all these cultures were recorded on the first, second, third and tenth days of incubation at 37° C. At the same time sub-cultures were also made in milk and in broth and gelatin slopes inoculated. Cultures were examined for motility after 24 hours' incubation, and a broth culture was tested for indol on the seventh day. For this purpose the para-dimethyl-amido-benzaldehyde test was used. The gelatin slope cultures were kept at room temperature for a month. They were examined at frequent intervals."

Classification of bacilli, which do not ferment lactose or liquefy gelatin.

"When acid production, with or without gas formation, occurred the reaction was usually well marked after 24 to 48 hours' incubation. In some cases, however, several days elapsed before the reaction became definitely acid. It was found that in some cases the formation of acid was followed by a return to alkalinity. In tabulating the results a culture which produced acid at any time was recorded as acid, whether it subsequently became alkaline or not, except in the case of milk cultures. The changes in the latter medium were fully recorded.

"The writer found great difficulty in comparing the results of investigators who had recently worked on the non-lactose fermenting bacilli in fæces, owing to the different methods of classification which had been adopted. Lewis (1911) classified the bacilli he isolated into groups according to their actions on the fermentable substances used. O'Brien (1911), Ross (1911), and Orr (1911) used the same general classification.

"With the concurrence of Dr Lewis and Dr Moore Alexander this classification has been amplified, each group being divided into sub-groups in such a manner that all the known organisms can be tabulated and compared, and those subsequently discovered can be added in their proper places. The scheme may be readily comprehended from the following table."

TABLE 18. *Showing the method of classifying bacilli which do not ferment lactose or liquefy gelatin into Groups and Sub-groups according to their fermenting properties.*

Group	Sub-group	Glucose	Mannite	Dulcite	Saccharose	Salicin	Sorbite	
A	a	O	O	O	O	O	O	*
B	a	A	O	O	O	O	O	*
	b	A	O	A	A	A	A	
	c	A	O	A	A	A	O	
	d	A	O	A	A	O	A	
	e	A	O	A	A	O	O	
	f	A	O	A	O	O	O	
	g	A	O	A	O	A	A	
	h	A	O	A	O	A	O	
	i	A	O	A	O	O	A	
	j	A	O	O	A	A	A	*
	k	A	O	O	A	A	O	*
	l	A	O	O	A	O	A	*
	m	A	O	O	A	O	O	*
	n	A	O	O	O	A	A	*
	o	A	O	O	O	A	O	*
	p	A	O	O	O	O	A	*
C	a	A	A	O	O	O	O	*
	b	A	A	O	A	A	A	*
	c	A	A	O	A	A	O	*
	d	A	A	O	A	O	A	*
	e	A	A	O	A	O	O	*
	f	A	A	O	O	A	A	*
	g	A	A	O	O	A	O	*
	h	A	A	O	O	O	A	*
D	a	A	A	A	O	O	O	*
	b	A	A	A	O	A	A	*
	c	A	A	A	O	A	O	
	d	A	A	A	O	O	A	*
E	a	A	A	A	A	O	O	*
	b	A	A	A	A	O	A	
F	a	A	A	A	A	A	O	*
	b	A	A	A	A	A	A	

A = Acid. A + G = Acid and Gas. O = No change.
* = Described Sub-group.

TABLE 18—(*continued*).

Group	Sub-group	Glucose	Mannite	Dulcite	Sac-charose	Salicin	Sorbite	
G	a	A+G	O	O	O	O	O	*
	b	A+G	O	A+G	A+G	A+G	A+G	*
	c	A+G	O	A+G	A+G	A+G	O	
	d	A+G	O	A+G	A+G	O	A+G	
	e	A+G	O	A+G	A+G	O	O	
	e (*a*)	A+G	O	A	A	O	O	*
	f	A+G	O	A+G	O	O	O	*
	f (*a*)	A+G	O	A	O	O	O	*
	g	A+G	O	A+G	O	A+G	A+G	
	h	A+G	O	A+G	O	A+G	O	
	i	A+G	O	A+G	O	O	A+G	
	i (*a*)	A+G	O	A	O	O	A	*
	j	A+G	O	O	A+G	A+G	A+G	
	j (*a*)	A+G	O	O	A	A	A	*
	k	A+G	O	O	A+G	A+G	O	
	k (*a*)	A+G	O	O	A	A	O	*
	l	A+G	O	O	A+G	O	A+G	
	m	A+G	O	O	A+G	O	O	*
	m (*a*)	A+G	O	O	A	O	O	*
	n	A+G	O	O	O	A+G	A+G	
	o	A+G	O	O	O	A+G	O	
	o (*a*)	A+G	O	O	O	A	O	*
	p	A+G	O	O	O	O	A+G	*
	p (*a*)	A+G	O	O	O	O	A	*
H	a	A+G	A+G	O	O	O	O	*
	b	A+G	A+G	O	A+G	A+G	A+G	*
	c	A+G	A+G	O	A+G	A+G	O	*
	c (*a*)	A+G	A+G	O	A	A+G	O	*
	c (*b*)	A+G	A+G	O	A	A	O	*
	d	A+G	A+G	O	A+G	O	A+G	
	e	A+G	A+G	O	A+G	O	O	*
	e (*a*)	A+G	A+G	O	A	O	O	*
	f	A+G	A+G	O	O	A+G	A+G	*
	g	A+G	A+G	O	O	A+G	O	*
	h	A+G	A+G	O	O	O	A+G	*
I	a	A+G	A+G	A+G	O	O	O	*
	b	A+G	A+G	A+G	O	A+G	A+G	*
	c	A+G	A+G	A+G	O	A+G	O	*
	d	A+G	A+G	A+G	O	O	A+G	*
J	a	A+G	A+G	A+G	A+G	O	O	
	b	A+G	A+G	A+G	A+G	O	A+G	*
	b (*a*)	A+G	A+G	A+G	A	O	A+G	*
K	a	A+G	A+G	A+G	A+G	A+G	O	
	b	A+G	A+G	A+G	A+G	A+G	A+G	*

A=Acid. A+G=Acid and Gas. O=No change.
*=Described Sub-group.

"It is obvious that each sub-group may be further divided into 20 possible varieties according to the reactions of the milk cultures, the formation or non-formation of indol, and the presence or absence of motility. The method adopted for differentiating the varieties, according to numbers which always indicate the same reactions, is given in Table 19.

TABLE 19.

Milk	Indol	Motility	Indicating Number
No change	O	O	1
	O	+	2
	+	O	3
	+	+	4
Alkaline	O	O	5
	O	+	6
	+	O	7
	+	+	8
Acid, later Alkaline	O	O	9
	O	+	10
	+	O	11
	+	+	12
Acid	O	O	13
	O	+	14
	+	O	15
	+	+	16
Acid and Clot	O	O	17
	O	+	18
	+	O	19
	+	+	20

"It will be seen that by adopting such a scheme the characters of an organism can be very easily recorded, for example G a 8 signifies a bacillus producing acid and gas in glucose, but no change in the other fermentable substances. Milk becomes alkaline, indol is produced and the bacillus is motile.

"This scheme seems to give the greatest differentiation which is possible by means of the media employed. The bacilli composing a sub-group are probably specifically distinct from those composing other sub-groups. To what extent each variety represents a different species is a matter which cannot be decided at present. The varieties within sub-groups which produce no change or an alkaline reaction in milk are probably specifically different from those which produce permanent acidity. The production of acid followed by the formation of alkali is also perhaps a specific character. The capacity to produce indol is possibly a racial character. Undoubtedly the presence or absence of motility is the least important of the differentiating characters. The presence of well marked motility is easily ascertained. On the other hand the absence of motility cannot be so readily determined. In many cultures only a few of the organisms possess motility at the time of examination, and prolonged observations with cultures of different ages may be necessary before it can be definitely stated that the organism in question is non-motile.

"By the use of a larger number of fermentable substances the bacilli might no doubt be further differentiated, but for the purpose of preliminary examination the method which has been adopted ought to suffice until it has been definitely ascertained that some of the bacilli belonging to certain groups possess important pathogenic properties and cannot be differentiated without the use of other media.

The results of the cultural examinations of flies.

"The results of these examinations are considered under three headings: (1) the distribution in flies from different localities of lactose fermenting and non-lactose fermenting bacilli; (2) the distribution of varieties of bacilli which do not ferment lactose and do not liquefy gelatin in flies from different localities, and (3) the relative frequency of the occurrence of such varieties in flies and in the excreta of children."

(1) *The distribution in flies from different localities of lactose fermenting and non-lactose fermenting bacilli.*

Out of the 642 flies from diarrhœa infected houses examined, 209 (32 %) were infected with bacilli which do not ferment lactose or liquefy gelatin, 283 (44 %) with lactose fermenting bacilli of the colon type, and 43 (7 %) with non-lactose fermenting bacilli which liquefy gelatin. Of the 600 flies examined from non-diarrhœa infected houses, 125 (20 %) contained bacilli which do not ferment lactose or liquefy gelatin, 212 (35 %) bacilli of the colon type, and 9 (1·6 %) non-lactose fermenting bacilli which liquefy gelatin. From these figures it can be seen that all three classes of bacilli are more often found in flies from diarrhœa infected houses.

"Further analysis of the results shows that during the whole period (July 14th to October 16th) covered by these examinations at least 20 % of flies from all sources were infected with colon bacilli. The degree of infection with both colon bacilli and non-lactose fermenters was greatest during August and the first three weeks of September. In the series of flies from diarrhœa infected houses the greatest degree of infection with non-lactose fermenters (51 %) was reached in the third week in August. After the second week in September very few of the flies were found to be infected.

"It is of interest and importance to note that the percentage of infection in flies of separate batches obtained from one place on different occasions varied greatly. For example, from one non-diarrhœa infected house (Series G) 11 batches of flies were obtained. On two occasions only 5 % were infected with non-lactose fermenting bacilli, while on three occasions nearly 40 % were infected. Of the whole series 24 % were infected. In the same series the infection with colon bacilli varied from 25 % to 78 % (mean 44 %). The degree of infection with non-lactose fermenting bacilli in batches of flies (Series C) obtained from the diarrhœa infected farm house near Cambridge varied from 5 % to 69 %, with colon bacilli from 50 % to 93 %.

"Similar variations were seen in batches from different diarrhœa infected houses in Birmingham (Series A). In this series the infection with non-lactose fermenting bacilli varied from 0 % to 86 %, and with colon bacilli from 0 % to 87 %.

"According to the writer's observations a high degree of infection with non-lactose fermenting bacilli cannot be inferred from a high degree of infection with colon bacilli."

(2) *The distribution of varieties of bacilli which do not ferment lactose or liquefy gelatin in flies from different localities.*

In Table 21 the varieties of non-lactose fermenting bacilli which occurred in the flies of the different series are recorded. In many cases the percentage of flies infected is given.

TABLE 20. *Showing the general results of the bacteriological examinations of flies.*

	Flies from diarrhœa infected houses, of series				Flies from non-diarrhœa infected houses, of series						
	A	B	C	Total	D	E	F	G	H	Total	Total
Flies examined	471	97	74	642	147	51	157	155	90	600	1242
Flies infected with non-lactose fermenters	149 (31 %)	27 (28 %)	33 (44 %)	209 (32 %)	45 (30 %)	7 (13 %)	18 (11 %)	37 (24 %)	18 (20 %)	125 (20 %)	334 (26 %)
Flies infected with colon bacilli	183 (38 %)	48 (49 %)	52 (70 %)	283 (44 %)	47 (32 %)	19 (37 %)	52 (33 %)	68 (44 %)	26 (29 %)	212 (35 %)	495 (39 %)
Flies infected with liquefying bacilli	26 (16 %)	7 (8 %)	10 (13 %)	43 (7 %)	2 (1 %)	0	7 (4 %)	0	0	9 (1·6 %)	52 (4 %)

Table 21 available for download from www.cambridge.org/9781107458017

From this table it will be seen that 77 varieties of bacilli which do not ferment lactose or liquefy gelatin were isolated. Of these, 45 were isolated only once, seven twice and eight three times.

The varieties isolated belong to 6 groups and 20 sub-groups. Bacilli belonging to groups A and H were found with equal frequency (about 2 %) in flies from diarrhœa infected and non-infected houses. Bacilli belonging to groups B and C were met with twice as frequently in flies from diarrhœa infected houses. These slight differences in the degree of infection appear to be of little importance. On the other hand bacilli belonging to group G, sub-group a (Morgan's bacillus), were found much more frequently (nine times as often) in flies from diarrhœa infected houses than in flies from non-infected houses.

Up to the present a sufficient number of observations have not been made on which to determine definitely the relative frequency of the various types of bacilli in flies at different times during the season. The observations made on Birmingham flies showed that from August 14th to October 1st the weekly relative proportions of bacilli belonging to groups B, C and H varied very slightly. Members of group A were found relatively more frequently during the last three weeks, whereas members of group G, sub-group a, were much more frequently present during the first five weeks. No member of this group was isolated from this series after September 16th. The observations on the seasonal occurrence of this group are given in the following table:

TABLE 22. *Showing the weekly percentage of infection with bacilli of the Ga type (Morgan's bacillus) of flies from diarrhœa infected houses.*

	Birmingham flies	Cambridge flies	Total
	%	%	%
August 14th to August 20th ...	2·6	5·4	3·8
,, 21st ,, ,, 27th ...	12·0	15·6	12·8
,, 28th ,, September 3rd ...	1·8	3·6	2·3
September 4th ,, ,, 10th ...	—	—	—
,, 11th ,, ,, 17th ...	4·5	·0	3·4
,, 18th ,, ,, 24th ...	·0	14·3*	2·3
,, 25th ,, October 1st ...	·0	—	·0
October 2nd ,, ,, 8th ...	·0	—	·0
,, 9th ,, ,, 15th ...	·0	—	·0

* Only a few flies could be obtained for examination.

From this table it is evident that during the year 1911, both in Cambridge and in Birmingham, a much higher proportion of flies were infected with Morgan's bacillus (Ga) during the fourth week in August than at any other time.

(3) *The relative frequency of the occurrence of varieties of bacilli which do not ferment lactose and do not liquefy gelatin in flies and in the excreta of children.*

In order to show the relative frequency of the occurrence of varieties of non-lactose fermenting bacilli in the excreta of children, healthy and suffering from diarrhœa, and in flies Table 23 has been constructed. As far as possible from the data given the bacilli described by Lewis (1911 and 1912), O'Brien (1911), Orr (1911), Ross (1911) and Alexander (1912) in fæces have been tabulated according to the scheme which has been explained. The results of the examinations of flies have also been recorded.

It will be seen that bacilli belonging to group A are occasionally found in the fæces of healthy children, and of those suffering from diarrhœa. They occur in about 2 % of flies from all sources. Bacilli belonging to group B, sub-group a, seem to occur more commonly in the fæces of children suffering from epidemic diarrhœa than in the fæces of healthy children, and they are twice as often found in flies from infected houses as in flies from non-infected houses. Bacilli belonging to sub-group m have seldom been found in fæcal material, but occur in about 1·5 % of flies from all sources. Bacilli belonging to sub-groups j, k, l, n, o, and p are very rare.

Bacilli belonging to group C, sub-group a, occur moderately frequently in the fæces of children suffering from epidemic diarrhœa, but are very frequently found in flies (11 %; from infected houses 14 %, from non-infected 8 %). Bacilli belonging to sub-groups b, c, d, e, f, and h are seldom met with. Bacilli belonging to sub-group g have rarely been isolated from fæces, but are very common inhabitants of the fly's intestine (12 %). (See p. 117.) Bacilli belonging to groups D, E and F are very rarely encountered.

As already seen bacilli belonging to group G, sub-group a, are of special interest, and will be discussed later. Those belonging to sub-groups b, e (*a*), f, f (*a*), i (*a*), j (*a*), k, k (*a*), m, m (*a*), o (*a*), p, and p (*a*) are seldom met with. Bacilli belonging to group H, sub-group a, are occasionally found in the fæces of children, and occur in about 2 % of flies from all sources. Those belonging to sub-groups b, c, c (*a*), c (*b*), d, e, e (*a*), f, g, and h are uncommon.

Bacilli belonging to groups I, J and K are sometimes found in fæces, but have never been isolated from flies.

It will be seen from the foregoing account that flies often harbour bacilli which are found in the excreta of children, and it is probable that they often infect food materials with bacilli belonging to groups A, B (sub-groups a and m), C (sub-groups a and g) and H (sub-group a). There is at present, however, little evidence that any of these varieties produce pathogenic effects in children, though Lewis (1911, 1912) and Morgan and Ledingham (1909) have shown by feeding experiments that some members of all these groups are pathogenic for rats and mice.

In regard, however, to the varieties of bacilli composing the sub-group a of group G, evidence to show that they are very frequently present in the fæces of children suffering from epidemic diarrhœa, in some outbreaks, has already been quoted.

Through the kindness of Dr Robertson I was enabled to examine flies caught in 53 houses in Birmingham in which cases of epidemic diarrhœa had occurred. Dr Lewis examined the fæces of the patients living in 49 of these houses. I am, therefore, fortunate in being able to compare, through the courtesy of Dr Lewis, the varieties of bacilli in the fæces of the patients with those isolated from flies caught in the houses in which they lived. Dr Lewis obtained bacilli of the Ga type (Ga 8 = 34, Ga 4 = 1, Ga 7 = 1) from the fæces of patients living in 36 (74 %) of these houses. The present writer found bacilli of this group in flies from 10 of these houses. In the fæces of patients living in the other 13 houses Dr Lewis did not find bacilli of this type.

If the data are further analysed the results are found to be still more remarkable. No satisfactory examinations could be made of the flies from 10 of the 36 houses in which the patients were infected with Morgan's bacillus. Either all the flies were dead on arrival, or only a few were still alive. Deducting these cases we find that this type of bacillus was found in flies from 10 (38 %) out of 26 of these houses. Further, it is of importance to note that no bacilli of this type were isolated from flies received after September 16th. Previous to that date satisfactory cultures from flies from 24 infected houses were made and Morgan's bacillus isolated from flies from 10 (42 %).

Satisfactory cultures were obtained from flies received from 11 of the 13 non-Morgan infected houses mentioned. Flies from one (9 %) yielded a bacillus of the Morgan type (Ga 6). Flies from three houses yielded bacilli of the types discovered by Dr Lewis in the fæces of the patients.

Flies from four other Birmingham houses, in which cases of epidemic diarrhœa had occurred, were examined. All the flies from two houses were dead on arrival, but from a fly from one (50 %) of the remaining two batches Morgan's bacillus (Ga 8) was isolated.

Batches of flies (series B) from seven houses in Cambridge, in which cases of epidemic diarrhœa had occurred, were examined between 18th and 31st August. Morgan's bacillus (Ga 8) was isolated from the flies from three (43 %) houses. Batches of flies (Series C) from the diarrhœa infected farm house near Cambridge were examined on six occasions. Morgan's bacillus was isolated from the flies of three batches.

On the other hand 10 batches of flies from Birmingham houses (series D) in which no cases of epidemic diarrhœa had occurred, were examined. Cultures were made from 147 flies, but from only one fly was a bacillus of the Morgan type (Ga 6) isolated. From four Cambridge houses (series E, F, G, H), in which no cases of diarrhœa had occurred, 452 flies were examined. From three flies bacilli of this type (Ga 5, Ga 7, Ga 8) were isolated (0·6 %).

Taking the results of all the examinations made, it is found that bacilli of the Morgan type (86 % of which belong to the variety Ga 8) were isolated from 5·3 % of flies (32 out of 642 flies) from diarrhœa infected houses and from 0·6 % of flies (4 out of 600) from houses in which no cases of diarrhœa had occurred.

Taking into consideration the following facts—that in tabulating the results cultures from dead flies which seldom yielded non-lactose fermenting bacilli are included, that the patients, in some of the houses from which the flies were sent, were convalescent, that from most of the infected houses only a single batch of flies was received, that only a small number of flies from each batch was examined and further that only three colonies of non-lactose fermenting bacilli were isolated from each infected fly—the results are interesting and suggestive. They show that flies obtained from diarrhœa infected houses in Birmingham and in Cambridge during the summer of 1911 harboured Morgan's bacillus at least nine times as often as flies from non-infected houses. Experiments previously quoted (p. 109) have demonstrated that non-spore producing bacilli can survive for several days in the intestines of flies, and that during that period the flies can infect the materials on which they feed and on which they settle. If the larvæ are allowed to eat food contaminated with Morgan's bacillus, this organism is sometimes present in a small proportion of the flies which eventually emerge from them (p. 121).

Similar investigations, which will be published in the Report of the Medical Officer to the Local Government Board, were carried on by the writer during the summer of 1912, which was unusually cold and wet. Very few cases of summer diarrhœa occurred either in Cambridge or in Birmingham, and flies were difficult to obtain. Though non-lactose fermenting bacilli of various kinds and bacilli of the colon type were isolated from the flies, not a single example of the Morgan type was met with. In regard to the presence of Morgan's bacillus in flies obtained from these two towns the contrast between the severe diarrhœa year, 1911, and the non-diarrhœa year, 1912, is very striking and suggestive.

Morgan and Ledingham (1909, p. 142) examined batches of flies from diarrhœa infected and non-infected houses, and obtained Morgan's bacillus from nine (25 %) out of 36 batches from infected and from one (3 %) out of 32 batches from non-infected houses.

Nicoll (x, 1911) found that certain varieties of bacilli "seem to be able to establish themselves in the fly's intestine, to the exclusion sometimes of other forms, and to remain there for a considerable time. Amongst these may be mentioned Morgan's bacillus No. 1." Orr (1911, p. 380) isolated non-lactose fermenting bacilli from 16 out of 74 batches of flies. Morgan's bacillus was found twice.

Before the exact part played by flies in the dissemination of Morgan's bacillus can be finally decided the sources from which they obtain the infection must be demonstrated. Up to the present very little information on the possible sources of infection has been obtained. In certain outbreaks the organism is present in the excreta of a large proportion of children suffering from epidemic diarrhœa, and no doubt flies which can settle on such material become infected. Morgan and Ledingham (1909, p. 142) isolated Morgan's bacillus once from fresh cows' fæces (18 animals examined) but not from the fæces of the horse (13 animals examined). Lewis (1912) isolated this bacillus from the fæces of five out of twenty healthy mice. Possibly more extended observations will reveal that this type of bacillus is commonly present in certain materials which attract flies and to which they have access. It must be remembered however that all organisms giving the cultural reactions of Morgan's bacillus do not necessarily belong to one species since Lewis (1912, p. 276) has shown that bacilli of this type may be separated into groups by means of agglutination tests.

SUMMARY.

Recent epidemiological investigations strongly suggest that house-flies play a not unimportant part in the dissemination of summer diarrhœa. More extended observations on the correspondence between the numbers of flies and the numbers of cases of diarrhœa occurring in several districts, and on the effects of exterminating flies in limited areas, may aid in deciding the exact part played by flies.

The bacteriological investigations made up to the present show that flies can obtain and carry in their intestines most of the bacteria of the non-lactose fermenting types found in the fæces of children suffering from summer diarrhœa, and probably infect articles of food with them. Whether Morgan's bacillus is a causative agent in this disease or not, the facts relating to its presence in flies well illustrate the powers of these insects of acquiring and carrying organisms of this type, for in outbreaks associated with the presence of Morgan's bacillus in the stools of infants this bacillus is often found in flies caught in houses in which cases have occurred, but it is rarely present in flies from other situations.

The epidemiological and bacteriological evidence is so suggestive, and the disease is of such importance, that an attempt to definitely settle the connection between flies and summer diarrhœa by preventive measures against flies in a selected area seems now justifiable.

CHAPTER XV

CHOLERA

Experiments.

Maddox (1885) was the first to carry out experiments on the relation of flies to cholera by feeding *C. vomitoria* and *E. tenax* with cultures. He states that he found these organisms in their fæces, but his methods were not very satisfactory. Sawtchenko (1892) fed flies on broth cultures and found the vibrios in their fæces two hours later. He also found the vibrios in the flies' intestines and gained the impression that they multiplied in their bodies. Simmonds (1892) placed flies on opened intestines of persons who had died of cholera, and then transferred them singly to large flasks in which they could fly and move about freely. Roll cultures of these flies made at intervals from five to ninety minutes all gave positive results. Uffelman (1892) allowed two flies to feed on liquid gelatin cultures of *V. choleræ*, and after keeping them separately for an hour and two hours respectively, made cultures from them. The first yielded 10,000, and the second 25 colonies. He also demonstrated that flies infected in this way could contaminate milk on which they fed. Tsuzuki (1904, p. 77) showed that infected flies could contaminate media over which they walked, and Chantemesse (1905) and Ganon (1908) isolated the vibrios from flies 17 and 24 hours respectively after infection. Graham-Smith (1910, p. 35) experimenting with old laboratory cultures found that the vibrios soon died on the legs and wings, and that even in the crop and intestine their numbers rapidly diminished, all cultures made more than 48 hours after infection yielding negative results. Infected fæces were passed for 30 hours.

Isolation of V. choleræ from 'wild' flies.

Simmonds (1892) isolated the vibrios from a fly caught in the post-mortem room of the Old General Hospital in Hamburg, where autopsies were being made on the bodies of persons dead of cholera. When antiseptic precautions were observed and the autopsies conducted as rapidly as possible the vibrios could no longer be obtained from the flies in the room. Tsuzuki (1904) succeeded in isolating the vibrios from flies captured in a cholera house in Tientsin.

Observations during cholera epidemics.

Moore (1853) first drew attention to the necessity of guarding food against flies in cholera outbreaks, adding: "flies in the East have not far to pass from diseased evacuations or from articles stained with such excreta, to food cooked and uncooked." Nicholas (1873) describing the epidemic at Malta in 1849 writes: "My first impression of the possibility of the transfer of the disease by flies was derived from the observation of the manner in which these voracious creatures, present in great numbers, and having equal access to the dejections and food of the patients, gorged themselves indiscriminately and then disgorged themselves on the food and drinking utensils." Flügge (1893), Simmonds (1892), Tsuzuki (1904), Chantemesse (1905), Ganon (1908) and others, from their personal experiences, have all expressed the opinion that flies play an important part in the spread of cholera under favourable conditions.

The two most interesting observations are those of Macrae (1894) and Buchanan (1897) in India. Macrae describes an outbreak in a jail at Gaya, when flies were present in great numbers. "They were present in swarms when the disease broke out, and it was an observation of daily occurrence to see them settling on cholera stools whenever possible." At feeding time there was "a struggle between them and the prisoners for the food." In the female department, shut off from the male side by a high wall, which apparently prevented the access of flies from the other side, no cases occurred. On the male side there were several cases and boiled milk exposed there and in the cow shed became infected with *V. choleræ*. This infection could only have been carried by flies. Macrae considers that the well-known erratic behaviour of cholera in certain outbreaks may be explained by fly infection, and thinks that the fly "should be considered as one of the most important agencies in the diffusion of the disease." Buchanan describes a jail outbreak which occurred at Burdwan in 1896. Flies swarmed, and outside the prison were some huts in which cholera prevailed. A strong wind blew large numbers of flies from the direction of the huts into the prison enclosure. Only those prisoners who were fed at the jail enclosure nearest the huts acquired the disease, whilst all the others remained healthy.

It will be noticed that most of the observations quoted were made more than ten years ago, when the methods of bacteriological diagnosis were less perfect. Consequently further bacteriological investigation during cholera outbreaks is necessary before the exact part played by flies in the spread of the disease is ascertained, though the evidence at present available seems to indicate that flies are often responsible for infecting food with the vibrios.

CHAPTER XVI

TUBERCULOSIS

Experiments.

Spillman and Haushalter (1887) seem to have been the first to investigate the possible relation of *M. domestica* to the dissemination of *B. tuberculosis.* They found tubercle bacilli in the intestinal contents and fæces of flies which had fed on tubercular sputum. Hofmann (1885) fed flies on tubercular sputum and found the bacilli in their fæces. He also inoculated three guinea-pigs with emulsions of the intestines of these flies, and one of them developed tuberculosis. He found, however, that fly fæces six to eight weeks old gave negative results on inoculation. Celli (1888) reported on some experiments by Alessi who inoculated the fæces of flies which had fed on tubercular sputum into rabbits. Some of these animals developed the disease.

Lord (1904) made a number of careful investigations.

In one experiment he placed about 30 flies in an inverted jar together with a small dish containing tubercular sputum showing about 10 tubercle bacilli in the field, and around it some clean cover-glasses. "Examination of many specks on the cover-glasses showed that the number of bacilli in each microscopic field had increased from about 10 in the original sputum to 150 in the specks. Each speck contained 3000 to 5000 bacilli. About 2000 specks had been deposited by 30 flies within three days, thus from 6,000,000 to 10,000,000 tubercle bacilli had been transferred from the sputum to the inner side of the cage during this period." By inoculation experiments he proved that the bacilli in these fæcal deposits, when protected from the direct sunlight, were virulent for guinea-pigs up to the 15th day, but not on the 28th and 55th days. He also made sections of flies which had fed on tubercular sputum, and found the bacilli in their intestinal contents. "No invasion of other parts of the body could be determined."

Hayward (1904) also made a series of interesting observations.

"Flies caught feeding on the bottles containing tuberculous sputum that came to the laboratory for examination" were placed in a cage, and deposited fæces on clean cover-slips. Ten out of sixteen cover-slips examined showed tubercle bacilli. Control examinations of fæces of flies had shown that no acid-fast bacilli were present in them. Other flies were fed on tuberculous sputum placed in watch-glasses and covered with a fine wire screen. "On this screen the fly could walk without getting its feet or wings in sputum and could feed through the meshes." Tubercle bacilli were found in the fæces and in the intestines of these flies, and guinea-pigs injected with emulsions of their fæces died of tuberculosis. He further states "culture plates made of the fæces on glycerine agar and incubated two weeks, showed a growth of tubercle bacilli."

Hayward seems to have been the first to notice that "flies apparently suffer from diarrhœa after feeding on sputum."

Cobb (1905) writing on this subject says:—"I have demonstrated that the fly carries the bacillus," but does not quote his experiments.

Buchanan (1907) made the following investigations:

"To test the power of flies in relation to expectoration a specimen of tuberculous sputum rich in *Bacillus tuberculosis* was spread in a thin film in the bottom half of a Petri capsule. A house-fly was introduced into the capsule, and caused to walk over the film for a few minutes. It was then transferred to another Petri capsule containing a layer of agar. On washing the surface of the agar with a cubic centimetre of bouillon and inoculating a guinea-pig intraperitoneally therewith, tuberculosis was induced which killed the guinea-pig in 36 days."

Graham-Smith (1910, p. 27) carried out elaborate experiments with cultures of *B tuberculosis* and with sputum containing this organism.

Experiments with B. tuberculosis (Culture).

"A large number of freshly-caught flies were allowed to feed on an emulsion of a culture of human tubercle bacilli in syrup. After feeding, the flies were transferred to a clean cage and fed daily on syrup. After varying intervals of time flies were caught and dissected. Smear preparations were made from the crop and intestinal contents and stained in the usual way for tubercle bacilli. Smears were also made from vomit and fæcal material and stained in the same way. Each of the preparations was very carefully examined for tubercle bacilli by two observers."

TABLE 24. *Showing the results of an experiment with a culture of B. tuberculosis.*

Time after infection	No. of fly	Crop	Intestine	Fæces
17 hours ...	1	+	+ (many)	−
22 ,, ...	2	+	+ ,,	−
55 ,,	3	+	+ ...	+
	4	+	+ ...	
58 ,, ...	5	+	+ ...	+ in 6 out of 6 samples
78 ,,	6	+	+ ...	+ in 3 out of 3 samples
	7	+	+ ...	also in vomit
96 ,,	8	−	+ ...	+ in 5 out of 6 samples
	9	−	+	
5 days ...	10	o	+ (few) ...	+ in 3 out of 7 samples
	11	o	+ ,,	
6 ,, ...	12	o	+ (many)	+ only 1 tubercle bacillus found in several samples
	13	−	+ (several)	
7 ,, ...	14	−	+ ,,	−
	15	−	+ ,,	
8 ,, ...	16	−	+ (8 found)	+ several
	17	−	+ (2 ,,)	
9 ,, ...	18	−	+ (several)	o
	19	−	o	
10 ,, ...	20	−	+ (several)	o
	21	−	+ ,,	
11 ,, ...	22	−	+ (2 found)	+ 1 tubercle bacillus found
	23	−	+ (few)	
12 ,, ...	24	−	+ (1 clump)	o
	25	−	+ (2 found)	
13 ,, ...	26	−	o ...	+ 3 tubercle bacilli in 2 samples
14 ,, ...	27	−	o	
15 ,, ...	28	−	o	
	29	−	o	
	30	−	o	
	31	−	o	
16 ,, ...	32	−	+ 1 tubercle bacillus found	

"These experiments show that, under experimental conditions, tubercle bacilli, derived from a culture, may be present in the crop for three days. In the intestine, however, they may be found for much longer periods, being present in considerable numbers for at least 6 days. Subsequently their numbers diminish, but they may be discovered by careful search for 12 days or even longer. In the fæces they are numerous up to the 5th day, and occasional specimens may be found in fæcal material deposited between the 6th and 14th days after infection. A number of preparations made from the crop and intestinal contents of normal flies were examined but acid-fast bacilli were never found."

Experiment with B. tuberculosis in sputum.

"A large number of flies were allowed to feed for 30 minutes on sputum, rich in tubercle bacilli, which they took up greedily. Subsequently they were fed on non-tuberculous sputum. In other respects the experiment was conducted in the same way as the previous one, except that the contents of the crop were not examined."

TABLE 25. *Showing the results of an experiment with sputum containing B. tuberculosis.*

Time after infection	No. of fly	Intestine	Fæces
20 hours	1	+ ...	+ (few)
	2	+	
50 "	3	+ (few) ...	+ in 3 out of 6 samples
	4	+ "	
69 "	5	+ ...	+ in 2 out of 6 samples
	6	o	
90 "	7	+ ...	+ in 1 out of 3 samples
	8	+	
4 days	9	+ (1 found)	o in many samples
	10	o	
5 "	11	o ...	+ 1 tubercle bacillus in many samples
	12	+ (2 found)	
6 "	13	o ...	o in many samples
	14	o	
7 "	15	+ (few) ...	o " "
	16	o	
8 "	17	o ...	o " "
	18	o	
9 "	19	o ...	o " "
	20	o	
10 "	21	o	
13 "	23, 24, 25	Intestinal contents emulsified and injected into a guinea-pig. The animal was kept under observation for 8 weeks. After that time it was killed and found to be healthy	

"This experiment shows that under more natural conditions tubercle bacilli may be found in the intestinal contents of flies for at least four days. The fæces passed during that period are also infected. The experiment is not, however, quite comparable with the previous one since continual feeding on sputum gives the flies diarrhœa."

Wild Flies. Hofmann (1888) appears to be the only observer who has examined 'wild' flies for the presence of tubercle bacilli. He examined six flies caught in the room of a tuberculous patient and found acid-fast bacilli in four of them. Similar bacilli were also found in fly-fæces scraped from the walls, door and furniture of the room.

SUMMARY.

In making observations on 'wild' flies it must be remembered that acid-fast bacilli closely simulating *B. tuberculosis* are frequently present in milk and other substances, and consequently may be found in flies. The nature of these bacilli can only be proved by animal inoculations.

The experiments quoted, however, conclusively indicate that flies may carry *B. tuberculosis*, and distribute it for several days after feeding on infected material. No doubt under suitable conditions they frequently infect articles of food, and in the rooms of phthisical patients may infect the food daily. In the production of tuberculosis the influence of dose, especially the initial dose, is probably a most important factor (Cobbett, 1907, p. 1028), and in most cases the number of bacilli deposited cannot be very great. Only the actual number of bacilli deposited are ingested with the food, since even under the most suitable conditions these bacilli multiply very slowly. In this connection, however, the fact that flies feeding on sputum suffer from diarrhœa may be of some importance.

The experimental evidence clearly proves the desirability of protecting sputum from flies, which according to all observers are greatly attracted to it, but in considering their relation to infection in the human subject the influence of dose must be taken into consideration.

CHAPTER XVII

ANTHRAX

Though anthrax is not uncommon in cattle, sheep, and some other animals, it is not a disease which occurs very frequently in man, except amongst those engaged in certain trades.

Experiments.

Raimbert (1869) and Davaine (1870) placed flies on infected material, and proved by inoculation experiments that the bacilli were present on their limbs. Celli (1888) showed that the bacilli recovered from the fæces of infected flies still retained their virulence. Sangree (1899) demonstrated that if a fly walked over an anthrax culture, and was then placed on a sterile agar surface the latter became infected. Buchanan (1907) carried out similar experiments, and also found that a specimen of *C. vomitoria* could infect Petri dishes of agar by walking over them after having walked over the skinned and gutted carcase of a guinea-

PLATE XX

FIG. 1.—Photograph ($\frac{2}{3}$ nat. size) of an agar plate before incubation, inoculated with the organs of four flies infected with *B. anthracis*. The cultures from each fly are separated from each other by lines drawn on the bottom of the plate, and are numbered I, II, III, IV. In each case the parts inoculated with the crop and gut contents and the fluid expressed from the proboscis are surrounded by circles and marked C, G and P respectively. The legs, wings and heads have been separately inoculated in each case.

FIG. 2.—Photograph of the same plate after 24 hours' incubation at 37° C. Large anthrax colonies have developed in the places inoculated with the crop and gut contents of fly III. Colonies of *B. anthracis* and other organisms have grown round several of the other inoculated portions of the plate.

FIG. 3.—Photograph of a plate culture made from the legs, head and contents of the abdomen of a fly, which died of infection with *E. muscæ* 14 days after feeding on syrup infected with the spores of *B. anthracis*. The body was subsequently kept in a glass bottle, and the culture made 155 days after death. Colonies of *B. anthracis* have developed round the legs and several portions of the abdominal contents. (From Graham-Smith, *Reports to Local Government Board,* No. 40, 1910.)

Plate XX

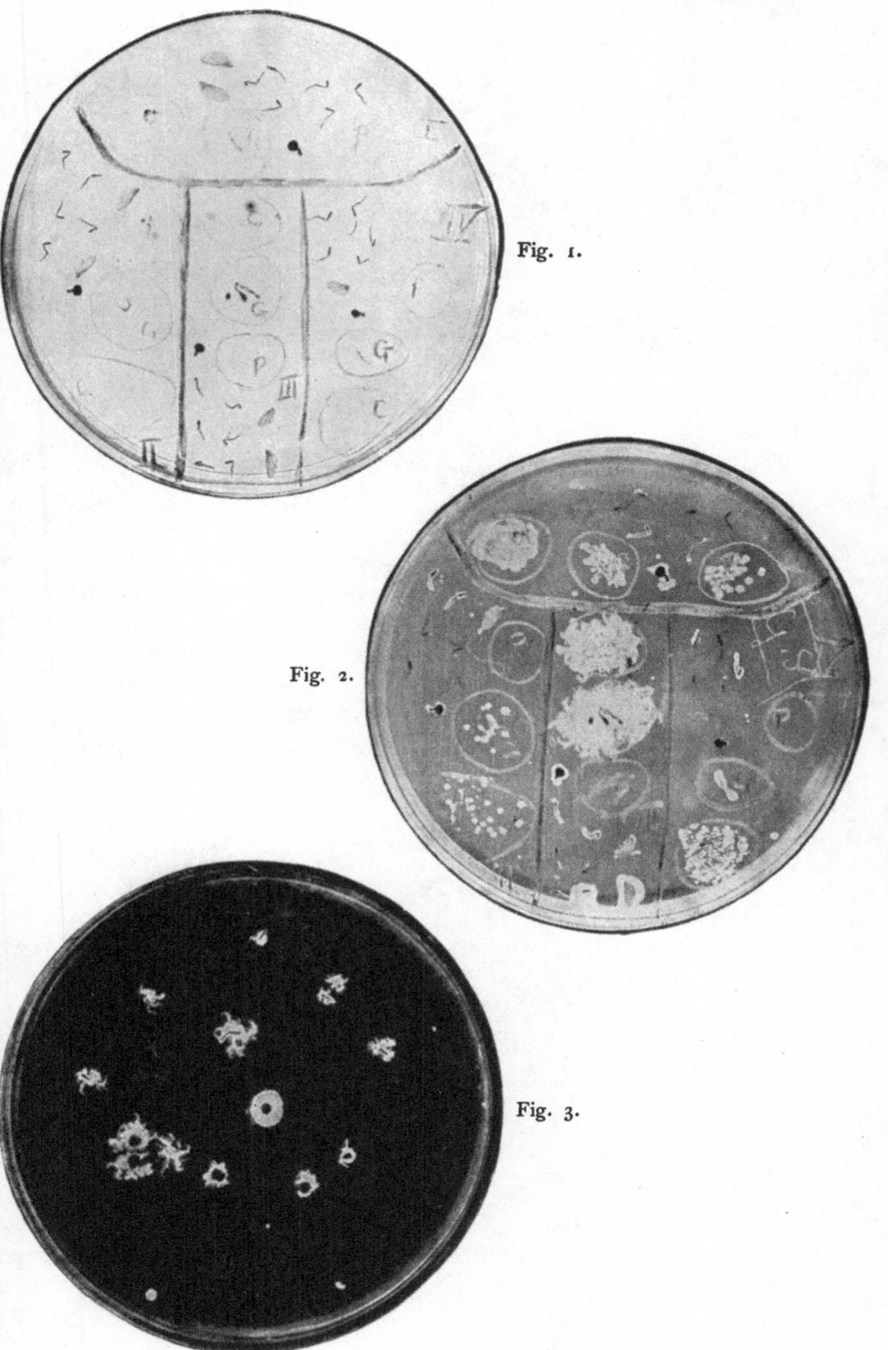

Fig. 1.

Fig. 2.

Fig. 3.

pig, which had died of anthrax. House-flies placed on anthracic meat, seized in the market, also became infected. Graham-Smith (1910, p. 29) carried out experiments with non-spore-bearing anthrax bacilli in blood and with spore-bearing cultures.

(*a*) *Experiment with B. anthracis in blood* (Non-spore-bearing).

"Twenty-four flies were placed in a cage for one hour together with the body of a mouse just dead of anthrax. The latter had been opened so that the flies could feed on the blood. The flies were then transferred to a clean cage. The next morning the cage contained numerous red spots of vomit, and several masses of yellowish fæces. In the former *B. anthracis* was found both microscopically and by cultures. The flies were transferred daily to fresh cages and fed on syrup. At intervals specimens were caught and dissected and cultures made, on agar, from their legs, wings, heads, and crop and intestinal contents. Cultures were also made from the fæcal deposits."

TABLE 26. *Showing results of experiments with B. anthracis* (Non-spore-bearing).

Time after infection	No. of fly	Cultures from													
		Legs						Wings			Crop		Intestine		
		1	2	3	4	5	6	1	2	Head	M.	C.	M.	C.	Fæces
18 hours	1	o	o	o	o	o	o	o	o	o	+	+	+	+	−
	2	o	o	o	o	o	o	o	o	+	−	−	+	+	
24 "	3	+	+	o	o	o	o	o	o	o	−	−	+	+	+
	4	o	o	o	o	o	o	o	o	+	+	+	−	+	
	5	o	o	o	o	o	o	o	o	−	−	−	+	+	
	6	o	o	o	o	o	o	o	o	o	−	−	+	+	
48 "	7	o	o	o	o	o	o	o	o	+	o	+	+	+	+
	8	o	o	o	o	o	o	o	o	o	o	o	o	o	
	9	o	o	o	o	o	o	o	o	+	−	+	−	+	
	10	o	o	o	o	o	o	o	o	o	−	o	−	o	
3 days	11	o	o	o	o	o	o	o	o	o	+	+	−	+	o
	12	o	o	o	o	o	o	o	o	o	−	+	−	+	
	13	o	o	o	o	o	o	o	o	o	o	o	−	o	
	14	o	o	o	o	o	o	o	o	o	−	o	−	+	
4 "	15	o	o	o	o	o	o	o	o	o	o	o	−	o	
	16	o	o	o	o	o	o	o	o	+	+	+	−	o	Crop full of apparently coagulated blood.
	17	o	o	o	o	o	o	o	o	o	−	−	−	o	
5 "	18	o	o	o	o	o	o	o	o	o	−	−	−	o	
	19	o	o	o	o	o	o	o	o	o	−	−	−	o	
	20	o	o	o	o	o	o	o	o	o	+	+	−	o	" "
	21	o	o	o	o	o	o	o	o	o	−	o	−	o	

From crop and intestinal contents both Microscopic preparations (M) and Cultures (C) were made.

"This experiment shows that non-spore-bearing anthrax bacilli do not remain alive on the external parts of flies for more than 24 hours. They may, however, remain alive in the intestine for three days, and in the crop for five days, especially when partially coagulated blood remains in that organ. Film preparations made at various times from the crop and intestinal contents showed no spore-bearing forms. Plate XVIII, fig. 3, is a reproduction of a photograph of a smear made from the crop of a fly (No. 11). The bacilli are present in the fæces deposited 48 hours after infection."

TABLE 27. *Showing the results of experiments with anthrax spores.*

Time after infection	No. of fly	Cultures from: Legs 1	Legs 2	Legs 3	Legs 4	Legs 5	Legs 6	Wings 1	Wings 2	Head	Crop	Intestine	Fæces	Vomit
2·5 hours...	1	o	o	o	o	o	o	+	o	++	++	++	–	–
4 ,, ...	2	+	+	+	+	+	+	+	+	++	++	++	o	+
19 ,, ...	3	o	+	+	+	+	+	+	+	++	++	++	+(3 out of 4)	+(5 out of 5)
24 ,, ...	4	+	+	+	+	+	+	+	+	+	+	++		
28 ,, ...	5	+	+	+	+	+	+	+	+	+	–	++	+(3 out of 4)	
30 ,, ...	6	+	+	+	+	+	+	+	+	+	–	++	+(8 out of 8)	+(5 out of 5)
48 ,,	7	+	+	+	+	+	+	+	+	+	–	++		
	8	+	+	+	+	o	o	o	o	++	–	++		
54 ,, ...	9	+	+	+	+	+	+	+	+	+	++	++		
3 days	10	+	o	o	o	o	o	+	o	+	++	++	+(1 out of 5)	+(1 out of 4)
	11	+	+	+	+	o	o	+	o	+	++	++		
	12	+	+	+	+	o	o	+	+	+	–	++		
4 ,,	13	+	+	o	o	o	–	+	+	+	+	++	+(3 out of 5)	+(4 out of 5)
	14	+	o	o	o	o	o	+	+	+	+	++		
5 ,,	15	o	o	o	o	o	o	o	o	o	++	++	+(3 out of 7)	o out of 3
	16	o	o	o	o	o	o	o	o	o	++	+		
6 ,, ...	17	+	+	o	o	o	o	o	o	+	++	+	o out of 4	+(1 out of 5)
7 ,, ...	18	o	o	o	o	o	o	o	o	o	++	++	o	
8 ,, ...	19	+	+	o	o	o	o	o	o	o	+	o		
9 ,, ...	20	o	o	o	o	o	o	o	o	o	o	o	+(1 out of 7)	
10 ,, ...	21	+	o	o	o	o	o	+	o	o	–	+	o	
11 ,, ...	22	o	o	o	o	o	o	o	o	+	o	o	o	
12 ,, ...	23	o	o	o	o	o	o	o	o	o	o	o	o	
13 ,, ...	24	o	o	o	o	o	o	o	o	o	o	o	–	
15 ,, ...	25	o	o	o	o	o	o	o	o	o	o	o	–	
16 ,, ...	26	o	o	o	o	o	o	o	o	o	+	o	–	

"Cultures were also made from drops of syrup after the flies had been allowed to feed on them. Anthrax bacilli were cultivated on the 3rd, 4th, 6th, 7th, 8th, and 10th days, but not later."

(*b*) *Experiments with anthrax spores.*

"An emulsion of an old anthrax culture was made and heated to 70° C. for 15 minutes, and subsequently a number of flies were allowed to feed on it. These flies were transferred to fresh cages daily and fed on syrup. Specimens were caught and dissected at intervals. Cultures were made, on agar, from their legs, wings, heads, crop and intestinal contents and fæcal deposits. Although numerous smears were made from crop and intestinal contents at various times, no anthrax bacilli were seen microscopically, showing that the spores do not develope into bacilli in the fly."

"This experiment shows that flies infected with anthrax spores may carry the spores on their legs and wings for at least 10 days, and that the spores are present in considerable numbers in the crop and intestinal contents for at least 7 days. The vomit and fæcal deposits contain living spores for 6 days or longer. In another experiment, which was intended to confirm and prolong the one just described, a number of flies were allowed to feed on syrup infected with anthrax spores. Unfortunately an epidemic of *Empusa muscæ* killed off these flies after 20 days."

This experiment, however, confirmed the previous one and showed that anthrax spores may remain alive on the legs and wings and in the intestinal contents for at least 20 days. Fæces passed 14 days after infection contained living spores.

The experiment differed slightly from the last since the flies were kept in one cage all the time and were not transferred to fresh cages daily.

"In order to ascertain how long spores will retain their vitality in dried fæces and vomit the following experiment was made.

"After feeding on infected material the flies were placed for 24 hours in a fresh cage (A), and then removed to another. At intervals (1, 3, 4, 5, 7, 8, 12, 13 and 20 days) cultures were made both from the vomit and fæces deposited on cage A and, in every case, numerous colonies of *B. anthracis* grew. At the end of 20 days the cage was sterilized by mistake. Probably the spores would have remained alive for a much longer period."

In order to ascertain how long anthrax spores may remain alive in dead infected flies some infected flies, dead of empusa disease, have been kept in a bottle. From time to time cultures have been made from them. At the time of writing, nearly three years later, the spores are alive and virulent.

Experiments on Larvæ.

Graham-Smith (1911, p. 43) allowed the larvæ of blow-flies (*C. erythrocephala*) to feed on meat artificially infected with the spores of *B. anthracis.*

"Altogether about 70 flies emerged. Of these 17 were dissected and cultures made from these organs a few hours after emerging. From four specimens *B. anthracis* was not cultivated, but from the other 13 cultures were obtained. It was present in the intestinal contents of 10; on one or both wings of 8; on one or more legs of 12, and on the heads of 8.

"Three specimens were dissected after living two days in a cage. From the legs, wings, crop and intestinal contents of all *B. anthracis* was obtained. One specimen three days old was dissected, and *B. anthracis* was obtained from one wing. *B. anthracis* was cultivated from a leg and from the head of a specimen 6 days old." Three specimens were dissected after living 10 days in a cage. *B. anthracis* was obtained in culture from two of them. Six specimens 11 days old were dissected, and *B. anthracis* obtained from three. Three flies 15 days old were dissected and *B. anthracis* cultivated from two of them. *B. anthracis* was cultivated from one leg of one of three flies 19 days old, which were dissected. Several of these cultures, including that obtained from a fly 15 days old, were proved to be fully virulent.

Two flies 22 days old, three 23 days old, two 29 days old, three 30 days old and two 33 days old were dissected, and cultures made from their limbs and organs, but *B. anthracis* was not found.

"A few other experiments were carried out with these flies. Four flies were allowed to walk over agar plates a few hours after emerging. Numerous colonies of *B. anthracis* developed on these plates.

"Twelve flies a few hours old were kept in a glass cage, and fed on syrup. Shortly after their first meal some of the remains of the syrup on which they had been feeding was smeared on the surface of agar plates. Numerous colonies of *B. anthracis* developed on these plates. Nearly every fly very shortly after emerging deposited a large quantity of whitish, semi-fluid material. Cultures made from this material were negative. The fæces deposited by flies two days old contained *B. anthracis* in considerable numbers, as also did the remains of syrup on which they had fed.

"*B. anthracis* was not found in cultures made from the fæces of flies 22 and 23 days old, nor in those made from the remains of syrup on which they had been feeding, but a single colony of *B. anthracis* was obtained from the remains of syrup on which flies 21 days old had fed."

Not infrequently anthrax-like colonies occur on plate cultures made from flies, but these can usually be distinguished in subcultures from *B. anthracis* without any difficulty.

Another series of experiments (Graham-Smith, 1912, p. 333) was conducted with the larvæ of house-flies (*M. domestica*) fed on material infected with anthrax spores.

"Cultures were made on agar from 95 flies which emerged."

Cultures from	11	out of	14	newly hatched flies	showed	*B. anthracis*	(78 %)
,,	,,	48 ,,	62	flies 1 day old	,,	,,	,,
,,	,,	2 ,,	8 ,,	3 days ,,	,,	,,	(25 %)
,,	,,	1 ,,	6 ,,	4 ,,	,,	,,	(16 %)
,,	,,	1 ,,	5 ,,	6 ,,	,,	,,	(20 %)

"Positive results were obtained from 63 (66 %) out of the 95 flies examined. A few of the flies which emerged were kept in a clean cage without food and died in a few days. After they had been dead for some weeks cultures were made from three of them. *B. anthracis* was found in cultures from two."

In another series of experiments (p. 332) half grown larvæ of *C. erythrocephala* and *L. cæsar* were allowed to feed on the bodies of guinea-pigs which had died of anthrax.

"The larvæ pupated in 10—15 days and the flies began to emerge in 20 days. In order to avoid the possibility of the flies re-infecting themselves after emerging the pupæ were removed to clean cages and placed on clean sand. In some cases before the preparation of cultures the flies were sterilized in various ways, while in other cases no sterilization of the exterior was attempted. Sometimes the flies were killed shortly after emerging, while on other occasions they were kept for some hours or days. In the latter case they were fed on syrup.

"Cultures on agar were prepared in the way previously described from the intestinal contents of 511 flies, 170 *C. erythrocephala* and 341 *L. cæsar*, which emerged from larvæ which fed on the body of a guinea-pig dead of anthrax. Only three colonies were met with which resembled in any way those produced by *B. anthracis*. By subcultures they were proved not to be those of *B. anthracis*."

These experiments show that flies (*M. domestica* and *C. erythrocephala*) which hatch out from larvæ which have fed on material contaminated with anthrax *spores* are heavily infected on emerging, and remain infected for several days. They can infect surfaces on which they walk, and fluids on which they feed and deposit infected fæces. On the other hand flies (*C. erythrocephala*) which develop from larvæ which have fed on non-spore bearing anthrax bacilli are not infected.

Wild Flies. Dickinson states that "Billings (1898) found anthrax bacilli in the stomachs and intestines of flies collected from the body of an infected steer."

SUMMARY.

Experiments have shown that flies (*M. domestica* and *C. erythrocephala*) infected with the spores of *B. anthracis* may carry and distribute the organism for many days, and that the spores may remain alive in dead infected flies for an indefinite period. Flies, which emerge from larvæ, which have fed on spore contaminated materials, are also infected, and can distribute the organism. The fæces deposited by infected flies certainly remain infective for 20 days, and probably for a much longer time.

It is evident, therefore, that under suitable conditions, which are not infrequently fulfilled, the bacillus may be distributed by flies in many ways, though no definite evidence of infection either in men or animals has yet been obtained.

CHAPTER XVIII

OTHER BACTERIAL DISEASES

Diphtheria.

Smith (1898) allowed flies to walk over material infected with *B. diphtheriæ* and then over sterile media. "Naturally he obtained a positive result." Graham-Smith (1910, p. 33) carried out two series of experiments with cultures of *B. diphtheriæ.*

"In the first, a number of flies were allowed to feed for 30 minutes on an emulsion of *B. diphtheriæ* in saliva, and were then transferred to a fresh cage. At intervals flies were killed and cultures made on transparent serum medium (Nuttall and Graham-Smith, 1908, p. 150), from their legs, wings, heads, and crop and intestinal contents."

"These experiments seem to indicate that *B. diphtheriæ* seldom remains alive for more than a few hours on the legs and wings, but may live in the crop and intestine for 24 hours or occasionally longer. The fæces passed during the first few hours are frequently infected. It is very probable that these experiments under-estimate the vitality of *B. diphtheriæ*, since in many cases film-forming bacilli overgrew the cultures."

There is no evidence that under natural conditions flies are concerned in the spread of this disease, which is usually not prevalent when flies are numerous, but, under suitable conditions, it is possible that the disease may be occasionally conveyed by them.

TABLE 28. *Showing results of experiments with B. diphtheriæ emulsified in saliva.*

Time after infection	No. of fly	Cultures from: Legs 1	Legs 2	Legs 3	Legs 4	Legs 5	Legs 6	Wings 1	Wings 2	Head	Crop	Intestine	Fæces
1 hour	1	o	o	o	o	o	o	o	o	+	–	+	o
	2	o	o	o	o	o	o	o	o	+	–	++	
2 hours	3	o	o	o	o	o	o	o	o	o	–	++	++
	4	o	o	o	o	o	o	o	o	+	–	++	
3 ,, ...	5	o	o	o	o	o	o	o	o	o	–	++	
4 ,,	6	o	o	o	o	o	o	o	o	o	o	o	
	7	o	o	o	o	o	o	o	o	o	–	o	
6 ,,	8	o	o	o	o	o	o	o	o	o	–	o	
	9	o	o	o	o	o	o	o	o	o	+ (1 colony)	o	+ (2 colonies)
24 ,,	10	o	o	o	o	o	o	o	o	o	+	o	
	11	o	o	o	o	o	o	o	o	o	++	+	
	12	o	o	o	o	o	o	o	o	o	o	o	
48 ,,	13	–	–	–	–	–	–	–	–	o	o	o	
	14	–	–	–	–	–	–	–	–	o	o	o	
72 ,, ...	15	–	–	–	–	–	–	–	–	o	o	o	o

"In the second series of experiments the flies were allowed to feed for 1 hour on an emulsion of *B. diphtheriæ* in broth. The subsequent proceedings were the same as in the first series."

TABLE 29. *Showing the results of experiments with B. diphtheriæ emulsified in broth.*

Time after infection	No. of fly	Cultures from: Legs 1	Legs 2	Legs 3	Legs 4	Legs 5	Legs 6	Wings 1	Wings 2	Head	Crop	Intestine	Fæces
5 hours ...	1	+	o	o	o	o	o	o	+	o	o	o	+
27 ,, ...	2	o	o	o	o	o	o	o	o	o	o	o	o
51 ,, ...	3	o	o	o	o	o	o	o	o	o	o	o	+ (2 colonies)
77 ,, ...	4	o	o	o	o	o	o	o	o	+(1)	+	+	
101 ,,	5	o	o	o	o	o	o	o	o	o	o	o	
	6	o	o	o	o	o	o	o	o	o	o	o	
	7	o	o	o	o	o	o	o	o	o	o	o	
116 ,, ...	8	o	o	o	o	o	o	o	o	+	+	+	
6 days	9	o	o	o	o	o	o	o	o	o	o	o	
	10	o	o	o	o	o	o	o	o	o	+	o	
	11	o	o	o	o	o	o	o	o	o	o	o	
7 ,,	12	o	o	o	o	o	o	o	o	o	+ (1 colony)	o	
	13	o	o	o	o	o	o	o	o	o	o	o	
8 ,,	14	o	o	o	o	o	o	o	o	o	o	o	
	15	o	o	o	o	o	o	o	o	o	o	o	

Ophthalmia.

As early as 1862 Budd considered that Egyptian ophthalmia was carried by flies, and Laveran (1880), at Briska, was of the same opinion. Howe (1888) gave an interesting account of his observations on the subject. "He referred to the extraordinary prevalence of purulent ophthalmia among natives up and down the river Nile, and to the extraordinary abundance of the flies in that country. He spoke of the dirty habits of the natives and of their remarkable indifference to the visits of flies, not only children but adults allowing flies to settle in swarms about their eyes sucking the secretions, and never making any attempt to drive them away. He called attention to the fact that the number of cases of this eye disease always increases when the flies are present in the greatest numbers and that the eye trouble is most prevalent in the place where flies are most numerous. In the desert where flies are absent, eyes as a rule are unaffected. He made an examination of the flies captured upon diseased eyes, and found on their feet bacteria which were similar to those found in the conjunctival secretion" (Howard, 1911, p. 168).

"Welander (1896) observed an interesting case wherein an old bedridden woman in a hospital became infected. This patient's bed was alongside of that of another patient who had blennorrhœa, but a screen, which did not reach to the ceiling separated the beds. All means of infection, except through the agency of flies, appeared to be excluded. Welander found that flies bore living *gonococci* upon their feet three hours after they had been soiled with secretion, for they infected ascites agar plates with which they came in contact" (Nuttall and Jepson, 1909, p. 21).

Nuttall and Jepson (1909) consider that "the evidence regarding the spread of Egyptian ophthalmia by flies appears to be conclusive, and the possibility of gonorrhœal secretions being conveyed by flies cannot be denied."

Plague.

In the light of modern investigations relating to the dissemination of plague it seems most improbable that flies play a part of any importance. Yersin (1894) and Nuttall (1897) have, however, both shown that when opportunities for infection occur flies may contain living and virulent plague (*B. pestis*) bacilli for at least 48 hours after infection.

Staphylococcal infections.

Staphylococci of various kinds have been isolated from the external parts and from the alimentary canal of the fly by various observers, and there can be little doubt that flies can carry these organisms from the pus in which they occur to open sores on healthy individuals.

CHAPTER XIX

NON-BACTERIAL DISEASES

Infantile paralysis or acute anterior poliomyelitis.

Though the precise nature of the virus of this disease has not been demonstrated, Flexner and his colleagues and other observers have shown that it is present in the throat and nose and also sometimes in the intestinal discharges. Flies can, therefore, often gain access to infectious material, and Flexner and Clark (1911) and Howard and Clark (1912) have investigated the subject experimentally. Some experiments by the latter observers are quoted.

"After being allowed to feed on infected cord the flies (*M. domestica*) were placed in fresh receptacles from which certain numbers were removed at intervals, killed with ether, ground up with sand in physiological salt solution, and passed through a Berkefeld filter. The filtrate was injected as usual into the brain of *Macacus rhesus* monkeys." One monkey (*A*) received "3 c.c. of a filtrate of the bodies of 7 flies which had had an opportunity to feed on infected cord for 5 hours, and had then lived in clean surroundings for 24 hours before they were killed." On the sixth day the monkey became weak and showed typical symptoms of the disease on the eighth day, when it was killed. "At autopsy the cord showed the characteristic macroscopic lesions of experimental poliomyelitis. The microscopic sections were also typical." Another monkey (*B*) which had received "4 c.c. of the filtrate of the bodies of 10 flies which had fed on infected cord 48 hours previously," showed marked symptoms on the twelfth day and was killed. "The autopsy showed characteristic lesions of experimental poliomyelitis in the spinal cord, and the sections typical histological lesions." A third monkey (*C*) received "5 c.c. of filtrate representing the viscera of 9 flies which had had an opportunity to feed on infected cord for 18 hours. They were then removed to a clean receptacle for 6 hours, when they were etherized, and their legs, wings and heads removed. The viscera were then taken out with sterile instruments, ground and filtered as usual and injected as above." The animal died with marked symptoms on the 14th day and "at autopsy the gross lesions of the cord were characteristic and the microscopic sections were also typical."

The writers conclude that "the domestic fly (*M. domestica*) can carry the virus of poliomyelitis in an active state for several days upon the surface of the body, and for several hours within the gastro-intestinal tract."

Flexner (1912) who has very closely studied the subject writes as follows: "The preponderance of cases in the late summer and autumn months early suggested an insect carrier of the infection. House-flies can act as passive contaminators, since virus survives on the body and within the gullet of these insects."

The observers quoted have undoubtedly proved that under experimental conditions non-biting flies can convey the virus, but up to the present we have little knowledge of what part they play in the dissemination of the disease. Biting flies, such as *Stomoxys calcitrans*, may also play a part.

Small-pox or *variola.*

The only published account of the possible relation of flies to small-pox is that of Hervieux (1904). He states that Laforque at Tamorna-Djedida, in the Province of Constantine, observed that during an epidemic of small-pox the children who were attacked lived in the south-west of the village, the northern part of the village remaining free from the disease. He thought that this was due to the distribution of flies and mosquitoes by the prevailing wind. Laforque himself believed that flies played an important part in the spread of the virus of small-pox.

Tropical sore.

Hirsch (1886, p. 681) states that Seviziat (1875) believed that this disease might be spread by *winged insects.* Laveran (1880) considered that flies might carry the disease. No recent observations on the subject have been published.

Trypanosomiasis.

It is well known that biting flies of the genus *Glossina* are responsible for the spread of sleeping sickness, the most important human trypanosome disease, and possibly other biting flies may transmit other forms of trypanosomiasis. It appears, however, from Darling's (1912) work that *M. domestica* may be responsible for the spread of a trypanosome disease in mules in the Panama Canal Zone. He found that mules and horses were equally susceptible to the disease, caused by *Tr. hippicum*, but that "when they were stalled together, mules developed the disease, but saddle horses never became infected." "The mules, from the nature of their work, frequently suffered from 'scraper cuts,' galls, and other injuries in which the skin became broken, while such injuries were rarely noted on the saddle horses." Darling thought that flies visiting the excoriated patches carried the disease, and proceeded to confirm his view by experiments.

"Three lots of *Musca domestica* were caught and each was placed in a biting jar. A guinea-pig richly infected with *Trypanosoma hippicum* was bled from the ear. Two or three drops of blood were placed on the centre of a glass plate which was inverted over the biting area of the jar containing the flies. Jar *A* contained about eighteen flies, jar *B* nine, and jar *C* six. A number of the flies in each jar were seen to feed on the guinea-pig's blood, those in jar *A* being hungrier than the others.

"The glass plate with the guinea-pig blood was carefully replaced by a towel that was used to wipe away any possible droplet of blood that might have touched the rim of the jar, or that might have been deposited near the rim by the flies. This was done to prevent any possible inoculation of the mule by guinea-pig blood that might be on the margin of the jar. The towel was replaced by a clean glass plate that was slipped out when the biting area of the jar was placed over the recently shaved, scratched skin of the mule. In each experiment the flies were exposed to the guinea-pig blood for three or four minutes, and then, after an interval of about thirty seconds, were placed over the scratched skin of the mules where they remained for about five minutes. As the flies were not hungry they fed with some difficulty, and, as the experiment was conducted out of doors in bright sunshine, they sought the opposite end of the jar, and could be made to visit the scratched skin only by covering the jar and making it quite dark. On this account the conditions of the experiment were probably not as favourable for infecting as they would have been under natural conditions in a corral, yet after a period of ten days, the usual incubation period in mules for the strain of *Trypanosoma hippicum* employed, the temperature of one of the animals rose to 103° F., and its blood contained *Trypanosoma hippicum*. The other two mules have shown no signs of infection.

"The mule that became infected had been exposed to the flies in jar *A*, which contained about eighteen active, vigorous specimens that had been caught about two hours before the experiment."

The writer points out that as the disease was not epidemic at the time of the experiment the possibility of the mule having become infected in any other way is "too remote to be considered," and further that the strain of trypanosome used had a longer incubation period, namely ten days, than most strains. Also the mules had been under observation several days before the experiment in a screened stable; and their blood had been examined daily.

It is evident that this subject is an important one and requires very careful investigation.

Yaws (*Frambœsia tropica*).

Yaws, which is a contageous and inoculable disease of the tropics, characterized by ulcers of the skin, is caused by an extremely delicate spirochæte, *Sp. pertenuis.*

Bancroft (1769) writing of Guiana, S. America, nearly 150 years ago, made the following remarks. "A small quantity of yellowish pus is common seen adhering to the surface (of the pustules) which is commonly covered with flies through the indolence of the negroes."..."It is usually believed that this disorder is communicated by the flies which have been feasting on the diseased object to those persons who have sores or scratches which are uncovered; and from many observations I think this is not improbable, as none ever receive this disorder whose skins are whole; for which reason the whites are rarely infected; but the backs of negroes, being often raw by whipping, and suffered to remain naked, they scarce ever escape." Wilson (1868) a hundred years later says the belief prevails in the West Indies that the disease is conveyed from one individual to another by flies.

More recently Hirsch (1896), Cadet (1897), Castellani (1907), Robertson (1908) and Nicholls (1912) have all expressed the opinion that, though the disease is usually communicated by direct contact, flies not infrequently distribute it. Hirsch (1896) quotes two very doubtful instances of the disease being carried by flies, but Castellani and Robertson quote investigations by modern methods.

Castellani (1907, p. 567) working in Ceylon thinks that yaws is generally conveyed by actual contact, but under certain conditions may be conveyed by flies and possibly by other insects. "In my opinion, there can be no doubt that in certain cases insects may carry the disease. It is very noticeable that flies eagerly crowd on the open sores of yaws' patients. In the hospitals, as soon as the dressings are removed the yaws' ulcerations become covered with flies sucking with avidity the secretion, which they may afterwards deposit in the same way on ordinary ulcers on other people. Ants are also occasionally found on yaws' ulcerations as well as on ordinary ulcers.

"I may quote some experiments I have made to prove that flies are instrumental in the dissemination of the disease.

"*Experiment I.* Some scrapings were collected from slightly ulcerated papules of a yaws' patient. The *Sp. pertenuis* was present, together with various other thicker spirochætes (*Sp. obtusa*; *Sp. acuminata*), but no bacteria. The scrapings were placed in a sterile Petri dish. Ten flies (*Musca domestica* and allied species), caught in the rooms of the Bacteriological Institute, were placed inside the Petri dish, and left there for half an hour. They fed greedily on the material; then their mouth parts and legs were examined for spirochætes, extracts and films being made: in nine flies the spirochætes of the thicker type were found; in two also the *Sp. pertenuis*. As a control five flies were caught the same day, in the same room and examined at once, with negative results as regards the presence of spirochætes.

"*Experiment II.* Twenty flies were collected from the rooms of the Bacteriological Institute. The buccal apparatus and legs of five were removed and examined by making extracts and films: no spirochætes of any kind were present. The other 15 flies were divided into several groups and placed on various semi-ulcerated papules of three yaws' patients presenting the *Sp. pertenuis*, and spirochætes of the thicker type which are often found in semi-ulcerated lesions. The flies were kept in place by covering the papules with a piece of gauze made to adhere to the skin by means of collodion all round the margin. After two hours the mouth parts were removed, extracts and films made and stained. Out of 15 flies so examined, in 14 it was possible to detect the coarse spirochætes, and in two, the *Sp. pertenuis*, as well as the thicker ones.

Transmission of Yaws to monkeys by means of flies fed on Yaws' material.

"*Experiment III.* Thirty flies were fed in a sterile Petri dish for half an hour on scrapings from non-ulcerated papules of a case of yaws, containing only the *Sp. pertenuis.* Three *Semnopithecus priamus* and two *Macacus pileatus* were then infected in this way; over the left eyebrow of each monkey, very numerous deep scarifications were made; then five flies, deprived of their wings, were applied to the scarified spots and kept there by means of a piece of gauze smeared with collodion at the margins; the monkeys were prevented from removing the gauze by tying their legs. After two hours the gauze and flies were removed. Of these monkeys, one *Semnop. priamus* after 45 days developed a small infiltrated spot, which soon became enlarged and covered with a thick crust. The microscopical examination of the lesion showed the presence of *Sp. pertenuis*. The other four monkeys gave negative results.

"*Experiment IV.* Twenty-eight flies (*Musca domestica* and similar species) were caught in one of the rooms of the Bacteriological Institute. The legs and buccal organs of five were removed and examined for spirochætes, numerous preparations being made, with negative results. The remaining flies, deprived of their wings, were placed on two slightly ulcerated lesions of a yaws' patient. The flies were kept on the ulcers by means of pieces of gauze, the margins of which were made to adhere to the skin with a little collodion. The flies readily sucked the secretion of the ulcers. After one hour the flies were removed. Meanwhile seven *Semnopithecus priamus* had been deeply scarified over their eyebrows, and several flies which had fed on the ulcerated yaws' lesions were placed on the scarified areas of each monkey and kept in place there for two hours by using the device already described.

"One of the monkeys, 46 days later, developed a slightly infiltrated spot, which slowly enlarged into a frambœtic nodule covered with a thick crust; the microscopical examination of films taken from this nodule showed the presence of *Sp. pertenuis*. In another monkey, 67 days after inoculation, three tiny papules developed at the place of inoculation; they soon fused together into an infiltrated mass covered by a thick crust. Films made from scrapings of the lesion contained the *Sp. pertenuis*. The remaining five monkeys have given negative results."

Robertson (1908) asked patients in a yaws' house in Tarawa Hospital to catch the flies settling on yaws' lesions, and to place them in sterile glass jars which were given to them. Later the jars were filled with sterile water and well shaken. After standing for 24 hours the water was centrifugalized and smears made from the precipitate. About 200 flies were used, and in four slides "well-formed examples of *Spirochæte pertenuis* of Castellani" were found.

Nicholls (1912) working in St Lucia, Windward Islands, made the following statement: "I believe that the majority of cases of yaws (frambœsia) in the West Indies are caused by the inoculation of surface injuries by this fly (*Oscinis pallipes*). They feed only on the skin discharges of man and other animals, and though rare in the town of Castries, they are very numerous in the country districts of St Lucia, and can be seen hovering round the bare legs and arms of labourers, searching for abrasions or the secretions of the sweat and sebaceous glands. The persistence of these little flies is extraordinary; they must be brushed off by actually touching them, and they will immediately return. If undisturbed, they engorge themselves with pus, blood, serum or sebaceous secretion, until their abdomens are greatly distended."

SUMMARY.

All observers agree that flies swarm round the ulcers of yaws, and some consider them to be important agents in spreading the disease. It is remarkable, however, that Castellani's experiments, which appear to have been carried out under ideal conditions for fly infection, only yielded a small proportion of positive results. Further careful investigations and experiments are required.

CHAPTER XX

ON THE PART PLAYED BY FLIES IN THE DISPERSAL OF THE EGGS OF PARASITIC WORMS

Experiments.

Grassi (1883) was the first to demonstrate that flies could ingest the eggs of parasitic worms (*Tænia solium*, and *Oxyuris*), and that these eggs could pass through their intestines, and be deposited in the fæces apparently unaltered and undamaged. By placing sheets of white paper on the floor on which the flies defæcated he showed that the flies could deposit the eggs of *Trichocephalus* 10 metres from the place at which they had fed. Stiles (1889) "placed the larvæ of *Musca* with female *Ascaris lumbricoides*, which they devoured, together with the eggs they contained. The larvæ, grubs, as also the adult flies, contained the eggs of *Ascaris*. The experiment being made in very hot weather, the Ascaris eggs developed rapidly, and were found in different stages of development in the insects, thus proving that the latter may serve as disseminators of the parasite" (Nuttall and Jepson, 1909, p. 28). Galli-Valerio (1905) found that flies could carry on the surface of their bodies, not only the eggs but also the larvæ of *Necator americanus.* Calandruccio (1906) observed a number of flies, which had fed on material containing the eggs of *Hymenolepis nana*, deposit fæces containing the eggs on sugar. A girl who had eaten some of this sugar was found twenty-seven days later to be infected with the tape-worm. Other sources of infection were carefully excluded. Léon (1908) fed flies on honey mixed with the eggs of *Dibothriocephalus latus*, and found the eggs in their fæces.

Nicoll (1911) has carried out by far the most extensive investigations on this subject, experimenting with ten different species of parasites infesting men or animals.

Nature and life-history of parasitic worms.

"In order to indicate the precise relationship which flies and other insects may bear to the dissemination of parasitic worms, it may be advisable here to recapitulate briefly the principal facts which are known concerning the mode of life and means of transmission of these worms. They belong to three principal classes, namely Trematodes or flukes, Cestodes or tape-worms and Nematodes or round-worms. These worms in their adult state live for the most part in the alimentary canal of vertebrate animals. Practically speaking all tape-worms live in the intestine, the great majority of round-worms and flukes live in the intestine, stomach or œsophagus, but certain varieties live in the lungs, the liver, the kidneys, the bladder, the blood and lymphatic vessels. In whatever situation they live, however, they all possess the common characteristic of being unable to multiply without some intermediate external influence. They all produce a large number (in many cases an enormous number) of eggs, but before the latter can grow into adult worms, they must pass part of their life outside their host under certain definite conditions, which vary according to the particular kind of worm. In most cases the eggs are conveyed out of the body in the fæces, in some cases in the urine or expectoration. Some tape-worms throw off a segment containing eggs, which may pass out independently of the fæces. The chief exceptions to this method are the *Filaria* worms and their allies. With these, however, the present investigation is not concerned. The conveyance of the eggs to the outside is only a short stage in the life of the parasite. Thereafter a more or less lengthy and complicated career awaits them before they are suited to re-infect their original host. This portion of their life-history follows one of two broad lines: 1. The egg develops and in time produces a larva, which may be retained in the egg-shell or set free, but in either case the larva is ready to re-infect. 2. The egg gives rise to a larva which enters an animal (intermediate host) different from that in which the egg was produced. In this second animal it passes a short part of its life and, in the event of this animal being devoured by the first, the parasite is enabled to complete its life-cycle and cause infection again.

"The avenue by which the first animal is infected is in the great majority of cases its food; in a few instances it may be infected by the larva penetrating its skin. It is evident, therefore, that there must be some means by which the food is contaminated with excremental matter in the first of the above-mentioned categories, and, in the second, some means by which the eggs of the parasite are conveyed to the second animal. Water is by far the most important vehicle of transit. A certain amount of moisture is necessary for the development of the eggs although many of them can resist drying for long periods. In closely-associated communities, however, mechanical transit on the feet of individual animals is a common mode of dispersing the eggs. It is here that the agency of flies has to be reckoned with, especially such flies as divide their attention between excremental matter and food-stuffs. The common house-fly is well known to have such habits and it is thus with reason that it has been suspected of conveying the eggs of parasites from fæcal material to food. There are many flies, other than *Musca domestica*, which display like habits, and though they do not bear such a close relationship to man several of them are commonly associated with the domesticated animals.

"With regard to their life-histories, the parasites of man may be divided into two classes, excluding the *Filaria* worms, and mentioning only the best known species, as follows:

I. Those not requiring an intermediate host.

(*a*) Those in which the larval worm remains within the egg-shell.

Ascaris lumbricoides.
Toxascaris limbata.
Belascaris mystax.
Oxyuris vermicularis.
Trichuris trichiurus.
Hymenolepis nana.

(*b*) Those in which the larva is liberated from the egg-shell and spends its life in water.

Ankylostoma duodenale.
Necator americanus.
Schistosomum hæmatobium.
Schistosomum japonicum.

II. Those requiring an intermediate host.

(*a*) Those encysting in animals which are commonly eaten by man.

Trichinella spiralis in the pig.
Tænia solium in the pig.
Tænia saginata in the ox.
Dibothriocephalus latus in fresh-water fishes.

(*b*) Those encysting in animals which may be swallowed accidentally by man.

Fasciola hepatica in pond snails and eventually on grass.
Dicrocœlium lanceatum in slugs and pond snails.
Hymenolepis diminuta in fleas and other insects.
Dipylidium caninum in fleas.

"There are several other common human parasites of which the life-history is entirely unknown. Of those in the above list, the mode of infection of *Schistosomum hæmatobium* has not been definitely proved, but it is probably similar to that of *Schistosomum japonicum*, the free-swimming larva of which is capable of infecting directly. *Trichinella spiralis* is peculiar in being viviparous and its larvæ are shed into the blood-stream or lymphatics. The house-fly can therefore take no part in its dissemination. The species in II (*b*) are, as might be expected, but very occasional parasites of man.

"In addition to the above-mentioned worms of which man is the final or adult host, there are a few others for which man figures as the intermediate host. By far the most important of these is *Tænia echinococcus*, a tape-worm of the dog, the larva of which gives rise to hydatid disease. Man is also an intermediate host of *Tænia solium* and *Trichinella spiralis*.

"It is evident from this short summary of the life-histories that the only parasites with which it is possible that flies can directly infect man are those in Section I, along with *Tænia echinococcus* and *T. solium*. In other cases and in the case of *Tænia solium* also, the infection is conveyed to some other animal, e.g. pig, ox, etc. The nature of the problem is therefore not the same in every instance."

The nature and size of the eggs of parasitic worms.

"These factors have an important bearing on the present question, for it is obvious the eggs must bear some definite proportion to the vehicle which carries them. In most cases the eggs are ovoid in shape. Sometimes they are more elongated, and become almost spindle-shaped. Frequently they are nearly globular. Occasionally they are cuboid while a few other shapes occur more rarely. Appendages are not uncommon. They may take the form of slight roughnesses or small knobs scattered irregularly over the surface of the shell. There may be a small spike projecting from one end, or from the side. In some cases one end of the shell tapers to a point and is prolonged as a spiral filament, which may be much longer than the egg itself. In certain other cases there may be button-like projections from either end of the shell.

"The shell may be of various degrees of thickness and hardness. In some cases it is quite thin and transparent, in others it is much thicker and opaque. In most cases it possesses a considerable amount of flexibility, so that it can be compressed to a certain extent without breaking. In this way a globular egg can be pressed into an ovoid shape. This is of importance in relation to the ingestion of eggs by flies.

"The general surface of the shell may be either smooth or slightly roughened. It is usually covered by a layer of mucus when it is being extruded by the worm, and it may receive an additional coating of mucus in the intestine of the host. This imparts to it a certain degree of adhesiveness. In some cases the eggs are laid in batches surrounded by a gelatinous or mucous investment.

"The size of the eggs varies in different worms. They are rarely smaller than ·01 mm. or larger than ·15 mm. in length. The breadth is most commonly half to two-thirds the length. Even in the same worm the eggs vary considerably in size although they usually approximate towards a definite size and shape, which is more or less characteristic for the species. On that account the eggs of most species of human parasites can be recognized very readily. In the following list the parasites of man are arranged according to the size of their ova, the sizes given being approximate averages. They are divided into three sections, the first of which contains those whose eggs do not exceed ·045 mm. in both diameters, the second comprises those with eggs of which the breadth is less than ·045 mm., while in the third the minimum diameter exceeds ·045 mm. The reason for this division is, as will appear later, that *Musca domestica* is apparently unable to ingest particles of larger size than about ·045 mm.

		Length	Breadth
I.	Opisthorcis felineus	·030 ...	·010
	Clonorchis sinensis	·025 ...	·015
	Heterophyes heterophyes ...	·030 ...	·015
	Opisthorcis noverca	·035 ...	·020
	Oxyuris vermicularis ...	·050 ...	·020
	Tænia saginata	·035 ...	·025
	Trichuris trichiurus	·050 ...	·025
	Tænia solium	·035 ...	·030
	Tænia echinococcus ...	·035 ...	·030
	Dicrocœlium lanceatum ...	·040 ...	·030

		Length.	Breadth.
	Hymenolepis nana	·040 ...	·040
	Dipylidium caninum ...	·040 ...	·040
	Davainea madagascarensis ...	·040 ...	·040
II.	Ankylostoma duodenale ...	·060 ...	·040
	Ternidens diminutus ...	·060 ...	·040
	Necator americanus ...	·065 ...	·040
	Trichostrongylus subtilis ...	·065 ...	·040
	Schistosomum japonicum ...	·075 ...	·040
	Ascaris lumbricoides ...	·060 ...	·045
	Eustrongylus gigas	·065 ...	·045
	Dibothriocephalus latus ...	·070 ...	·045
	Schistosomum hæmatobium	·115 ...	·045
III.	Diplogonoporus grandis ...	·065 ...	·050
	Dibothriocephalus cordatus	·075 ...	·050
	Hymenolepis diminuta ...	·070 ...	·065
	Paragonimus westermanni ...	·090 ...	·065
	Belascaris mystax	·075 ...	·070
	Toxascaris limbata	·080 ...	·070
	Gastrodiscus hominis ...	·150 ...	·070
	Fasciolopsis buski	·125 ...	·075
	Fasciola hepatica	·130 ...	·080

"The resistance of eggs to external conditions is also of importance. All do not withstand similar conditions equally well. For many, moisture is absolutely essential, and in its absence they rapidly die. This is true for the eggs of practically all Trematode worms. Many of these can survive only in sea water, others only in fresh water, and changes in the composition of the water affect them injuriously. Drying is usually fatal within a few hours; the shell becomes crumpled and shrivelled up, the embryo dies and the subsequent application of moisture does not resuscitate it. On the other hand, eggs of some tape-worms and round-worms can survive desiccation for comparatively lengthy periods. For instance, I have kept the eggs of *Hymenolepis diminuta* in dry powdered fæces for as long as 17 days, at the end of which time many of them were still alive. In the presence of even a small amount of moisture, other conditions being suitable, the eggs of most parasitic worms will remain alive for a great length of time. Thus it is stated by Davaine that the eggs of *Trichuris trichiurus* may remain alive for as long as five years. With regard to other conditions, temperature is probably the most important. A fairly high temperature (80—90° F.) hastens development, but temperature much above that will destroy the eggs in many cases. Continued exposure to cold is also fatal, although freezing, if not too prolonged, is not necessarily fatal. Little information, however, is available on this point except in regard to a few species.

The feeding of flies and their larvæ in relation to the ingestion of eggs.

"It is a matter of common observation that fresh and moist fæces attract flies much more readily than old and dried fæces. Flies feed on warm fresh fæces with considerable avidity, and they will do so even although they have been previously feeding on other material. To flies which have not fed for some time the presence of fresh human fæces acts as an immediate source of attraction, and in some of my experiments the eagerness with which they attacked it was most striking. When the portion of fæces was so small that all the flies could not find standing room upon it or around it, they struggled together and pushed each other aside, and more than once I have seen them so closely packed together that each fly could find room for only the tip of its proboscis, the flies on top practically 'standing on their heads,' supported by the bodies of those around. Their behaviour towards older fæces, however, is very different. When the material has become cold it does not attract flies nearly so readily. So long as it remains moist it continues to attract and does so quite as much as moist bread, although very much less so than moist sugar. When it has become dry it possesses little or no attraction, but this is increased when it is moistened again. It is evident therefore that the presence of moisture plays an important part in a fly's attitude towards fæces as an article of food.

"When the alternatives of fresh fæces, sugar and bread were offered, the flies did not confine their attention to any one of these articles, but made repeated excursions from one to the other.

"Some interesting observations were made in regard to flies feeding on segments of tape-worms. As already mentioned, such segments may be deposited along with fæces or independently, and in the case of several tape-worms their eggs are conveyed to the exterior in this way instead of being shed singly into the gut. In the course of the present experiments it was rather surprising to find that such segments possessed a great attraction for flies. When an intact segment of a tape-worm (*Tænia serrata*, *Tænia marginata*, *Dipylidium caninum*) mixed with moderately fresh fæces was presented to some flies they appeared to select the tape-worm and feed upon it in preference to the fæces. The observation was made on several occasions. Further when an isolated tape-worm segment, some fæces and some sugar, were separately introduced into the fly cage, the flies showed a decided preference for the tape-worm, which they attacked with much assiduity. This trait was displayed not only when the tape-worm was in a fresh state, but even when it had lain for a day or longer. Tape-worms usually possess a faint characteristic, musty odour, but whether it is this or simply the juicy nature of the body which proves the attraction, it is, at present, impossible to say.

"The action of flies feeding on tape-worms was studied in close detail. Applying their proboscis to the surface of the worm they suck with considerable vigour for as long as half a minute on end. Having selected a spot they continue there for some time. From time to time a small drop of fluid was seen to be extruded from the proboscis, and this apparently was used to moisten the surface of the worm. The vigorous sucking efforts were kept up, with intermissions, for several hours. Flies examined within two or three hours after the beginning of such an experiment were found to have very little fluid in their crops, which contained, however, numerous large bubbles of air. Later, when the flies had been feeding on the tape-worm for 5—10 hours their crops were found greatly distended with white milky juice recognizable as the juice of the tape-worm. In such flies, too, several tape-worm eggs were found in the intestine. It is evident, therefore, that house-flies, although they possess no piercing or biting mouth-parts, are able in course of time to penetrate the fairly tough external covering of tape-worms and to extract the internal contents. In this they are helped to a considerable extent by the fact that tape-worms undergo a process of decomposition (autolysis) independent of putrefaction. This is further hastened by the action of putrefactive bacteria. Dead tape-worms will remain soft and 'juicy' for 48 hours after exposure to the air. Later their fluids evaporate and they begin to shrivel up and become dark brown in colour. Living tape-worms or their segments will remain alive on exposure to air for two or three days, and in suitable media (saline solution, etc.), they may be kept alive for over a week. There can be little doubt, therefore, that living tape-worm segments when expelled from their host may remain a source of attraction to flies for several days.

" Similar observations were made in the case of round-worms (*Toxascaris limbata, Ascaris megalocephala*). These appeared to possess much less attraction for flies. Not infrequently they were attacked with some readiness and in the same manner as tape-worms. The extremely thick cuticular investment of round-worms, however, is much more resistant than the covering of tape-worms, and in no case were the flies able to penetrate this even after the lapse of three or four days, by which time the worms had become dry and shrivelled up.

" It seems worthy of note that solid particles were rarely found in the crops of flies dissected in the course of these experiments. The intestine, however, except in flies which have been feeding for several days on nothing but fluid food, invariably contains a large number of particles. After feeding on fæces, for instance, the intestine becomes filled with the debris of which the fæces are composed, but none of this is found in the crop. The particles met with are of various sizes and irregular shapes, but they rarely exceed ·04 mm. in diameter. It would thus appear that when flies feed on fluids or soluble solids such as sugar, the food is first sucked into the crop, and when this is full it passes into the intestine directly, as noted by Graham-Smith. Insoluble solid food, however, is probably taken directly into the intestine. This suggests that the fly is able to exercise some voluntary control over the passage of food into the crop or the intestine respectively.

"The feeding of fly larvæ was studied specially in regard to their behaviour towards round-worms. The voracity with which larval flies feed is well known, and the increase in their size from day to day is remarkable. They appear to be as omnivorous as adult flies. When fresh round-worms were offered to the larvæ, they were at once attacked. The larvæ swarmed over the worms, nibbling at them with great vigour. They seemed, however, quite unable to penetrate the tough cuticle unless there were a crack or a small tear, and, if other food were not provided, the larvæ died. On the other hand, when the worms were cut or broken before being introduced, the larvæ devoured the internal parts with extraordinary rapidity. Starting at one end of a broken piece, they would eat their way right through to the other end leaving nothing but a tube of cuticle. In this way half a dozen larvæ would devour, within two or three days, a large worm 20 or 30 times their own bulk. On examining larvæ which had fed on female egg-bearing worms, large numbers of eggs were found surrounding the larvæ but not actually sticking to them. On examining the intestine of the larvæ no intact eggs were ever found, but numerous fragments of shells were always recognizable. No embryonic worms in any stage were seen. From these experiments I am convinced that even full grown larvæ are unable to swallow unruptured eggs as large as those of the worms used (·07 mm.).

Methods.

"The common house-fly, *Musca domestica*, was used almost exclusively. Only a few experiments were made with the lesser house-fly, *Fannia canicularis*, and the blow-fly, *Calliphora erythrocephala*. In most cases the flies were obtained from the surrounding locality, but artificially-reared flies were used on several occasions.

"For the experiments a large cage was constructed. All the sides were made of perforated zinc, except one, which consisted of a large sheet of plate-glass; this was fixed in two grooves and could be removed. The bottom was of plain zinc. The dimensions of the cage were 3 ft. × 1½ ft. × 1 ft. It was divided into two by a partition of perforated zinc in which was a sliding panel, by which communication could be made between the two compartments. Each compartment was further furnished with a sliding door at the bottom of one side for the admission of flies, and another door at the top, through which they could be removed. For the latter purpose a small square cage with a sliding door was used. This fitted the door in the top of the large cage, and the two sliding panels could be drawn out simultaneously. The object of the cage was to afford the flies as much space, light and air as possible, and it was found that they could be kept alive in it for over a month. The plate-glass side was of use in allowing the experiments to be accurately watched. A few experiments were conducted in a large bell-jar, and in a considerable number of cases glass chimneys, similar to those described by Graham-Smith (1910) were employed.

"Infective material was offered to the flies in four different ways: 1. Fæces containing ova. 2. Complete worms or intact parts of them. 3. Broken or damaged segments of worms. 4. Suspensions of ova in water.

"The flies which were removed for examination were killed with chloroform vapour. Their bodies and legs were examined for eggs. The legs and wings having been removed, the body was carefully washed in order to get rid of any adhering eggs. The intestine, ventriculus and crop were then dissected out separately. No eggs were ever found in the crop, so that the positive results in the following records refer to the intestine or ventriculus only."

The carriage of eggs in the intestine of the fly.

Nicoll's results which are carefully set out in tables, showing the times at which the flies were examined, may be tabulated in the following way.

TABLE 30. *Showing the results of feeding experiments with adult flies.*

Parasite	No. of flies used	No. of flies negative	No. of flies in which eggs found	Examinations of fly fæces
Hymenolepis diminuta ...	35	35	0	0
Toxascaris limbata ...	20	20	0	0
Ankylostoma caninum ...	8	8	0	0
Trichuris trichiurus ...	12	11	1 (8%)	+
Tænia marginata ...	16	12	4 (25%)	−
Dipylidium caninum ...	11	7	4 (36%)	−
Tænia serrata	46	28	18 (39%)	+

In most of these experiments curiously uneven results were obtained. For example in one series of experiments seven flies were fed on ruptured segments of *T. serrata* and 400 ova were found in the intestines of two flies, two ova in one fly and none in the other four. A possible explanation of this phenomenon has already been given (p. 66).

Nicoll concludes "that *M. domestica* is quite unable to ingest eggs as large as those of *Hymenolepis diminuta*." The fly, however, "can suck out" the eggs of *D. caninum* and carry them for at least 43 hours in its intestine. The eggs of *T. marginata* "are fairly readily ingested not only by Musca but also by *Fannia canicularis*," and may be found in the intestines of the flies after an interval of nearly three days.

The longest and most important series of experiments were carried out with *T. serrata* and show "unmistakably that *Musca domestica* can quite readily ingest the ova of *Tænia serrata*, not only from the fæces, but also from intact segments of the worm." The eggs when suspended in a liquid may be ingested in enormous numbers, as many as 312 having been found in one fly. "Large numbers can remain in the intestine of the fly for one or two days, without visible change." By feeding experiments Nicoll showed that young rabbits may be infected by ova received from flies, and he further demonstrated "the very important fact that fæces containing tape-worm segments may continue to be a source of infection, from which such food as sugar may be contaminated (by flies), for as long as a fortnight."

The body and legs as carriers of eggs.

Nicoll also investigated the length of time during which eggs may adhere to the body and legs. "On flies caught during the act of feeding, or immediately afterwards, I have found numerous particles of fairly large size, and in many instances the eggs of parasites as large as those of *Ascaris megalocephala*. These were found chiefly on the distal segments of the legs and on the proboscis. When, however, the flies were allowed to clean themselves before being examined, few particles were found and only occasionally were eggs observed. On examining the spot where flies had rested while cleaning themselves, eggs were found quite frequently. Apparently, therefore, the eggs are got rid of at the spot where the fly first alights after feeding. How far flies can convey eggs in this way depends on the distance they may traverse in their first flight after feeding. In the experimental cage I was only able to demonstrate this up to a distance of three feet." When they have finished feeding flies usually walk a short distance away to a convenient dry spot, or, especially if disturbed, they fly off to the nearest place of safety. They generally do not fly to a great distance under such circumstances. Occasionally eggs which have been rubbed off may again adhere to the fly. Nicoll showed that the longest interval after which eggs were found adhering to flies was about three hours.

"The possibility of flies in this way contaminating food was demonstrated by allowing some to feed on fæces containing eggs of *Hymenolepis diminuta*, and subsequently affording them access to some moist sugar placed at the other end of the experimental cage. After 24 hours the sugar was examined and found to contain a few eggs. Now, as has already been shown, the eggs of *Hymenolepis diminuta* are too large to be ingested by the fly, so that in this experiment they must have been carried on the legs or body."

Feeding experiments with larvæ.

Larvæ were allowed to feed on ripe segments of *Tænia serrata*, and some of them were examined from time to time. In some the ova were found but in every case broken. Flies which hatched did not contain eggs or larvæ of the parasite. Larvæ allowed to feed on dog fæces containing mature female *Toxascaris limbata*, and on horse fæces containing female *Ascaris megalocephala* with numerous eggs did not show eggs in their intestines. Nicoll, therefore, concludes from these experiments, which were repeated several times, "that the eggs are not transmitted through the larvæ to the fly." He points out that these results are "entirely at variance" with the already quoted observation of Stiles in the case of *Ascaris lumbricoides*.

'Wild' flies.

Nicholls (1912) in St Lucia made observations on *Limosina punctipennis*, which he considers as "by far the most objectionable" of all the flies he investigated "as on every occasion on which it was caught its abdomen was found to be distended with pure fæcal matter." "In 26 out of 100 specimens, taken in different situations," he obtained the ova of the worms *Ascaris lumbricoides*, *Necator americanus*, or *Trichocephalus dispar*.

SUMMARY.

It is evident from the investigations which have been quoted that house-flies and other species are greatly attracted to the ova of parasitic worms contained in fæces and other materials, and make great efforts to ingest them. Unless the ova are too large they often succeed, and the eggs are deposited uninjured in their fæces, in some cases up to the third day at least. The eggs may also be carried on their legs or bodies. Under suitable conditions food and fluids may be contaminated with the eggs of various parasitic worms by flies, and in one case infection of the human subject has been observed. Fæces containing tape-worm segments may continue to be a source of infection for as long as a fortnight. Up to the present, however, there is no evidence to show what part flies play in the dissemination of parasitic worms under natural conditions.

CHAPTER XXI

INFECTION BY NON-BITING FLIES OF THE WOUNDS CAUSED BY BITING FLIES

Patton seems to have been the first to recognize that the wounds produced by biting flies might be infected subsequently through the agency of non-biting flies. His observations relate to a species of Indian Musca, named by Austen (1910) *M. pattoni*. "This fly has peculiar habits, in that it sucks the blood which oozes from the bites inflicted on cattle by *Hæmatopota*, and other Tabanids, *Stomoxys*, and *Philæmatomyia*. It likewise sucks the juice out of vaccine vesicles of calves, and also the blood after the vesicles are scraped. The species breeds in cow dung and its pupæ are *dirty white*."

Musca pattoni.

Austen (1910) gives the following description of this fly:

"*Length of ♂ 5·6 to 8·5 mm., ♀ 6·8 to 7·8 mm.; width of head ♂ 2·4 to 3 mm.; ♀ 2·8 mm.; length of wing ♂ 5·4 to 7·6 mm., ♀ 6·25 mm.*

"*Eyes in ♂ almost in contact in centre of front, separated by little more than the greatest width of stoutest thoracic macrochæta; side of face in ♂, and of lower part of front, viewed from above, brilliantly white; front in ♀ of moderate width, its sides (parafrontals) each at least half as broad, or more than half as broad, as frontal stripe; thorax bronze-black, greyish or yellowish-grey pollinose, dorsum longitudinally striped as in M. domestica L., median grey stripe rather brighter in front; abdomen ochraceous-buff, or buff, with shimmering yellowish pollinose patches, and on dorsum a clove-brown or black median stripe, at least on second and third segments, and a more or less conspicuous and often triangular clove-brown mark on apex of fourth segment; in ♀ extreme hind margins of second and third segments also clove-brown on dorsum; wings hyaline; legs black.*

"*Head:* ground colour blackish-grey pollinose, side of front in ♀ with a slight yellowish tinge, distinctly grey right up to vertex when viewed somewhat from behind, posterior orbits conspicuous above (yellowish-grey) in ♀, but disappearing above in ♂; occiput black; frontal stripe black in ♀, decidedly narrower than in ♀ of *M. domestica* L., the sides being slightly curved; first and second joints of antennæ black or blackish, third joint clove-brown, shimmering grey or yellowish-grey, elongate, relatively narrower and distinctly larger than in *M. domestica*, arista (except buff band behind thickened portion) and its hairs clove-brown, all hairs and bristles on head, as also on body and legs, black. *Thorax:* dark stripes on dorsum narrower in ♀ than in ♂, in which sex the two dark stripes on each side of the median grey stripe are sometimes more or less confluent; median grey stripe on dorsum usually decidedly broader than each admedian dark stripe; scutellum sometimes entirely yellowish-grey pollinose, but when viewed from behind showing a bronze-black apical spot, which may be prolonged into a broad median longitudinal stripe. *Abdomen:* bright shimmering yellowish pollinose patches on dorsum not visible on first segment, but on the three following segments very conspicuous when viewed from certain directions, and varying in shape according to the angle from which they are seen; second and third segments each with a longitudinal elongate rectangular pollinose patch on each side of dark median stripe; on the fourth segment these patches coalesce into one; a transversely elongate, semi-rectangular or partially ovate pollinose patch on each side of the second, third and fourth segment; latero-ventrally these lateral patches curve round and reach the inner ventral edges of the dorsal scutes; extreme base of dorsum of first segment, beneath scutellum, clove-brown or black in ♂ connected by a clove-brown mark with median stripe on second segment; median stripe usually only about half as wide on third as on second segment, and often somewhat expanded on anterior margin of latter; hind border of third segment, a larger or smaller area on each side of this segment sometimes more or less infuscated in ♂; dark mark on apex of fourth segment sometimes connected with anterior margin, thus forming a continuation of the median stripe; hypopygium of ♂ blackish, greyish pollinose. *Alar squama* in ♂ cream coloured, *thoracic squama* in ♂ cream-buff; *squamæ* in ♀ waxen white. *Legs:* coxæ, posterior surface of front femora, and a streak on under surface of middle femora, bright grey pollinose."

Distinguishing features.

"From *Musca domestica* L., *M. pattoni* can be distinguished, *inter alia*, by its usually larger size, stouter habit of body, much narrower front in the male, the greater breadth of the sides of the front in the female, and the more sharply defined median stripe in the abdomen in both sexes. The fact that the first segment of the abdomen is in both sexes for the most part ochraceous-buff or buff, instead of entirely or for the most part black or bronze-black, will serve to distinguish *Musca pattoni* from *M. corvina* Fabr., and other species closely allied thereto. From *Musca nebulo* Fabr.—which, according to Captain Patton, is 'the common *Musca* of Madras, breeds in horse dung and other refuse, particularly in night soil, and has a reddish-brown pupa'—*M. pattoni* differs, *inter alia*, in its much larger size, in the front of the male being only half or less than half as wide, and in the presence of the clove-brown mark on the apex of the fourth abdominal segment. In *M. nebulo* the fourth segment of the abdomen, or at least its apex, is entirely pale."

CHAPTER XXII

MYIASIS

The term, myiasis, signifies the presence of dipterous larvæ in the living body, whether of man or animals, as well as the disorders, whether accompanied or not by the destruction of tissue, caused thereby. Though not strictly coming within this definition the sucking of blood by larvæ through punctures of the skin, which they themselves produce, may be included for the sake of convenience in classification.

Myiasis in man may be produced by dipterous larvæ

(*A*) Sucking blood through punctures in the skin

Auchmeromyia luteola.

(*B*)	Deposited in natural cavities of the body	*Chrysomyia.* *Lucilia.* *Sarcophaga.* *Calliphora.* *Œstrus.*
(*C*)	Deposited in neglected wounds ...	*Chrysomyia.* *Lucilia.* *Sarcophaga.* *Calliphora.*
(*D*)	Living in subcutaneous tissue ...	*Cordylobia.* *Dermatobia.* *Bengalia* (?). *Hypoderma.*
(*E*)	Passing through the alimentary canal	*Fannia.* *Musca.* *Eristalis.* *Syrphus.* *Gastrophilus.*

In the above list only the more common genera producing myiasis are mentioned. In England type *E* is fairly common, and types *B* and *C* are occasionally observed.

A. Blood-sucking larvæ.

The only dipterous larva, known to suck blood, is the 'Congo floor maggot,' which is widely distributed in both tropical and sub-tropical Africa. Lelean (I. 1904) described both the fly (*Auchmeromyia luteola*) and the maggot, and shortly afterwards Dutton, Todd and Christy (1904) gave a more detailed account of the life-history of this insect, and pointed out that in its larval stage it is a keen blood-sucker :—"When visiting a native village, we had the opportunity of seeing the natives collect these blood-suckers by digging with the point of a knife or scraping with a sharpened stick in the dust-filled cracks and crevices of the mud floors of their huts. We were soon able to find them ourselves as easily as the natives, and unearthed many larvæ which contained bright red blood. In collecting them the natives selected those huts in which the occupants slept on floor mats, saying that where people slept on beds or raised platforms the maggots were not so numerous." In some huts they collected twenty maggots from a small area of the floor. The natives think the maggot can jump some inches from the floor, but no evidence in support of this view has been obtained. Dutton, Todd and Christy describe the larva, which reaches the length of 15 mm., as follows:

"It is semi-transparent, of a dirty white colour, acephalous and amphipneustic. It resembles, when adult, the larva of bot-flies, and consists of eleven very distinct segments. The first or anterior one is divisible, owing to a slight constriction, into two portions, the foremost of which is small, bears the mouth parts, and is capable of protrusion and retraction to a considerable extent.

"The larva is broadest at the ninth and tenth segments, is roughly ovoid in section, and is distinctly divided into dorsal and ventral surfaces. At the junction of the two surfaces is a row of irregular protuberances, two or more being placed on each segment. On each protuberance is a small posteriorly directed spine and a small pit. The central part of the ventral surface is flattened, and at the posterior margin of each segment is a set of three foot pads, transversely arranged, each covered with small spines directed backwards. These aid the larvæ in their movements, which are fairly rapid and peculiar, in that the mouth parts are protruded to the utmost and the tentacula fixed, as a purchase, first on one side then on the other, while a wave of contraction runs along the body as each segment is contracted and brought forward.

"The last segment is larger than any of the others. Its upper surface is flattened and looks backwards and upwards at an angle of about 45° with the longitudinal axis of the larva. This surface is roughly hexagonal and bears anteriorly, one on either side, the posterior spiracles, which are seen with a pocket magnifying glass as three transverse, parallel brown lines. Around this flattened surface, towards its border, are placed groups of rather prominent spines. The ventral surface of the segment is also flattened, and is thrown into folds by muscular contractions. The anus is situated in the anterior portion of this segment in the middle line, and is seen as a longitudinal slit surrounded by a low ridge. Posterior to it and on either side is a long conspicuous spine. The anterior segment is roughly conical and bears the mouth parts in front. Posteriorly, on the dorsal surface, almost covered by the second segment, two spiracles, one on either side, are seen with a low power as small brown spots. Two black hooks, or tentacula, protrude from the apex of the segment. They are curved towards the ventral surface of the maggot. The apex of each hook is blunt, and its base surrounded by a fleshy ring. Between them is the oral orifice. The tentacular processes are continued for some distance into the body of the maggot as black chitinous structures with expanded bases. There is probably, as is *Œstrus ovis*, Linn., an articulation between the external and internal chitinous structures, since the arrangement of the mouth parts seems to be the same as in the maggot of that fly. Paired groups of minute spicular teeth are placed around the two tentacula so as to form a sort of cupping instrument. The arrangement of these teeth is as follows: A rather large tubercle is situated on either side of and above the tentacula ; each is surmounted by two or more groups of very small chitinous teeth. Just above each tentaculum is another small group of teeth. On either side of the black tentacula two irregular rows of small teeth are placed one above the other. The two latter groups are not placed upon tubercles. The integument of the larva is thick, and difficult to tear. The larva is able to withstand a good deal of pressure without injury."

They frequently noticed the fly, which is sluggish in its movements, in the huts, and were told that it often deposited its eggs on the ground of a hut, "particularly in spots where urine had been voided."

Lelean (1904) forwarded his flies to Austen, who gives the following description of them:

Auchmeromyia luteola.

"♂ ♀ length 10½ mm. to 12 mm.; length of wing 10⅝ mm. ; width of head 3½ mm. in ♂, 4 mm. in ♀.

"*A rather stoutly-built fly, orange-buff in general colour, but with the distal half of the abdomen blackish.*

"*Head,* orange-buff, with the eyes wide apart in both sexes; *thorax,* somewhat darker than the base of the abdomen, with a faint greyish bloom, and marked with two indistinct blackish longitudinal stripes, which do not extend to the hind margin of the thorax; *abdomen,* in the ♂ with the hind margin of the first segment more broadly, a more or less complete forwardly tapering median stripe, the whole of the third segment except the extreme base, and two large lateral blotches on the fourth segment, meeting, or nearly so, in the median line, blackish. In the ♀ the blackish area on the abdomen is greater, since it includes in addition the whole of the second segment, except a more or less narrow band at the base. A striking sexual difference is to be seen in the second abdominal segment, which in the ♀ is twice the length of the same segment in the ♂; *legs,* orange-buff; *wings,* faintly brownish, but entirely devoid of blotches or other markings, so that the veins are plainly visible."

B. Larvæ deposited in natural cavities of the body. Nose and ears.

Though various species of the genus *Sarcophaga* have been known to deposit eggs or young larvæ in natural cavities of the body opening on to the surface, the fly which most commonly does so is the screw-worm fly, *Chrysomyia macellaria.*

This fly occurs in many parts of America from Canada to Patagonia, but is especially common in the warmer regions. It measures 9—10 mm. in length, and bears a great resemblance to the common green-bottle, *Lucilia cæsar,* being of a dark metallic,

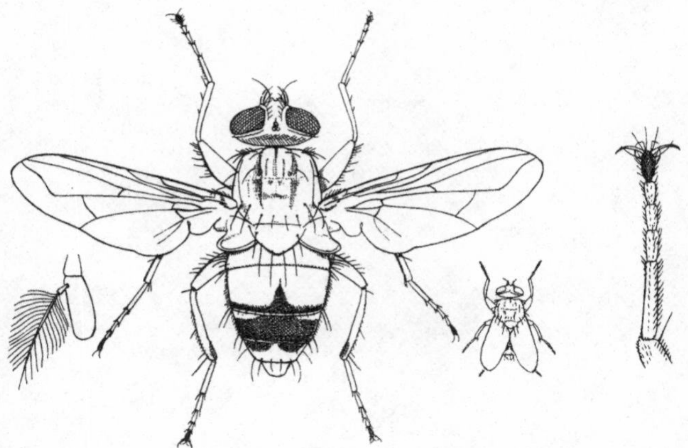

Fig. 1.

Congo floor-maggot fly, *Auchmeromyia luteola* (× 3). Antenna. Natural size, resting position. Tarsus to show dark terminal segment.

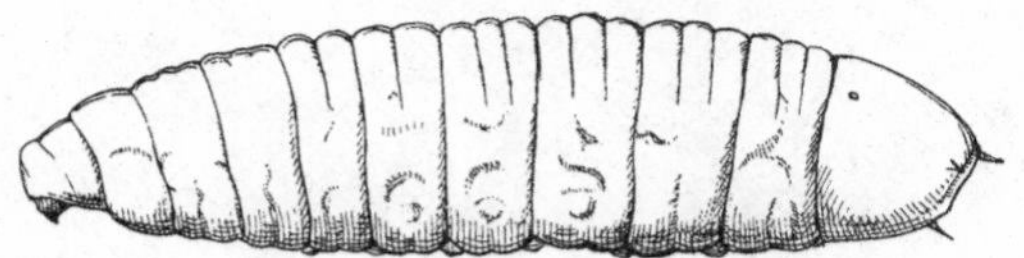

Fig. 2.

Congo floor-maggot (× 5).

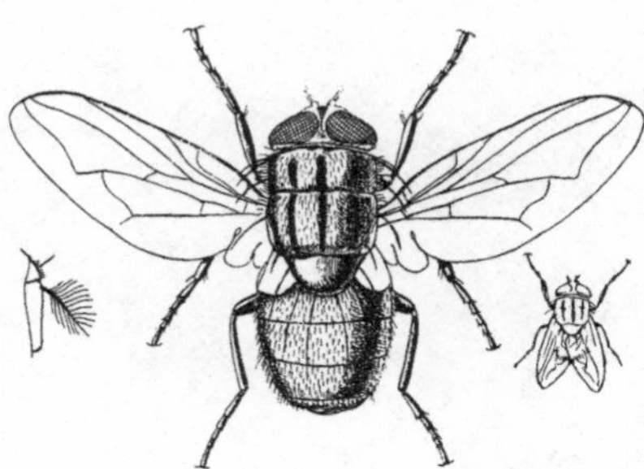

Fig. 3.

Screw-worm fly, *Chrysomyia macellaria* (× 3). Antenna. Natural size, resting position.

bluish green colour. On the thorax there are three longitudinal darker blue bands of a purplish tint. The larvæ usually live in decomposing animal matter. Hermes, who has carefully studied their habits, states that they behave in much the same way as the larvæ of *L. cæsar* (see p. 25).

The flies, however, occasionally deposit their eggs, or the young living larvæ, in great numbers in the ears or nasal fossæ of persons sleeping in the open air, especially if offensive discharges are present, which attract the fly. The larvæ burrow into the tissues, devouring the mucous membrane and underlying tissues, including the muscles, cartilages, periosteum, and even the bones, thereby producing terrible sores. Sometimes they invade the frontal sinuses, antrum and other cavities, causing serious loss of substance and mutilation. If the patient is left untreated they may penetrate into the brain and cause death.

The larvæ when full-fed measure 14—15 mm. in length. The twelve segments of the body carry circles of minute circularly arranged hooks, which give the larva a screw-like appearance, from which the popular name, screw-worm, is derived. The buccal cavity is armed with two powerful hooks, by means of which the larva attacks the tissue.

Pieter (1912) describes a case of infection of the vagina in an old beggar woman.

Animals are occasionally affected.

An interesting case of infection of the nose with the larvæ of the Blow-fly (*Calliphora erythrocephala*) is related by Lawrence (1909).

"Mrs B., aged 55, an asthmatic, while sitting sewing, felt a fly enter her right nostril. She at once tried to expel it by blowing her nose, but without success." Later the fly was discharged. Next morning there was a bloody nasal discharge. The nose began to smell. The day after she could not leave her bed. The third morning there was a foul sanious discharge, the swelling considerable, and the pain and distress severe. Soon the patient's condition was serious. A week from the time of infection some maggots were discharged and continued to come away for ten days. "As the right ala became very much swollen, and blocked the passage it was incised, and a small nest of maggots revealed. They spread into the right cheek up to the lower eyelid; they burrowed into the gums, and appeared in the mouth." Ultimately between 100—150 maggots passed out. "They left the nasal cavity disorganised and the bone exposed in many directions." A blow-fly was hatched from one of the maggots.

The extreme rapidity with which maggots deposited in the nasal cavity may cause serious trouble is well illustrated by an experiment carried out by Wellman (1906). He studied a fly of the genus *Sarcophaga*, near *regularis*, Wied.

"It is viviparous and I have seen it depositing its larvæ on decaying meat and fæces and, on one occasion, in wounds. The larvæ are small when first deposited (four to five millimetres long), but before pupating reach the length of fourteen millimetres or more." For the experiment a goat was used. "The method adopted was as follows: A large number of flies (seventy) were caught in an improvised fly trap baited with decaying meat. The goat was chloroformed and placed under a mosquito curtain, and tied in such a manner that it could not move its head or otherwise protect itself from flies. Then the edges of its nostrils were painted with water in which had been macerated pieces of putrid meat, and the flies liberated under the curtain. The flies could be seen entering the nostrils (which had been previously examined with a speculum, and were known to be in a healthy condition, and to contain no maggots) from time to time. The goat was untied at the end of an hour and tied where it could be watched.

"The goat seemed to experience little discomfort from the time of the experiment (3 p.m.) until next morning, although it could be heard sneezing in the night. The following morning, however, it could not eat, and was thirsty, feverish and seemingly in pain, as it bleated constantly. The odour from the nostrils was extremely fetid, although maggots could not be seen on external examination. By the evening it was very ill and would not stand up. It was killed on the morning of the third day and a post-mortem examination made at once. The post-mortem findings were as follows: The anterior nares unaffected. The posterior nares and frontal sinuses were extensively eroded and of a dark colour, in some places almost purple. In no instance were the lesions deep enough to involve the bone or even the periosteum. The maggots themselves were plentiful throughout the frontal sinuses and posterior nares, in some places being packed together in writhing masses." Two were present in the pharynx, but none in the trachea, bronchi, œsophagus, stomach or Eustachean tubes. "In all, one hundred and thirty-eight maggots were turned out, most of them of nearly full size."

Wellman thinks the severe inflammation and necrosis was entirely due to the maggots, as two other control goats with their nostrils similarly painted, but not exposed to flies, showed no symptoms.

Austen (1912) records a case of myiasis of the nose, attended with a profuse watery discharge of several weeks' duration and pain, due to the larvæ of *Piophila casei*. The case occurred in England, and the flies were bred from the larvæ.

The larvæ of flies of the genus *Œstrus* live in the nasal passages and neighbouring sinuses of sheep and some other ruminants. "The eggs are laid on the victim's nose, and the newly hatched maggots are said to creep up the nostrils. When the maggot is full grown it drops or is sneezed out" (Alcock, 1911, p. 182). The Sergents (1907) have described a similar type of human myiasis occurring in Algeria due to *Œstrus ovis*. They state that the fly deposits its ova while in flight, without settling, upon the eyes, nostrils or lips of shepherds, especially those who have eaten of fresh sheep or goat's cheese. The condition is also found in dogs fed on cheese.

Austen (1912) records a case of myiasis of the external auditory meatus, accompanied by deafness and pain due to a *Syrphus* larva.

Larvæ discharged from the urethra.

Although it would appear most unlikely for the larvæ of flies to be discharged from the urinary tract, yet there are a number of records of such occurrences. Chevrel (1909) has summarized the twenty-one cases of myiasis of the urinary tract which have been recorded; of these, including the one described by himself, he considers seven to be authentic, ten probable, and four doubtful.

In most cases the larvæ discharged, which were usually few in number, appear to have been those of *F. canicularis*. Chevrel himself, however, records an instance in which a woman, aged 55, suffered from albuminuria, and urinated with difficulty. Finally, during one day she passed between thirty and forty larvæ of *F. canicularis* of different sizes.

One case only is recorded in England by Palmer (1912, p. 12). In this case a larva of *F. scalaris* was passed by a male patient. The larva was identified by Austen (1912, p. 12).

C. Larvæ deposited on wounds.

Several species of flies have been known to deposit their ova, or living maggots, in neglected wounds in man, and many species do so on animals. The larvæ soon burrow into the surrounding tissues, often undermining the skin, and, unless removed in time, cause extensive and terrible sores. Many instances have been recorded from tropical countries, where the condition is fairly common, but cases are occasionally met with in temperate climates.

Chrysomyia macellaria is responsible for many cases in tropical America, where "the disease is rather common in persons who sleep in the open and in the sores of uncleanly individuals." In Paraguay, for instance, Lindsay (1902) says, "cases of myiasis are very common. The screw-worms are found in all conceivable situations." Harrison (1908) in Honduras, illustrates and describes two typical cases of the disease. In one case a chronic ulcer of the right cheek became infected.

"On admission a huge open foul ulcer was seen exposing the bones of the face and forehead and destroying the tissues of the cheek and face of the right side, and implicating also the right eye and orbit; any number of worms were seen wriggling about in this cavity, which was over 4 inches in diameter. Altogether upwards of about 300 worms were removed." In the other case extensive destruction of the nasal cavity had been produced.

In India the larvæ of *Sarcophaga carnaria*, *S. magnifica*, *S. ruficornis*, and of *Sarcophila* have been known to cause extensive destruction of tissue in wounds. The larvæ of several species of *Lucilia* have been detected in wounds in different parts of the world.

In England very few cases have been recorded. Andrewes records a case which "occurred in the summer of 1889 or 1890."

"The patient was a destitute person suffering from chronic Bright's disease and dropsy, who also had a chronic ulcer over the lower part of his leg. He slept out in Hyde Park, and the ulcer became fly-blown. When I saw him in the Surgery of St Bartholomew's Hospital, the larvæ had made a pretty clean dissection of the tibialis anticus and other muscles over the floor of the ulcer, which was some three or four inches in diameter. They had devoured the connective tissues, but spared the muscles and tendons. The ulcer was very foul and there were hundreds, perhaps thousands of maggots. The maggots were unfortunately not preserved but were probably those of *Calliphora* or *Lucilia*."

Lawrence (1909) records another case in which the species of the larva was not determined.

"An elderly lady had an epithelial tumour of the size of a small hen's egg growing in front of the left ear. It had begun to bleed. On examining its base, which was about 1½ inches by ¾ inch, I saw a few maggots. Evidently the bleeding was due to the destruction of the tissue where the vessels entered. In spite of strong applications for their destruction the maggots, which proved far more numerous than I thought, succeeded in riddling the tumour in 24 hours, causing pretty severe loss of blood. By the next day the tumour was fetid, the bleeding continuous and the face as far as the eye œdematous." "When the tumour was removed down to the line of the skin a large nest of maggots was found in the cheek and the whole centre was a mass of maggots."

Lucilia sericata commonly attacks young sheep, especially those suffering from diarrhœa, laying its eggs about the hind quarters of these animals. The larvæ burrow under the skin and cause considerable sores.

D. Subcutaneous myiasis.

In Africa the larvæ of the Tumbu-fly, *Cordylobia anthropophaga*, frequently penetrate under the skin of human beings and live there, giving rise to subcutaneous myiasis. Possibly the larvæ of *Bengalia depressa* behave in the same manner. In the tropical parts of America a similar disease is produced by the larvæ of *Dermatobia cyaniventris*. In many parts of the world, including the temperate climates, larvæ of flies of the genus *Hypoderma* form inflammatory tumours beneath the skin of various animals. "The eggs are laid on the hairs of the victim; and it has been supposed that the newly hatched maggots bore through the skin; but Curtice gives reasons for believing that the eggs or young maggots are ingested by the victim, and reach their destination under the skin by an internal route. The larva has no mouth-hooks. When the maggot is full grown it pierces the skin and leaves its host in order to pupate" (Alcock, 1911, p. 182). Very occasionally such larvæ are found causing subcutaneous tumours in man.

Tumbu-fly disease.

This is a disease caused by the larvæ of the Tumbu-fly, *Cordylobia anthropophaga*, living under the skin. According to Smith (1908) the larvæ attack several species of animals, including men, dogs, monkeys and rats. He thinks that "the flies deposit their offspring in the ground, commonly on the earthern floor of a hut, and the larvæ enter the skin of the person or animal sleeping on the ground." The larva burrows beneath the skin and becomes stationary. "The cavity in which it lives is not cut off from the external air; an opening is always left, and in or near this the posterior end of the maggot lies. When mature it drops out, burrows in the ground, and becomes a pupa." Austen (1908) suggests the fly may lay its eggs in flannel or woollen clothing hung out to dry. The fly hatches in sixteen or seventeen days. Blenkinsop (1908) states that "in the majority of cases a single larva is found in an individual at a time," but that in some cases as many as twenty-four are found. Marshall (1902), working in Rhodesia, makes the following remarks: "It has been a great scourge this year in Salisbury, especially among young babies, the maggots forming a painful boil-like swelling under the skin. One baby had no less than sixty maggots extracted from it, and there have been several cases in which there have been a dozen or more." Among Europeans the scrotum and upper part of the thigh and buttock are favourite sites, and "it is the generally received opinion that the parasites are often acquired at the latrine." Amongst natives "no special region seems to be selected." "In monkeys the tail is the favourite site of 'tumbu'" (Smith).

Smith (1908) gives the following description of the disease: "In the human being the appearance of the lesion produced by the larva is that of a raised reddish patch; on a clean, washed skin it looks something like an urticarial wheal. At some part of this swelling will be seen a tiny opening, or a moist spot, perhaps a blackish mark, according to how much, if any, of the larva is presenting at the opening and to the stage of growth. In some cases where the skin has not been washed, pus may have exuded or scabbed round the orifice, so that the appearance is that of a broken boil. There is intense itching in and around the spot. Strong pressure towards the opening forces the larva out easily enough, so that in adults familiar with the fly the larva does not get a chance to grow very big, unless it happens to be in a part where the sufferer cannot see what is wrong. In neglected children and helpless people the larva is able to grow to its full size. In such cases there is usually suppuration in the cavity, and it is common on ejecting the intruder to see a bleb of pus follow it out. I have not heard of any serious results from the attacks of this larva, but as affording an avenue of entry to germs, it seems likely that bad effects may occasionally follow a

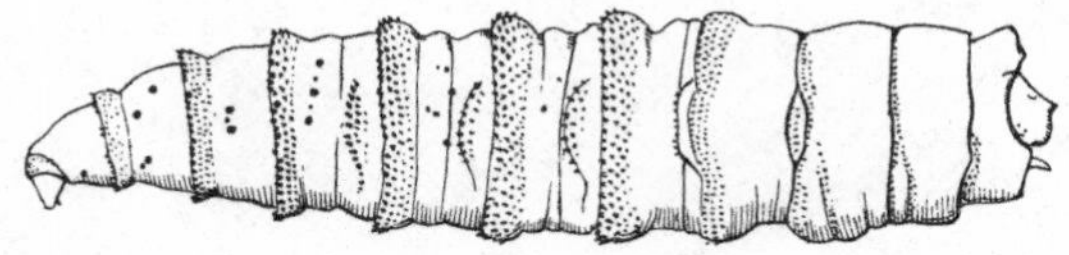

Fig. 1.

Screw-worm (× 5).

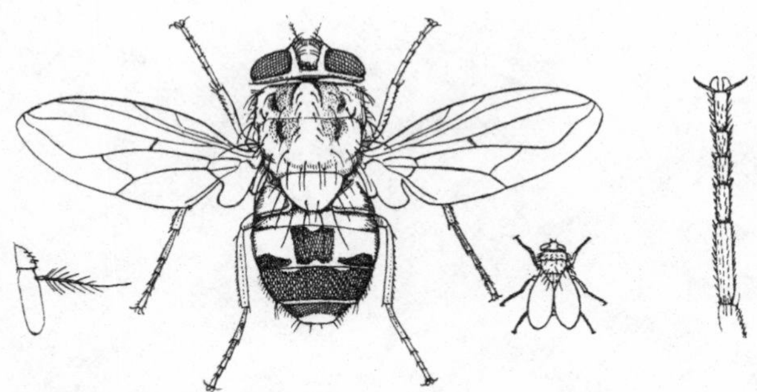

Fig. 2.

Tumbu fly, *Cordylobia anthropophaga* (× 4). Antenna. Natural size, resting position. Tarsus. (Compare Pl. XXI, Fig. 1.)

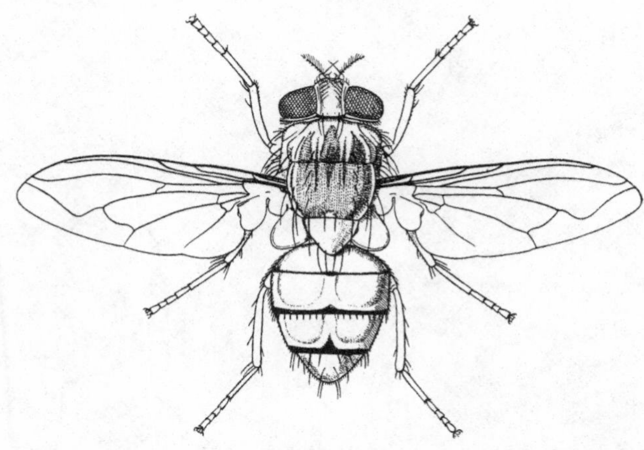

Fig. 3.

The maggot fly, *Bengalia depressa* (× 4).

'tumbu' lesion." Blenkinsop (1908) points out that "only the skin and subcutaneous tissue are affected, and the larva does not, like that of the screw-worm fly (*Chrysomyia macellaria* Fabr.) burrow in the deeper tissues."

Austen (1908) gives the following account of the fly and its larva:

"*Perfect insect.*—A thick set, compactly built fly, of an average length of about 9½ mm.; specimens as small as 6½, or as large as 10½ mm. in length are occasionally met with. Head, body and legs straw yellow; dorsum of thorax and of abdomen with blackish markings; wings with a slight brownish tinge. The eyes meet together for a short distance in the median line above in the case of the male, but are separated by a broad front in the female. On the dorsum of the thorax the dark markings, which are a pair of longitudinal stripes not reaching the hind margin, are covered with a greyish bloom, and, consequently, not very conspicuous; this bloom is also present on the abdomen, but here the markings are much more distinct, especially in the female, in which the third segment, as also the fourth segment, with the exception of the hind margin, is entirely black or blackish. In the female the second segment is marked with a blackish quadrate median blotch, and has a similarly coloured hind border, broadening towards the sides, while the first segment has a narrow dark hind margin. In the male these markings are not so extensive; the dark hind margin to the second segment is interrupted on each side of the median blotch, which is triangular in shape, and there is a yellow area of considerable size on the proximal half of the third segment, on either side of a blackish median quadrate blotch; the fourth segment is similarly but less conspicuously marked."

Care is necessary in order not to confuse *C. anthropophaga* with *Auchmeromyia luteola*, which is found in the same parts of Africa and presents a deceptive resemblance to the Tumbu-fly in colouration. "The two species may be distinguished by the fact that in *A. luteola* the eyes are wide apart in both sexes, the body is narrower and more elongate, the hypopygium of the male is in the form of a conspicuous, forwardly directed hook, for which the ventral half of the penultimate segment of the abdomen serves as a sheath; and lastly, by the fact that the second abdominal segment in the female is twice the length of the same segment in the male." *C. anthropophaga* has also been wrongly identified as *Bengalia depressa*.

"*Larva.*—The full-grown larva is a fat, yellowish-white maggot, 12 to 12½ mm. (about half an inch) in length, bluntly pointed at the anterior or cephalic extremity, and truncate behind; its greatest breadth (on the sixth and seventh segments) is 5 mm. The body consists of twelve visible segments, the divisions between which are strongly marked, except between the cephalic and first body-segment (the latter of which bears the anterior or prothoracic stigmata, or respiratory apertures), and between the eleventh and twelfth segments. On the under side of the cephalic segment the tips of the black paired mouth-hooks may be seen protruding, while in a slight depression in the flattened posterior surface of the twelfth segment are situated the paired posterior stigmatic plates. In the adult larva the slit-like apertures in these plates are not very easy to distinguish, but in a maggot in the second, or penultimate stage, it is seen that each plate bears three ridges of tawny coloured chitin; these ridges run obliquely downwards and outwards, at an angle of 45° from the median vertical line, and, while the median ridge on each plate is nearly straight, the other two ridges are characteristically curved, resembling inverted notes of interrogation, with the concavity directed towards the median ridge. The segments of the body are transversely wrinkled on the dorsal and ventral surfaces (especially on the latter), and puckered on the sides. From the third to the eleventh segment the body is thickly covered with minute recurved spines of brownish chitin (darker in the case of larvæ ready to leave the host), usually arranged in transverse series or groups of two or more, which can be seen to form more or less distinct, undulating or irregular, transverse rows. These spines will be described in somewhat greater detail below.

"Above and to the outer side of each mouth-hook is an antenna-like protuberance, which, as in the case of the larva of the blow-fly (*Calliphora erythrocephala* Mg.), exhibits a pair of light brown, ocellus-like spots, or rather papillæ, placed one above the other. In a small larva, 5 mm. in length, from Lagos, the papillæ are very clearly visible; each papilla is surrounded by a ring of pale brownish chitin, and its shape, when viewed from the side, is exactly that of the muzzle of an old-fashioned muzzle-loading cannon.

"This small larva also shows on the basal segment of each antenna, or antenna-like protuberance, below and a little to the outer side of the mouth-hook, a prominence bearing a series of about six small, brown-tipped, chitinous spines. In the same larva the spines on the body are most conspicuous, and most strongly developed and chitinized, on the fifth, sixth and seventh segments. The tenth and eleventh segments are also covered with spines, but, since the chitin of which they are composed is not tinged with brown, these segments appear bare. In the adult larva also, the spines on the tenth and eleventh are less conspicuous than those on the preceding segments; on the twelfth segment, which bears the posterior stigmatic plates, the spines are very minute. Fully chitinized spines are dark brown, but this colour is generally confined to the apical half of the spine, or may be absent from the extreme base. In shape each spine is a short cone, with the apex recurved, pointing towards the hinder part of the body. The spines are broad at the base in proportion to their length, and not infrequently, especially on the under side of the body, are bifid at the tip. They are closest together and most strongly developed on the anterior portion of each segment, becoming smaller and showing a tendency to disappear towards the hind margin. They are arranged in irregular transverse rows, which are usually seen to be composed of groups of from two to five spines, placed side by side.

"In the adult larva the median area of the ventral surface of the segments five (or six) to eleven inclusive is marked with a series of three transverse ridges, which are most prominently developed on the seventh and following segments. On each segment the foremost ridge is the shortest; next in length comes the hindmost, and the middle ridge is the longest of the three, curling round the posterior ridge at each end. Similar but less strongly marked ridges are seen on the dorsal surface.

"*Puparium.* Of the usual barrel-shaped Muscid type. Average dimensions: length $10\frac{1}{3}$ mm., greatest breadth $4\frac{2}{3}$ mm. Though at first of a ferruginous or light chestnut tint, the puparium gradually darkens until it becomes 'seal brown' or practically black."

"The 'floor-maggot' (p. 213) itself is devoid of the characteristic spines described above in the case of the Tumbu-fly larva, and the posterior surface of its last segment, instead of being vertical, as in the latter, slopes backwards at an angle of 45°, and has around its hind margin a series of fleshy spines; the stigmatic plates on this segment, too, are extremely small and wide apart (2 mm. apart in the adult larva), while in the Tumbu-fly maggot they are much larger and close together (at the nearest point separated by less than the diameter of a single stigmatic plate)."

The Maggot Fly. *Bengalia depressa.*

Theobald (1906) says, "the Maggot Fly (*Bengalia depressa* Walker) is a well-known human and animal pest in parts of Africa."..."The Bengalia occurs in numbers in Natal, but according to Fuller (1901) the range of this fly seems to be limited to the coast and no further inland than the 1000 feet elevation. It is common from the Tugela downwards, and is particularly abundant about Verulam and Durban, but not so much to the south of that port. It is also recorded further up the coast from Delagoa Bay." "Dr Balfour has had this insect sent him from the Bahr-el-Ghazal province, and has also given me a larva from the back of a native, which undoubtedly is the maggot of this fly." It is common in Rhodesia and ranges into British Central Africa and Uganda.

"The fly is half an inch long with wing expanse of about an inch. The head is large, with two prominent dark eyes, brown in colour with yellowish-brown between the eyes. The thorax is rusty to yellowish-brown with dark lateral and dorsal chætæ. The abdomen is pale brown, darker at the apex with two dusky bands, pale below. The legs of a similar tint to the pale colour of the thorax. The transparent wings are tinged, especially at their bases, with dusky brown. The fleshy mouth parts are not adapted to pierce the skin, on the other hand the female has a sharp needle-like ovipositor.

"The *ova*, according to Fuller, are elongated and white and about 3-50ths of an inch in length.

"The *larva*, which was obtained by Captain Lyle Cummins, is creamy white in colour with deep brown spines. (Fuller describes the maggot as 'of a white or dirty whitish colour and much besprinkled with minute black spots which, as a matter of fact, are really spines.') When mature it reaches half an inch in length. The cephalad area has two blunt processes, each of which bears a small blunt mammilliform process. The two mandibles, which project ventrally, are very thick, curved and black, there being apparently a serrated basal plate to each one. The first segment has on the dorsum short brown thorn-like spines on the anterior moiety, the posterior area being nude, and there are also two lateral pairs of short papillæ. At the base of this segment is noticed a small reddish-brown spot on each side; the second and third segments have short dark spines on their anterior moieties, especially pronounced on the second; the third, fourth, fifth and sixth segments have many similar spines all over them, the seventh has very much smaller, paler and scanty ones, the eighth and ninth have none. The anal segment bears two groups of spiracles, arranged three in a group; these are all curved, the two outer ones outwards, the middle curved towards the outer one; spiracular areas brown. The segments are deeply constricted and the spines are particularly prominent on the lateral borders. Ventrally the larva is spiny just as it is dorsally.

"The *puparium*, according to Fuller, is stout and oval, dark purple in colour, and as a rule covered with a mealy down."

"Fuller mentions that it is averred that the flies lay their eggs upon bedding. The sharp ovipositor seems to point to their being able to lay their eggs directly in the skin. The eggs when laid in the former position hatch out rapidly, and the larvæ bury themselves under the skin. They at first produce a boil or swelling which leads to inflammation, which becomes most painful owing to the accumulation of excreta and the rasping movements of the spiny maggot." "In the majority of cases, Fuller states, the scalp seems to be the part most subject to invasion, but the larvæ are found in other parts of the body." "Fuller was informed by a correspondent that he 'noticed a maggot fly in his tent on the Tuesday of one week, and on the following Saturday suffered from an itching in the arm and chest. On Monday the spots had taken the form of blind boils, with a black speck in the centre of each. A week later maggots measuring one-third of an inch were expressed from the boils. The fly observed was caught and living maggots extruded from the abdomen when squeezed.'"

"The adult fly is very sluggish in nature and does not move about on windy days. Pupation takes place on the ground just as in the Œstridæ. Besides man, *Bengalia depressa* attacks dogs, rabbits and other animals."

Austen (1908, p. 24), however, makes the following statement: "Within the last few years *C. anthropophaga* has been wrongly identified as *Bengalia depressa* Walk., under which name it is frequently referred to in reports on 'Economic Zoology' and other literature. The true *B. depressa*, however, is a very different insect, the life-history of which is unknown, and there is no evidence whatever to show that its larva is a subcutaneous parasite."

Dermatobia cyaniventris.

The larvæ of this fly cause subcutaneous myiasis in parts of America, where it is fairly common in some places throughout the tropical regions, especially near wooded lands. It also occurs in Tonquin. The fly measures 14—16 mm. in length. The head is yellow with prominent brown eyes, the thorax greyish, and the abdomen dark metallic blue. The larva penetrates the skin and produces an inflamed swelling with an aperture through which seropurulent fluid, containing the black fæces of the larva, exudes. In its earlier stages the larva is the shape of an elongated pear with the posterior part of the body much attenuated. The anterior border is ringed with several rows of strong, black, recurved hooks. In its later stages the larva is cylindrical, but stouter in its anterior half. Well marked hooks are present round the anterior segments, but not on the last five segments. The larva is known as the 'Macaw-worm.'

Infection of the orbital cavity has been described by Keyt (1900) and Gann (1902).

Various animals are also attacked.

Duprey (1906) says that in Trinidad myiasis due to these larvæ is not infrequent, and believes that the larvæ pass accidentally from leaves, etc., into men and animals.

Hypoderma.

Occasionally larvæ of flies belonging to the genus Hypoderma may produce subcutaneous myiasis in man. An interesting case is recounted by Miller (1910) in America. "In December 1907, the boy noticed a small round lump just below the left knee; this lump was slightly red and very tender, especially at night. About two days later the lump had disappeared from its original position and was found some three inches above the knee; the following day it was still higher in the thigh, and during successive days it appeared at different points along a course up the abdomen, under the axilla, over the scapula, up the right side of the neck, irregularly about the scalp, finally passing back of the ear and to the submental region, which it reached about two months after its first appearance; there it remained stationary." Another lump also migrated in the same manner about three or four inches a day.

One larva was extracted and identified by Stiles as "the larva of *Hypoderma lineata* in the second stage."

The larvæ of *H. bovis* and *H. diana* have also been observed in man.

E. Intestinal myiasis due to larvæ in the alimentary canal.

Dipterous larvæ may occasionally find their way into the alimentary canal, usually by accident, and may be vomited up or expelled in a living condition by the bowel. Many instances have been recorded in various parts of the world, especially in the tropics, and several have been recorded in England. Austen (1912) gives a list of cases in which the larvæ were submitted to him for determination, and from time to time other workers have published their experiences. The presence of the larvæ in the stomach is sometimes indicated by nausea, vertigo and violent pains; if present in the stomach the larvæ may be expelled by vomiting. If they occur in the intestine they are expelled with the fæces, and their presence is sometimes signalized by diarrhœal symptoms and abdominal pains, or more rarely by hæmorrhage. In several of the recorded cases the presence of the larvæ has not given rise to symptoms of any kind, and they have been noticed first in the stools by accident. Whether previous inconvenience is caused or not the patient is usually greatly alarmed by the passage of the larvæ.

Since the great majority of cases of intestinal myiasis in England are due to the presence of the larvæ of *F. scalaris* or *F. canicularis*, an account of infection with these larvæ will be given first, and then the cases due to other larvæ mentioned.

Mode of infection.

The larvæ of flies of the genus *Fannia* inhabit excrement and decaying vegetable products, and the females are attracted to such substances in order to lay their eggs. These facts render several modes of infection possible.

The eggs or young larvæ may be ingested with decaying fruit, vegetables, or other food eaten in a raw state, or the flies, which often deposit their eggs in the old-style privies, may deposit their eggs in or near the anus of persons using them (see Nicholson, 1910). In the same way babies left exposed in an uncleanly condition may become infected. The larvæ on hatching make their way into the rectum, and perhaps penetrate into the intestine.

Symptoms.

In some cases symptoms are marked as in the case described by Jenyns (1839):

"The patient in the case in question, to which reference has frequently been made in papers on the subject of myiasis, was an elderly clergyman living near Cambridge, whose symptoms prior to the appearance of the larvæ were 'general weakness, loss of appetite, and a disagreeable sensation about the epigastrium, which he described as a tremulous motion.' These symptoms commenced in the spring of 1836, and it was not till the summer and autumn of that year that the larvæ were observed in the motions. They then passed off in very large quantities on different occasions, the discharge continuing at intervals for several months. According to the patient's own statement, the chamber-vessel was sometimes half-full of these animals; at other times they were mixed with the stools. He thinks that altogether the quantity evacuated must have amounted to several quarts. The larvæ were nearly all of equal size, and, when first passed, quite alive, moving with great activity."

Austen (1912), who quotes this case, considers from the description given that the larvæ were those of *F. scalaris*.

Cattle (1906)[1] reports the case of a man, who had not been feeling well and complained of abdominal discomfort, who passed these larvæ for some months, and McCampbell and Cooper (1909) in America record a case in which a woman with gastric trouble passed larvæ in large quantities at intervals for seven years.

[1] Cattle considered the larvæ to be 'bots,' but Austen (1912, p. 12), from a consideration of his figure, thinks that they were the larvæ of *F. scalaris*.

On the other hand several recent writers, amongst them Soltau (1910) and Garrood (1910), have described cases in which no discomfort was produced, and the larvæ were noticed unexpectedly in the motions.

In England cases of intestinal myiasis due to the larvæ of *F. scalaris* have been recorded within the last few years, by Cattle (1906), Garrood (1910) and Austen (1912); and the latter writer, Stephens (1905), Hewitt (1909) and Soltau (1910) have described cases due to the larvæ of *F. canicularis*.

In England Austen (1912) has met with one case due to the larvæ of a *Thereva* (? *nobilitata*), two cases due to the larvæ of a *Syrphus* or hover-fly, one case due to the 'rat-tailed maggot'

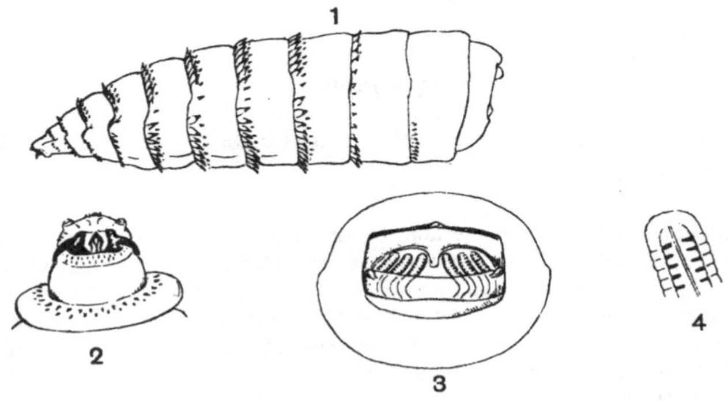

Fig. 24. 1, Bot, or full grown larva of *Gastrophilus equi* (× 3); 2, anterior extremity with mouth-hooks; 3, enlarged view of posterior extremity; 4, part of one spiracle greatly enlarged.

of *Eristalis tenax*, the drone fly, one due to the larvæ of *Anthomyia radicum*, and two due to the larvæ of *Musca domestica* in infants. Stephens (1905) has described a case in an infant in whose fæces the larvæ of both *M. corvina* and *F. canicularis* were found. Cases due to the larvæ of all these flies have been reported on the continent.

The larvæ of the 'Bot' flies are normally parasitic in domesticated and other animals. Though human cases of infection with Bot larvæ have been recorded not infrequently in Europe, Africa and America, no British cases of myiasis in man certainly due to these flies have been published.

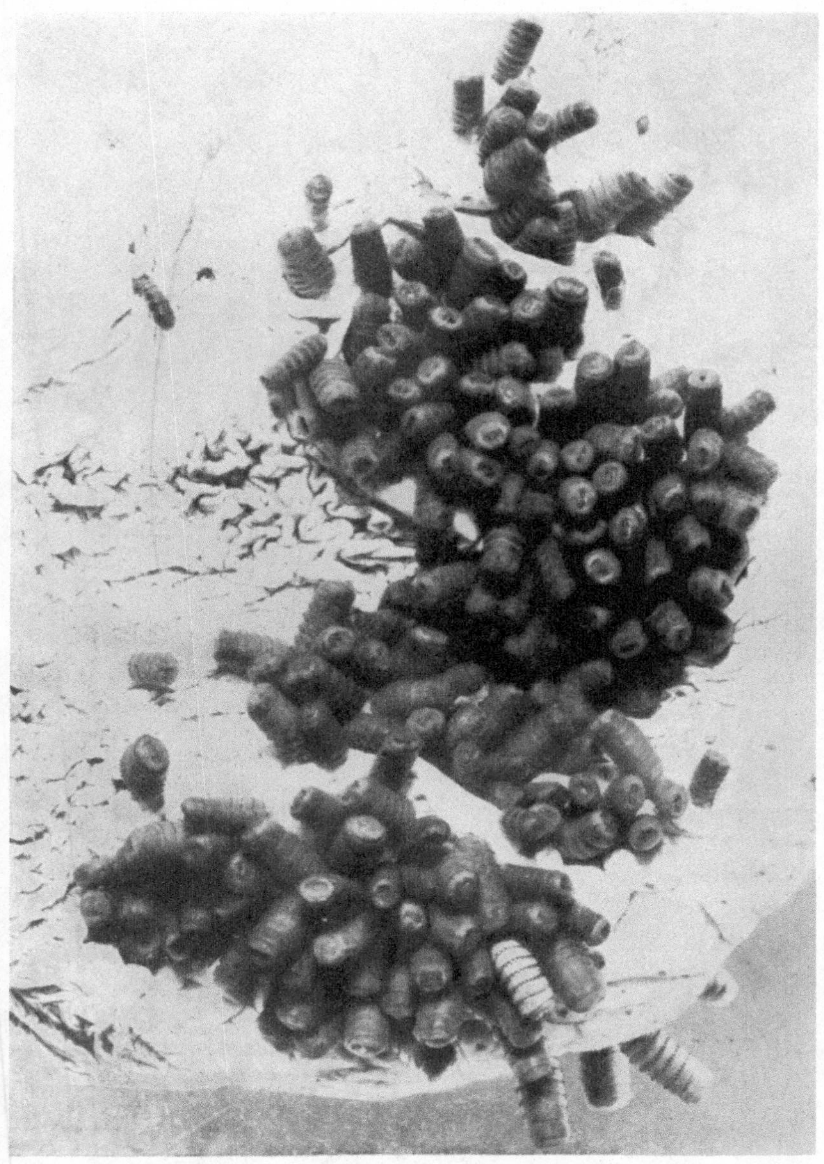

Photograph (natural size) of larvæ of horse-bot-fly, *Gastrophilus equi*, attached to the mucous membrane of the stomach of a horse.

These flies, one of the commonest of which is *Gastrophilus equi*, the horse-bot, attach their eggs to the hairs. The larvæ hatch and crawl on the skin, producing some itching, and cause the animal to lick the place. The larvæ are in this way introduced into the stomach, and attach themselves to the mucous membrane by means of their buccal hooks. They seem to subsist mainly on the inflammatory products resulting from the small wounds. When mature the larvæ become detached and are passed out of the body with the fæces, and pupate in the ground.

Up to the present, insufficient attention has been paid to the subject of intestinal myiasis, few of the cases which occur being recorded, and little trouble being taken to identify the larvæ.

CHAPTER XXIII

THE DISEASES OF FLIES

Flies seem to be totally unaffected by the bacteria, which produce disease in man, with the possible exception of the plague bacillus (*B. pestis*). The observations of Yersin (1894), Nuttall (1897) and Matignon (1898, p. 237) all seem to indicate that flies infected with this organism do not live as long as healthy flies.

Empusa Disease.

Under ordinary conditions adult flies (*Musca* and *Fannia*), so far as is at present known, appear to be subject to only one serious disease, that caused by the fungus, *Empusa muscæ* Cohn. The majority of flies which die in the late summer and autumn succumb to this disease. They are found attached to walls and ceilings, rigid but in life-like attitudes. On closer inspection it is often found that the abdomen is considerably swollen and "white masses of sporogenous fungal hyphæ may be seen projecting for a short distance from the body of the fly, between the segments, giving the abdomen a transversely striped black and white appearance."

"*Empusa muscæ* belongs to the group *Entomophthoreæ*, the members of which confine their attacks to insects, and in many cases are productive of great mortality among the individuals of the species attacked. In this country it may be found from about the beginning of July to the end of October, and usually occurs indoors. It appears to be very uncommon out of doors" (Hewitt, 1910, p. 372).

Mode of Infection.

The mode of infection is at present not well understood. Confinement of healthy flies with those which have died of the disease does not necessarily result in infection. The writer has occasionally been greatly hampered in experiments on the transmission of bacteria by empusa disease in the fly cages. In certain instances all the flies died of empusa infection within a few days. He has, however, been unable to infect from flies which had been dead of empusa for a few weeks either by confining living flies with dead infected flies, or by feeding with sugar syrup contaminated with the remains of dead flies, or by painting living flies with infected syrup. Brefeld (1873) successfully inoculated the spores under the skin and obtained germination of the gonidia on the surface of the fly. Olive's (1906) experiments with an allied species *E. sciara* indicate that infection may occur in the very young larvæ on the surface of the excreta, before they burrow into its depths.

It has generally been supposed that the empusa spore lodges on the surface of the insect and adheres, and that a small germinating hypha develops, pierces the chitin and eventually penetrates the fat-body. Here gemmæ are formed which penetrate to all parts of the body. After a few days the fly's body is completely penetrated by the fungus which destroys all the internal organs and tissues. "The whole body is filled with gemmæ, which germinate and produce ramifying hyphæ. The latter pierce the softer portions of the body wall between the segments and produce short, stout, conidiophores, which are closely packed together in a palisade-like mass to form a compact cushion of conidiophores, which is the transverse white ring that

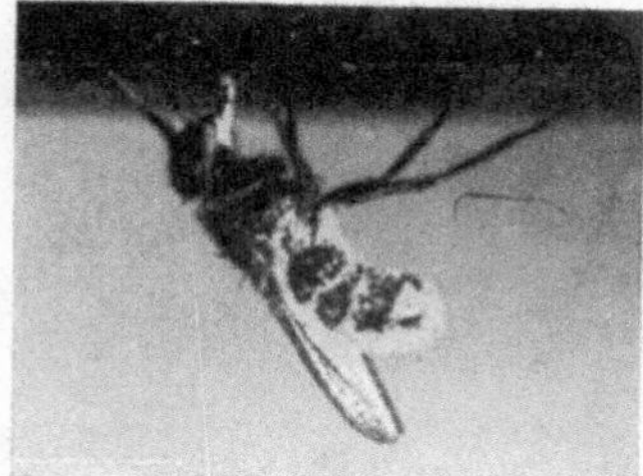

Fig. 1.

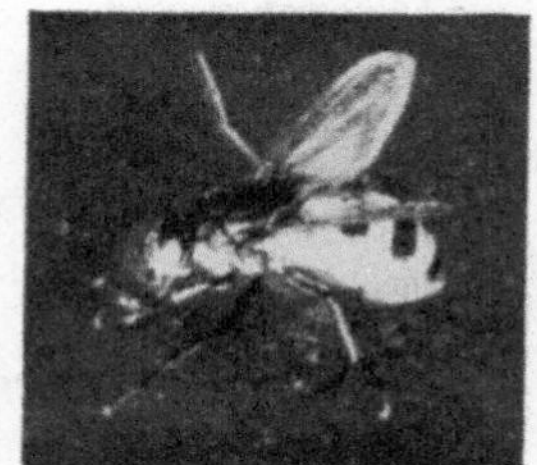

Fig. 2.

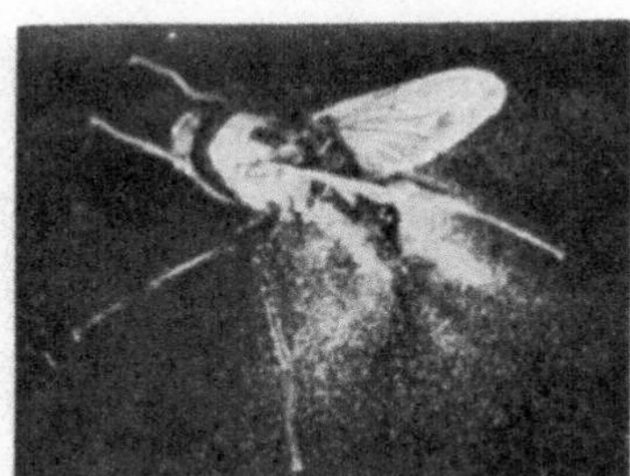

Fig. 3.

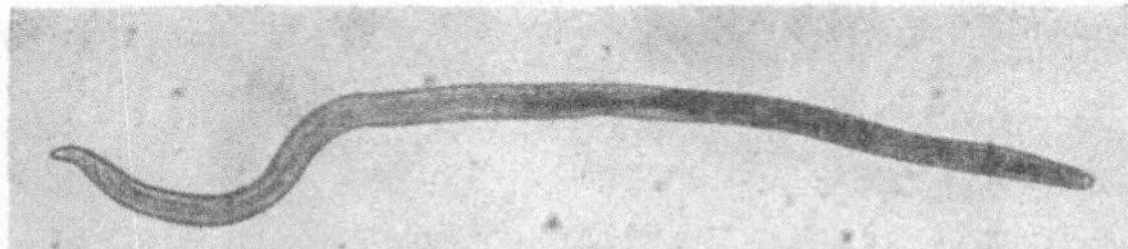

Fig. 4.

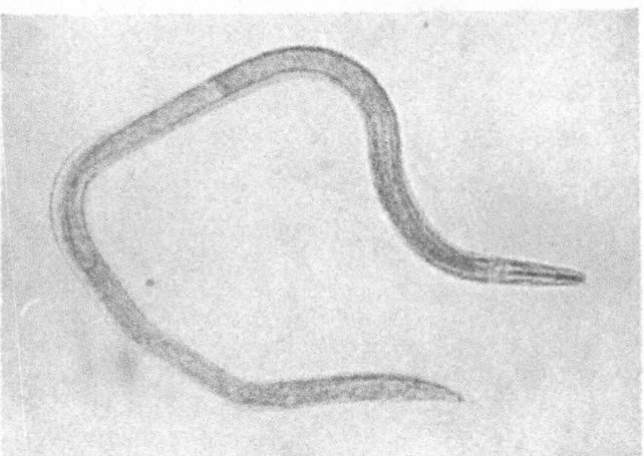

Fig. 5.

Fig. 1. Photograph of fly dead of *E. muscæ*, attached to the under surface of a shelf (× 3). The growth on the abdomen and proboscis can be clearly seen. Fig. 2. Photograph of fly dead of *E. muscæ*; abdomen distended and segments separated by growth of fungus. Fig. 3. Photograph of fly dead of *E. muscæ*, with spores scattered over surrounding surface. Figs. 4 and 5. Photographs of unstained specimens of *Habronema muscæ* (?) from proboscis of *Stomoxys calcitrans* (× 80).

one finds between each of the segments of a diseased and consequently deceased fly. A conidium now develops by the constriction of the apical region of the conidiophore. When it is ripe the conidium is usually bell-shaped, measuring 25—30μ in length; it generally contains a single oil globule. In a remarkable manner it is now shot off from the conidiophore, often for a distance of about a centimetre, and in this way the ring or halo of white spores, which is seen around the dead fly, is formed" (Hewitt, 1910). In many cases the fly is attached to the surface by its extended proboscis.

E. muscæ has been found on several species of *Syrphidæ*, and Thaxter (1888) records its occurrence in *L. cæsar* and *C. vomitoria*. The writer has on several occasions attempted to infect *C. erythrocephala*, *S. carnaria*, and *L. cæsar*, by confining them in cages together with infected flies but without success, and he does not remember to have seen naturally infected specimens. Thaxter (1888) states that two other species of empusa, *E. sphærosperma* and *E. americana*, occasionally attack house-flies and blow-flies. The former species destroys insects belonging to several orders.

Persistence of the fungus from season to season.

Some workers assert that they have observed resting spores, but the question of their production is still uncertain and needs further investigation. Without them it is extremely difficult to understand how the gap in the history of the empusa, between the late autumn of one year and the summer of the next, is filled up. It has been suggested, however, that the species may be kept alive in the few flies, which develop during the winter in stables, bake-houses, etc.

Artificial cultivation.

"If nature could be assisted in her methods, and the fungus brought into contact with the flies, or their larvæ, by scientific methods, it seems probable that the number of flies might thereby be brought under proper control. To this purpose a knowledge of the complete cycle of development, methods of infection, and the conditions which determine the persistence of the vitality of the fungus from the end of one fly season to the beginning of the next is necessary" (Bernstein, 1910, p. 41).

Knowledge on all these points is, however, very incomplete. Before the disease can be artificially reproduced on a large scale artificial cultures of the fungus must be obtained. Owing to the overgrowth of common harmless species of fungi on the bodies of flies dead of empusa great difficulty has been met with in attempting to grow *E. muscæ* on artificial culture media, and until recently little success has been reported.

Recently, however, Morgan (1912) very briefly reported that he had succeeded in cultivating the fungus "directly from the fly in liquid horse serum three months old, from which it can be subcultured on to blood agar." All the cultures were grown at 37° C. Hesse (29, XI, 1912), who lately published a short popular article on the subject, also believes that he has succeeded. In a letter to the writer he made the following statement. In May 1912 he contaminated the bodies of recently killed flies with a fly that had died of empusa in the previous autumn. Within four days a fungus of the mucor type appeared. The spores obtained from this growth he cultivated on egg-yolk in a jar containing sufficient water to maintain a saturated atmosphere. He later succeeded in infecting flies in a cage by allowing them to feed on a paper smeared with syrup containing spores. By the same means flies in a workshop and in an open room were also apparently infected. Experiments on larvæ were inconclusive; larvæ bred in manure, infected with spores from cultures, pupated but the imagines failed to appear.

Hesse therefore appears to have cultivated a fungus, which produces an empusa-like disease in flies, but further observations are necessary before its identity with *E. muscæ*, or its capacity for producing disease, is fully established. Should it be found that both adult flies and larvæ can be easily killed with this organism, a very effective means of reducing the number of flies will have been obtained.

CHAPTER XXIV

PARASITES OF FLIES

(A) *External parasites of adult flies. Mites.*

Small reddish mites are often found attached to the bodies of different kinds of flies. Unless very numerous they do not appear to affect the health of the fly, which usually seems to be oblivious of their presence. Mr Nathan Banks, an authority upon this group of creatures, gave Howard the following interesting information.

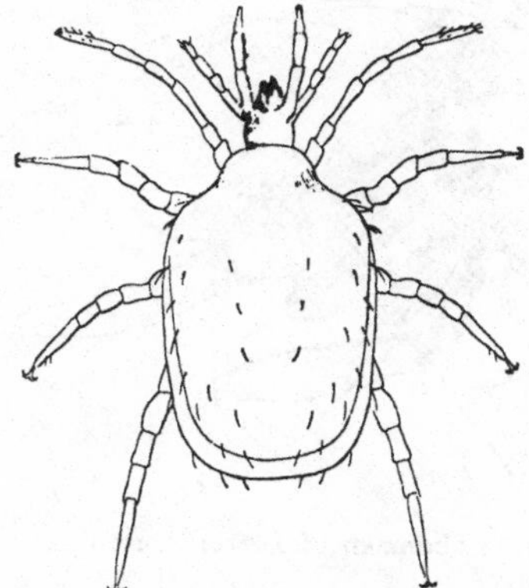

Fig. 25. Mite from *Stomoxys calcitrans* (× 50).

"Latreille based a new genus and species on mites from the house-fly, and he called it *Atomus parasiticum.* This is the young of one of the harvest mites of the family *Trombidiidæ*, but the adult has not been reared, and is still unrecognized in Europe. Riley found these harvest mites on house-flies in Missouri, in some years so abundantly, he says, that scarcely a fly could be caught that was not infested with some of them clinging tenaciously at the base of the wings. Later he succeeded in rearing the adult, and described it as *Trombidium muscarum.* All these forms are minute, six legged, red mites which cling to the body of the fly and with their thread-like mandibles suck up the juices of the host. When ready to transform, they leave the fly and cast their skins, the mature mite being a free-living, hairy, scarlet creature about one and five-tenths mm. long. The adults are usually found in the spring and early summer, while the larvæ are usually found in the autumn on house-flies and other insects.

"Mites of the genus *Pigmeophorus*, of the family *Tarsonemidæ*, have also been taken on house-flies. They cling to the abdomen of the fly, but it is uncertain whether they feed on the insect or use it simply as a means of transportation. The hypopus[1], or migratorial nymphal stage of several species of *Tyroglyphus*

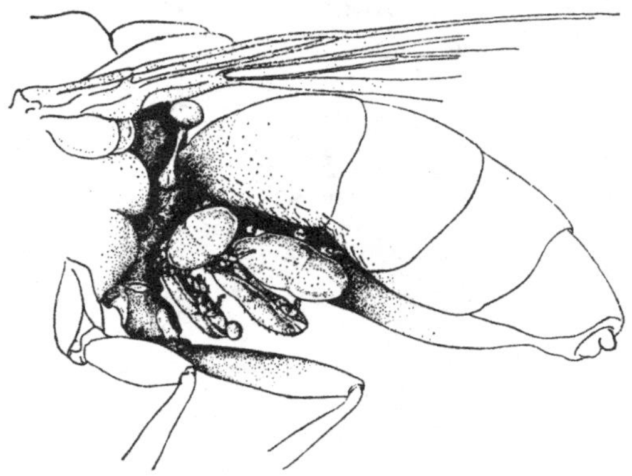

Fig. 26. Mites attached to abdomen of Lesser house-fly (from Hewitt, 1912, p. 61).

(mites destructive to cheese and other foods), has been found on house-flies. This hypopus attaches itself by means of suckers to the body of any insect that may be convenient. The mites do not feed on the fly, but when the fly reaches a place similar to that inhabited by the mites the latter drop off. The hypopi most commonly found on the house-fly are those of the common

1 "When the food supply becomes scarce or other unfavourable conditions prevail, instead of passing through the usual stages of development, the almost fully-grown mites develop hard protective cases or shells into which they can draw themselves for protection. This stage is known as the hypopus, and is in reality a migratorial stage. These hypopi attach themselves to flies and are carried away from the unfavourable conditions, under which probably most of the older mites together with the youngest have perished, to other places where they may encounter food" (Hewitt, 1912, p. 61).

household cheese-, ham- and flour-mites" (Howard, 1911, p. 75). Flies are, therefore, probably agents of some importance in spreading mites destructive to certain foods.

"Flies emerging from pupæ in a rubbish heap or hot-bed will frequently be found to be carrying numerous small brownish mites. Many of these belong to a group *Gamasidæ* which are rather flat and broad mites, and their larvæ occur in large numbers in such situations as rubbish heaps, etc. To these immature forms the fly serves as a most convenient transporting agent and assists in the emigration of the mites to new fields. Some of these forms are parasitic, as I have found them firmly attached by their mouth parts to the under-sides of flies" (Fig. 26) (Hewitt, 1912, p. 60).

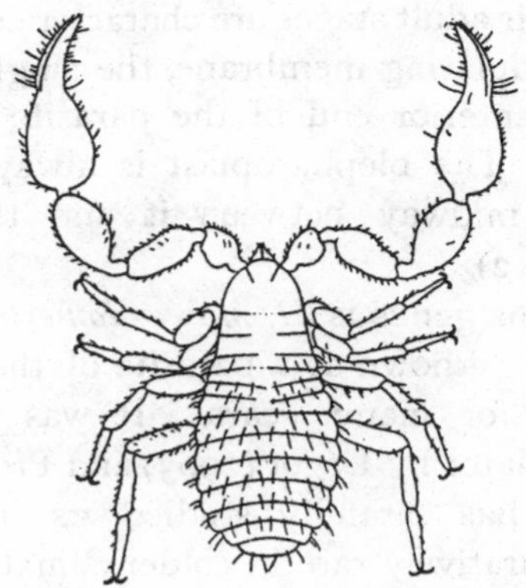

Fig. 27. Chelifer, *Chernes nodosus*.

False-scorpion. *Chernes nodosus* Schrank.

Small reddish scorpion-like creatures, often called *Chelifers*, belonging to the order *Pseudo-scorpionidea*, are frequently found attached to the legs of flies, the most common species being *C. nodosus*. This creature, which is about 2·5 mm. in length, possesses four pairs of legs, and a pair of large pincer-like appendages with which it clings firmly to the fly. It is reddish-brown in colour. The head and thorax are united in a single segment, and the abdomen is clothed with a large number of hairs. It commonly lives among refuse such as decaying vegetation, manure heaps and hot-beds. No doubt these creatures are distributed by flies, but it is at present uncertain whether they feed on the fly, or merely cling to it by accident. Occasionally more than one is found on a fly.

(B) *Internal parasites of adult flies.* (1) *Flagellates.*

(*a*) *Herpetomonas.*

Species belonging to two genera, *Herpetomonas* and *Crithidia*, of protozoon parasites have been found in the intestinal tracts of non-biting flies. They have also been found frequently in the intestinal tracts of biting flies.

The genus *Herpetomonas* "contains a large number of flagellates, which in their adult stages are characterized by the complete absence of an undulating membrane, the single flagellum being attached to the anterior end of the parasite by a short intra-cellular portion. The blepharoplast is always anterior to the nucleus usually midway between it and the anterior end" (Patton, 1909, p. 12).

The type of this genus is *H. muscæ-domesticæ* Burnett. This protozoon has been known as a parasite of the alimentary tract of the house-fly for many years. It was first described by Stein (1878), and later by Léger (1903) and Prowazek (1904), and Patton (1908–9) has carefully studied its life history. It is apparently comparatively rare in colder climates, but common in the tropics. Patton states that "in the case of non-blood sucking flies, which are foul feeders, it will be found that in certain localities, for instance house-flies caught in the Indian bazaars, 100 % are infected with *Herpetomonas muscæ-domesticæ*. The ingestion of a large number of parasites results in increased multiplication; examinations of house-flies, in which almost the whole alimentary tract is a living mass of young herpetomonads, can leave no doubt on this point."

"In order to simplify the study of these flagellates of the genus Herpetomonas, I have found it convenient to divide their life-cycles into three stages, preflagellate, flagellate and post-flagellate. In the preflagellate stages they are round or oval bodies with a large nucleus and round or rod-shaped blepharoplast; they multiply by simple longitudinal division...or by multiple segmentation. The flagellate stage is characterized by the formation of a flagellum and multiplication of the resulting flagellates.

The formation of the flagellum in *Herpetomonas muscæ-domesticæ* is preceded by the development of what appears to be a vacuole close to the blepharoplast, later the flagellum is seen lying in the vacuole, and when the vacuole ruptures it is extruded." The flagellate stages are found in the mid- and hind-guts of the adult insects. The post-flagellate stages are passed in the rectum. "The flagellates become attached to the intestinal epithelium, divide more than once, and at the same time the free portions

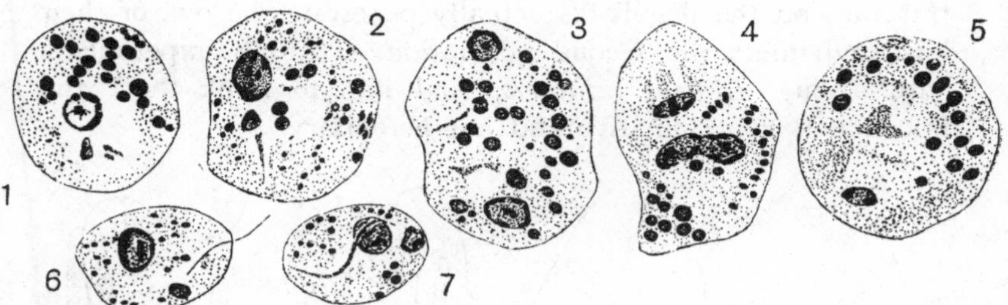

Fig. 28. Preflagellate stages of *Herpetomonas calliphoræ* in the crop of a fly.

1–2. Non-dividing forms; the nuclear karyosome shown in Fig. 1 was stained blue with Giemsa's stain. 3–4. Dividing forms; in Fig. 4 a pseudo-mitotic division of the blepharoplast. 5. Degenerated preflagellate; the nucleus has disappeared. 6–7. Forms with a short external flagellum.

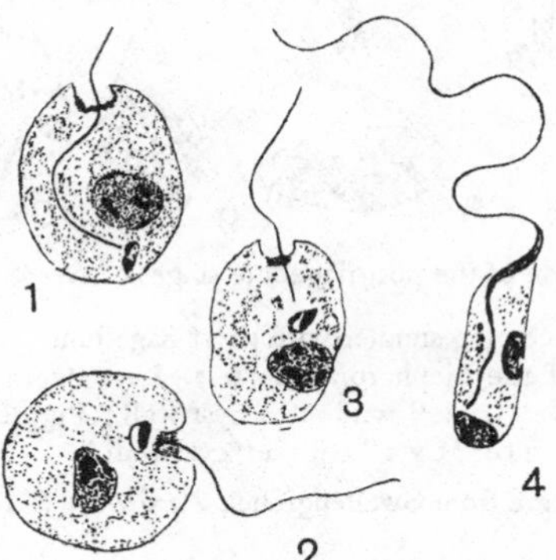

Fig. 29. 1–3. Preflagellate forms of *Herpetomonas calliphoræ* in the mid-gut. 4. Transitional stage towards the formation of a full-grown *Herpetomonas*.

of the flagellum become detached while the intracellular portion is absorbed. The parasites then become encysted and are attached loosely in masses to the rectal epithelium. The cysts are passed out in the fæces of the insects and again ingested." "I have had the opportunity of studying the flagellate in the house-fly and am unable to confirm Prowazek's view of its flagellar apparatus (who thought it had a double flagellum); in order to settle this point I carried out a number of feeding experiments in the hot weather of 1907, when flies were abundant in Madras, and as a result was able to study the early development of the parasite in the mid-gut of the fly."..."The majority of adult flagellates have the appearance of a double flagellum as figured by Prowazek, but this can only represent the commencing division of the flagellates."

It is generally believed that in addition to other methods of transmission the flagellates actually penetrate the ova of their host and infect the second generation. Patton's experiments with a bug, *Lygæus militaris*, lead him to think that "the infection is contaminative and not hereditary."

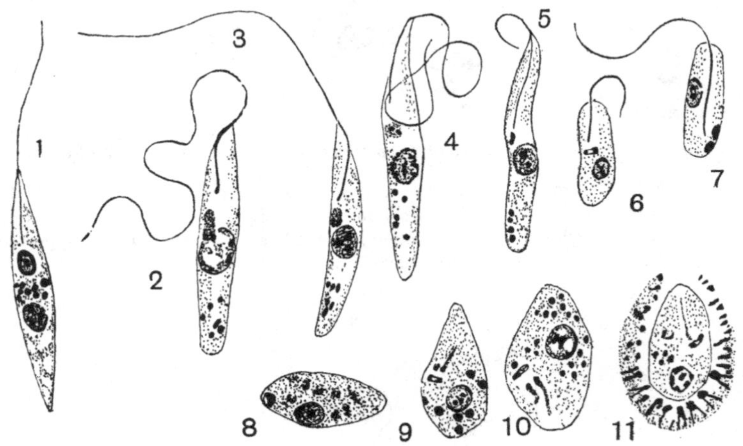

Fig. 30. Formation of the post-flagellate stages of *Herpetomonas calliphoræ*.

1. Normal flagellate becoming smaller with short flagellum. 2-5. Elimination of the achromatic part of the blepharoplast. 6-7. Last stages before the production of "cysts." 8-10. "Cysts" without a cyst-wall; Fig. 9 shows a "cyst" with double rhizoplast. 11. "Cyst" with a "cyst-wall."

(Figs. 28-30 are from Swellengrebel, *Parasitology*, 1911, p. 118.)

Wenyon (1912, p. 332) recently found that a large proportion of house-flies in Bagdad harboured Herpetomonas. The larger parasites he identified as *H. muscæ-domesticæ*, and the smaller as *Leptomonas*, a flagellate described by Flu. As he says, the latter may be a distinct flagellate as Flu claims, or it may be a stage in the life-cycle of *H. muscæ-domesticæ*.

Léger (1903) found *H. muscæ-domesticæ* in *F. scalaris* and *P. rudis*. Mackinnon (1910) discovered a species resembling

H. muscæ-domesticæ in three dung-flies, *Scatophaga lutaria* F., *Neuronecta anilis* Fallen., and *Fannia* sp. The larvæ of these species were also found to be infected, but it seems probable that the infection of the adult was freshly acquired.

Species have been described and named from several kinds of flies by different observers, Swingle (1911) and Swellengrebel (1912) in blow-flies, Swingle (1911) and Patton (1909) in flesh-flies, Patton (1908), Roubaud (1908) and Strickland (1912) in greenbottles, and Chatton and Alilaire (1908) in fruit-flies.

How far the forms described by these observers are different species it is at present difficult to ascertain. Mackinnon (1910) has suggested that there has been needless sub-division of this genus without consideration of the adaptability of one species to several hosts. This surmise is probably correct.

The species of Herpetomonas hitherto described in non-biting flies are given in the following table.

TABLE 31. *Species of Herpetomonas found in non-biting flies.*

Variety of Herpetomonas	Host	Observer
H. muscæ-domesticæ	*M. domestica*	
	F. scalaris	Léger (1903)
	P. rudis	,, ,,
	Lucilia sp.	Roubaud (1908)
	P. putorium	,, ,,
	S. lutaria	Mackinnon (1910)
	N. anilis	,, ,,
	Fannia sp.	,, ,,
	F. canicularis	Dunkerly (1911)
H. sarcophagæ	*S. hæmorrhoidalis*	Prowazek (1904)
	Sarcophaga sp.	Patton (1909)
H. lineata	*S. lineata*	Swingle (1911)
H. calliphoræ	*C. coloradensis*	,, ,,
	C. erythrocephala	Swellengrebel (1912)
H. (*Leptomonas*) *mesnili*	*Lucilia* sp.	Roubaud (1908)
H. Luciliæ	,, ,,	Strickland (1912)
H. mirabilis	*P. putorium*	Roubaud (1908)
H. (*Leptomonas*) *drosophilæ*	*D. confusa*	Chatton and Alilaire (1908)

The presence of these parasites seems to have little effect on the fly.

(*b*) *Crithidia.*

Under the name of *Crithidia muscæ-domesticæ*, Werner (1909) and Rosenbusch (1909) have each described a flagellate parasite in the intestinal tract of the house-fly, and more recently Swellengrebel (1912) has described a species *C. calliphoræ* in the blow-fly (*C. erythrocephala*). Patton speaking of the genus says:

"Crithidia in its adult flagellate stage is a very characteristic organism and can never be mistaken for a Trypanosome or a Herpetomonas, even in the fresh condition. Its body is pointed at both ends, the anterior (flagellar) end being always drawn out to a fine point; this end may be of considerable length or it may be short. The posterior end is usually pointed and may be markedly so, or it may be more or less blunt. The nucleus is situated at about the middle of its body and the blepharoplast, usually a large structure measuring as much as $1\ \mu$, is always situated close to the nucleus, either just anterior or a little distance posterior. Arising from it there is a well-marked flagellum which may be marginal or pass along the body depending how the parasite lies. In the majority of forms the undulating membrane is a narrow ectoplasmic band so that the flagellum exhibits very few undulations, in some species however the latter are quite marked....The flagellates of this genus have a characteristic developmental cycle; in those cases in which the infection is contaminative the cysts are ingested by the hosts;...the preflagellate stage is characterised by an increase in growth and possible multiplication by simple fission. In the next, the flagellate, stage, the flagellum develops at the margin of the parasite and instead of projecting freely is attached to the body by a narrow undulating membrane, as the flagellum becomes free, the anterior end of the parasite is drawn out. The flagellates multiply by simple longitudinal division or by multiple rosette formation. Owing to the irregularity exhibited in the method of divison flagellates of all sizes are produced. After remaining an indefinite time in the intestines they pass down and encyst in the rectum, and are then passed out in large numbers in the fæces. In the case of those *Crithidia* that are transmitted hereditarily the flagellates pass to the ova into which they penetrate and then round up."

The presence in the intestinal tracts of biting-flies of parasites belonging to the genera *Herpetomonas* and *Crithidia* has been the cause of considerable difficulty in the elucidation of the ways in which such flies transmit trypanosomes, pathogenic parasites, which in some respects resemble them.

(2) *Nematoda. Habronema muscæ.*

Carter (1861) appears to have been the first to describe a parasitic nematode worm in the house-fly. He found that in Bombay about half the flies were infected; the worms numbering two to twenty being found chiefly in the proboscis and head. He called the worm *Filaria muscæ* and described it as follows:

"Linear cylindrical, faintly striated transversely, gradually diminishing towards the head, which is obtuse, and furnished with 4 papillæ at a little distance from the mouth, two above and two below; diminishing towards the tail, which is short and terminated by a dilated round extremity covered by short spines. Mouth in the centre of the anterior extremity. Anal orifice at the root of the tail."

Generali (1886), Hewitt (1910, p. 381) and Ransom (quoted by Howard, 1911, p. 73) all describe a similar worm, which is now placed in the genus *Habronema*. Piana noticed that at certain seasons of the year 20–30% of flies in Italy might be infected, but Hewitt in England very rarely found infected flies. Ransom in the United States found the worm, mainly in the head, in nine out of thirty-four flies. Although he examined larvæ and pupæ for these worms with negative results he says "that infection with *H. muscæ* is acquired during some stage prior to the imago is proved by the discovery of the parasites in a fly caught just as it was emerging from the pupa." Since that time Ransom (1911) has further investigated the subject, and has apparently worked out the life-cycle of the parasite. It appears that the worm lives in the stomach of the horse, and that the embryos which pass out in the fæces enter the fly larvæ. When the flies emerge the larvæ are full-grown, but have to pass into the intestinal canal of the horse before reaching maturity.

The writer has examined several hundreds of *Stomoxys*, caught in various places, for similar worms, but has only found them in flies caught close to a certain farm near Cambridge. In 1908 4·3% were found to be infected, 9% in 1909, 13% in 1910, and 10% in 1911.

The degree of infection may be judged by a detailed account of the findings in 115 flies caught on July 15th, 1911. Each fly was carefully dissected, the proboscis, head, thoracic and leg muscles and abdomen being examined separately. In 100 flies no worms were found. Eight flies were infected with single worms; in four the worms were in the head, in two in the proboscis, and in two in the thorax. One contained two worms in the thorax, and one three worms in the head. In one fly two worms were found in the thorax and one in the proboscis; and in another two worms in the thorax, two in the proboscis and one in the head. Two flies were very heavily infected. In one of these twenty-three worms were present in the head and two in the thorax, and in the other four worms were present in the proboscis, eight in the thorax and ten in the head.

The flies do not seem to be affected in any way by the presence of the worms.

(C) *Parasites of the larvæ.*

Certain hymenopterous four-winged flies are accustomed to frequent excreta, especially cow dung, in order to lay their eggs in one of the many species of maggots that live there. Minute forms, belonging to the sub-family *Figitinæ* of the gall-fly family *Cynipidæ*, are parasitic upon other insects, and also in dipterous maggots. Some members of this group, *F. anthomyiarum* and *F. scutellaris*, have actually been bred from the larvæ of house-flies, and it is probable that others are parasitic on them.

A number of species belonging to the super-family *Chalcidoidea*, also live in the larvæ of flies. " In the family *Pteromalidæ* there is a genus *Spalangia*, which seems practically confined to dipterous larvæ. One species, *Spalangia niger*, was found by Bouché to lay its eggs in the pupæ of the house-fly, and to issue in April and May. The larvæ of the Spalangia are spindle-formed and white, almost transparent, and are to be found in the autumn in the puparia of the house-fly, where they destroy the pupæ " (Howard, 1911, p. 89).

Howard also states that Sanford observed a species named *S. muscæ* in the pupæ of house-flies, and that *Stenomalus muscarum* has also been recorded from house-fly pupæ. He also quotes the interesting observations of Girault and Sanders, of the University of Illinois, who obtained a species called *Nasonia brevicornis* from the pupæ of various flies. " It is a minute, dark, metallic, brassy-green fly, with clear wings and a rather stolid serious temperament. Girault and Sanders state that it heeds external influences very slightly, and quietly and persistently gives its whole attention to reproduction. They found that both sexes crawled rapidly. The female is able to fly; but the favourite means of locomotion appears to be crawling. The wings of the male appear to be non-functional. The parasite apparently attacks only the puparium, and that only after it has been formed for about twenty-four hours, and a number of them issue from the same puparium." They found that one female was able to parasitize twenty-two puparia, and another one sixteen. The average life-cycle was about twenty-two days. The parasite seems to hibernate as a full-grown larva in the puparium. In some of their observations they found that 90% of the puparia they examined were infected.

Girault and Sanders also studied two other species, *Pachycrepoideus dubius* and *Muscidifurax raptor.* The latter is a small clear-winged species, dark in colour, which was reared in some numbers from the pupæ of various flies in Illinois. The larva of this parasite lives in the puparium and feeds externally on the pupa of the fly, sucking its juices.

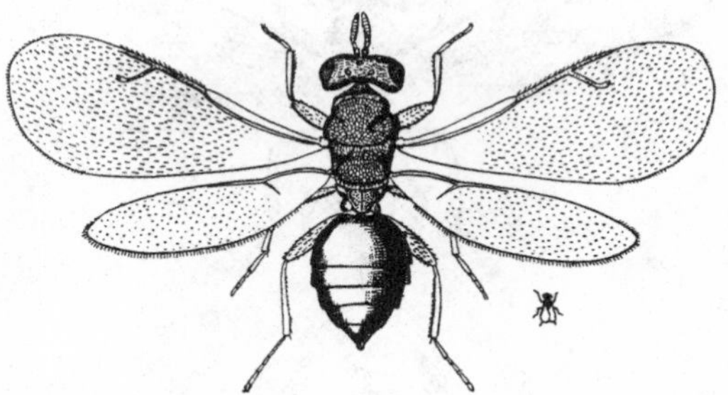

Fig. 31. *Pteromalus* sp. from pupa of blow-fly.

Nicholls (1912, p. 87), working in Saint Lucia, makes the following statement: "There are certain very small parasitic hymenoptera of the family *Chalcididæ* which are probably of some service in keeping down the numbers of some of the flies here considered. These insects deposit their eggs in the body of freshly hatched larvæ. This appears to have no effect on the growth or development of the host until it pupates, when the egg hatches and the resultant guest larva undergoes its development at the expense of the pupa. In a number of cases the period of time from laying the egg to the emergence of the hymenopteron varied from twenty-two to twenty-eight days. On one occasion

500 pupæ of three Tachinid families were placed in a vessel and 126 *Chalcididæ* hatched out." He gives a careful account of the process of egg laying.

Figure 31 represents a species of the genus *Pteromalus*, bred on several occasions by the writer from the pupæ of *C. erythrocephala.* Figure 32 represents an ichneumon-like fly belonging to the family *Braconidæ* from the pupa of a flesh-fly (*S. carnaria*). The larvæ of the flesh-fly pupated in the autumn of 1912, and flies emerged from some of the pupæ in the following

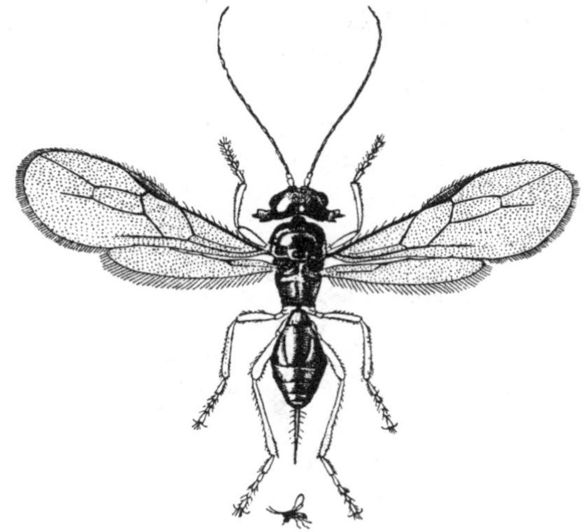

Fig. 32. Braconid from pupa of flesh-fly.

spring. From other pupæ large numbers of braconids appeared. Three of the parasitized pupæ contained 10, 13 and 14 braconids respectively.

Very little attention has yet been paid to this subject but careful study might reveal new and important facts, which might be utilised in the artificial control of flies.

CHAPTER XXV

ENEMIES OF FLIES

Certain vertebrate and invertebrate animals eat adult flies or larvæ or both, but the destruction wrought by them is probably insignificant in comparison with that produced by empusa disease, hymenopterous parasites of larvæ and cold and inclement weather.

Adult flies. (*a*) *Invertebrate enemies.*

Flies are caught and killed by various species of spiders, wasps and robber-flies belonging to the family *Asilidæ,* but their efforts seem to have little effect in reducing the swarms of flies. Howard (1911, p. 82) mentions that in many parts of the United States a small, rather fragile looking centipede, known as *Scutigera forceps* Raf., which is a constant inhabitant of the houses, lives on house-flies and other insects, and kills large numbers.

(*b*) *Vertebrate enemies.*

Some of the lizards which are found in houses in tropical countries feed upon flies. Outside houses, toads and birds, especially poultry, when they have access to manure piles, eat large numbers of larvæ as well as adult flies.

Larvæ.

The larvæ of certain Caraboeid beetles, especially those belonging to the genera *Harpalus*, *Platynus* and *Agonoderus*, and certain Rove beetles and their larvæ, of the family *Staphylinidæ*, are occasionally found in manure feeding on young fly larvæ, but apparently are not greatly attracted to places where fly larvæ flourish.

Howard (1911, p. 85) states that Jones, in the Philippines, found it impossible to raise flies unless the eggs and larvæ were protected from ants, as the latter carried off the eggs, larvæ, and even the pupæ. He also states that in some parts of America certain ants which are attracted to horse manure undoubtedly destroy some of the fly larvæ in it, but that reliable observers believe that they do not greatly reduce the numbers of flies bred from the manure. In Saint Lucia, Nicholls (1911, p. 87) says that ants are the worst enemies of the larvæ and pupæ of certain flies. "If these find a breeding place they will carry off all the larvæ and pupæ, and I have lost the entire number in several experiments in this way."

CHAPTER XXVI

FLIES BREEDING IN OR FREQUENTING HUMAN FÆCES

Howard seems to be the only investigator who has carried out systematic observations on the insects which breed in or frequent human fæces, though others have recorded the presence of the larvæ of certain flies in this material. This chapter is compiled from Howard's (1900) interesting paper, *A contribution to the study of the insect fauna of human excrement*, which contains an account of his observations, and descriptions and illustrations of most of the species mentioned.

He observed forty-four species of beetles and many hymenopterous parasites, "all of the latter having probably lived in the larval condition on the larvæ of Diptera or Coleoptera breeding in excrement. Neither the beetles nor the hymenoptera, however, have any importance from the disease-transfer standpoint. The Diptera alone were the insects of significance in this connection. Of Diptera there were studied in all seventy-seven species, of which thirty-six were found to breed in human fæces, while the remaining forty-one were captured upon such excrement. The following list indicates the exact species arranged under their proper families."

Reared (usually also captured)	Captured (not reared)
Family **Chironomidæ.**	
Ceratopogon sp. (scarce).	*Chironomus halteralis* Coq. (scarce).
Family **Bibionidæ.**	
Scatopse pulicaria Loew (mod. abundant).	
Family **Tipulidæ.**	
	Limnobia sciophila O. S. (scarce).
Family **Empididæ.**	
Tachydromia sp. (scarce).	*Rhamphomyia manca* Coq. (uncommon).
Family **Dolichopodidæ.**	
Diaphorus leucostomus Loew (scarce).	*Neurigonia tenuis* Loew (scarce).
Diaphorus sodalis Loew (uncommon).	
Family **Sarcophagidæ.**	
* *Lucilia cæsar* L.	*Chrysomyia macellaria* Fabr. (abundant).
* *Sarcophaga sarraceniæ* Riley (abundant).	* *Calliphora erythrocephala* Meig. (abundant).
* *Sarcophaga assidua* Walk. (abundant).	*Sarcophaga lambens* Wied. (scarce).
Sarcophaga trivialis V. d. W. (abundant).	*Sarcophaga plinthopyga* Wied. (scarce).
Helicobia quadrisetosa Coq. (abundant).	*Cynomyia cadaverina* Desv. (scarce).
	* *Phormia terrænovæ* Desv. (abundant).
Family **Muscidæ.**	
* *Musca domestica* L. (abundant).	*Muscina cæsia* Meig. (scarce).
Morellia micans Macq. (abundant).	*Muscina tripunctata* V. d. W. (scarce).
* *Muscina stabulans* Fall. ,,	* *Stomoxys calcitrans* L. (abundant).
Myospila meditabunda Fabr. (abundant).	*Pseudopyrellia cornicina* Fabr. (abundant).
	Pyrellia ochricornis Wied. (scarce).
Family **Anthomyidæ.**	
Fannia brevis Rond. (abundant).	*Hylemyia juvenalis* Stein (scarce).
* *Fannia canicularis* L. ,,	*Hydrotæa metatarsata* Stein (scarce).
* *Fannia scalaris* Fabr. (scarce).	*Cœnosia pallipes* Stein (scarce).
Hydrotæa dentipes Meig. (abundant).	*Mydæa palposa* Walk. ,,
Limnophora arcuata Stein ,,	
Ophyra leucostoma Wied. ,,	
Phorbia cinerella Fabr. ,,	
Phorbia fusciceps Zelt. ,,	
Family **Ortalidæ.**	
Euxesta notata Wied. (abundant).	*Rivellia pallida* Loew (scarce).

Reared (usually also captured)	Captured (not reared)
Family **Lonchæidæ.**	
Lonchæa polita Say (abundant).	
Family **Sepsidæ.**	
**Sepsis violacea* Meig. (abundant).	**Piophila casei* L. (scarce).
Nemopoda minuta Wied. (abundant).	
Family **Drosophilidæ.**	
**Drosophila ampelophila* Loew (abundant).	*Drosophila funebris* Meig. (scarce).
	Drosophila buskii Coq. ,,
Family **Oscinidæ.**	
Oscinis trigramma Loew (scarce).	*Hippelates flavipes* Loew (scarce).
	Oscinis carbonaria Loew (abundant).
	Oscinis coxendix Fitch (scarce).
	Oscinis pallipes Loew (scarce).
	Elachiptera costata Loew (abundant).
Family **Agromyzidæ.**	
Ceratomyza dorsalis Loew (scarce).	
Desmometopa latipes Meig. ,,	
Family **Ephydridæ.**	
Scatella stagnalis Fall. (scarce).	*Discocerina parva* Loew (scarce).
	Hydrellia formosa Loew ,,
Family **Borboridæ.**	
Limosina albipennis Rond. (abundant).	*Borborus equinus* Fall. (abundant).
Limosina fontinalis Fall. ,,	*Borborus geniculatus* Macq. (abundant).
Sphærocera pusilla Meig. ,,	*Limosina crassimana* Hal ,,
Sphærocera subsultans Fabr. ,,	
Family **Syrphidæ.**	
	Syritta pipiens L. (scarce).
Family **Phoridæ.**	
	Phora femorata Meig. (scarce).
Family **Scatophagidæ.**	
Scatophaga furcata Say (abundant).	*Scatophaga stercoraria* L. (abundant).
	Fucellia fucorum Fall (scarce).
Family **Micropezidæ.**	
	Calobata fasciata Fabr. (scarce).
	Calobata antennipes Say (abundant).
Family **Helomyzidæ.**	
	Leria pectinata Loew (scarce).
	Tephrochlamys rufiventris Meig. (scarce).

This list is an actual record of observations in America, and should not be considered as indicating definitely the habits of the species or their relative abundance under other conditions or in other places. Undoubtedly some of the species captured on excrement, but not reared from it, are excrement breeders, while the presence of others was probably accidental. Those species, which are found not uncommonly in houses, are marked *.

In India *M. domestica*, *M. enteniata*, *M. nebulo*, and several species of the genus *Pycnosoma* breed abundantly in trenches containing night soil.

Coquillet (1900) identified species of flies reared from cow manure. Several of these species also breed in human excrement.

CHAPTER XXVII

PREVENTION AND CONTROL OF FLIES

It is evident that the best method of controlling flies is to eliminate their breeding places. That they can be controlled is without question, but the work can only be done by united efforts in combination with suitable regulations. In many parts of the United States the requisite machinery has been established and considerable progress in the control of flies has been made, but up to the present nothing of the kind has been attempted in England, and some time must elapse before any noticeable results can be obtained. Before discussing the application of preventive measures to the breeding places it may be best, therefore, to consider the methods available for dealing with flies which enter houses.

Measures against adult flies.

Flies may be caught in considerable numbers on fly papers, of which the non-poisonous varieties should be preferred, or in balloon or other traps, baited with syrup or stale beer, or they may be destroyed by taking advantage of the fact that flies require large quantities of fluid, and usually seek something to drink early in the morning. A method which has often proved very successful, based on this fact, has been described by Hermes (1911).

Formalin, which, as purchased from the chemist, contains about 40% of formaldehyde in solution, is diluted by the addition of water to contain about 2% of formaldehyde, and the solution placed in saucers or shallow dishes on window sills or tables. During the day, in dining rooms, kitchens and other places, where there is plenty of fluid material for food and drink, many of the flies cannot be expected to drink the formalin solution, but if all other fluids are removed or covered up in the evening, the flies, which do not seem to object to the presence of the formalin, will greedily drink the solution in the morning. After doing so they usually die within a short distance of the vessel. This solution has the advantage of being non-poisonous to man, and may therefore be used with impunity around food.

Howard (1911, p. 184) records another simple method described in the Journal of the Department of Agriculture of Western Australia. "Flies may be effectively destroyed by putting half a spoonful of black pepper in powder on a teaspoonful of brown sugar and one teaspoonful of cream. Mix all together and place in a room where flies are troublesome, and it is said they will soon disappear."

Fumes created by burning pyrethrum powder and other substances have been recommended to stupefy flies, but could scarcely be used in sufficient concentration in living rooms. According to Hermes (1911, p. 540), "the fly-fighting committee of the American Civic Association recommends the following: Heat a shovel, or any similar article, and drop thereon twenty drops of carbolic acid; the vapour kills flies." In many places this method might be employed with advantage.

Food, especially substances, such as milk, condensed milk, sweets and fruit, which are consumed without cooking, should, when not in use, be protected against visits from flies. In many of these articles of food bacteria deposited by the fly multiply rapidly especially during warm weather, so that the initial dose deposited by the fly may be multiplied many times in the hours which elapse before consumption. To some extent protection is afforded by covering the dishes or jugs in which the food is contained, but flies are apt to crawl in or to feed on the remains adhering to the edges, and cause infection in this way. If possible, therefore, such articles ought to be placed in larders or cool places protected by gauze, with a mesh sufficiently small to prevent house-flies from penetrating through it. Some of the minute species of flies will penetrate almost any gauze, but their capacity for carrying disease-producing bacteria and their opportunities of acquiring them are probably much more limited. It should be remembered that house-flies will generally succeed in getting through any crevices which may be left.

Screening of the houses is adopted in some countries, especially in parts of the United States, where flies are very numerous during their season. The expense is considerable, but in some localities it is undoubtedly justified, as the majority of the flies is kept out. "No system of screening, however, seems to be so perfect as to keep them all out. They get in, one way or another, in spite of care; even when double doors are used they eventually gain entrance."

It is highly desirable, however, that sick rooms should be well screened, especially those occupied by persons suffering from transmissible diseases, and any flies that chance to find their way in should be killed to prevent them escaping and carrying the infection. Further, all soiled linen, bandages, sputum, etc., should be immediately disposed of in such a manner that flies cannot infect themselves from them.

It may be occasionally helpful to remember that flies are not so apt to find their way into darkened rooms, as into rooms to which sunlight has free access.

Hodge (1910) is of opinon that the fly problem can be effectively dealt with by catching adults at the breeding places, especially in the spring months, and thus diminishing the offspring of flies which have survived the winter. Even during the height of summer he thinks that this plan will be of great service, since there is a considerable period between the time the fly emerges from the pupa and the time it becomes sexually mature and lays eggs. He has devised several methods, the guiding principle being to attract flies to one spot and catch them. For example, he found that multitudes of flies could be caught in a garbage can, if the cover was held up slightly all round by strips of metal so that flies could easily crawl in, and a hole, covered by a wire trap, made in the lid. The flies entered the can, attracted by the odour, and, attempting to escape by the only opening through which light came, passed into the trap.

Measures against larvæ.

If it can be proved beyond doubt that house-flies are important transmitting agents in such serious and widespread diseases as epidemic diarrhœa and typhoid fever, the work of limiting their numbers should be undertaken seriously. The facts that they undoubtedly distribute fæcal bacteria, and that their presence is evidence of insanitary conditions, are in themselves sufficient justification for urging that the problem should be dealt with.

"The whole expense of screening should be an unnecessary one, just as the effort to destroy flies in houses should be unnecessary. The breeding should be stopped to such an extent that all these things should be useless" (Howard, 1911, p. 534).

"The work of control can be greatly furthered by the individual citizen ; indeed, the California State Board of Health, in Bulletin No. 11 (1909), makes the following statements : 'This work can be done only by an united effort. The citizen must do the work, and should do it willingly, but, if negligent, the strong hand of the law should compel it.' The citizen must, however, have instruction in the matter, since there is the greatest ignorance relative to the life history and development of the house-fly and disease transmitting agents in general. The writer finds that this ignorance is as prevalent among the educated as among the uneducated. Few ideas are more firmly rooted in the mind of the average man or woman than that Nature has brought forth nothing that is useless in the economy of the human family....Some have said that the house-fly acts as a scavenger, and is, therefore, a friend of man. *The house-fly is the poorest of scavengers, and one of the most dangerous of man's enemies—a veritable wolf in sheep's clothing.* There is no virtue in the house-fly; there is no reason why it should continue to exist, and its death knell is being sounded wherever communities care for the health of the individual. Dr E. P. Felt (1909) has said 'our descendants of another century will stand in amazement at our blind toleration of such a menace to life and happiness'" (Hermes, 1911, p. 533).

The methods employed in removing breeding places, or in rendering them unsuitable for the larvæ by chemical agents, or in preventing the deposition of eggs by mechanical means, must differ to some extent under the different conditions prevailing in various localities, but all must depend on an accurate knowledge of the habits of flies and their larvæ.

In this chapter it is not proposed to give specific and detailed instructions as to the methods which should be employed in each instance, but only to point out the main sources of flies.

Wherever a nuisance from flies prevails their breeding places must be searched for, and it should be remembered that numbers of flies may be bred from relatively small accumulations of filth, such as human excrement. In cities, however, the majority are probably bred from horse manure, though many of the larvæ live in the excreta of other animals, in ash-pits and in decaying vegetable matter. Search must therefore be made for accumulations of refuse. Fortunately to produce the requisite degree of fermentation for rapid breeding, quantities of most of the suitable materials, sufficient in amount to be readily noticeable, have to be accumulated, and the search for the breeding places of the bulk of the flies of a given neighbourhood need not be a very close one. At the same time no accumulations of rubbish of any kind ought to be ignored, since even rags and paper under proper conditions of moisture and temperature may afford breeding places.

The open manure heap ought to be abolished, and stables kept clean. House-flies breed in large numbers in the cracks of the stable and stall floors, where manure falls into them, and consequently floors with cracks ought not to be permitted. Receptacles may be constructed with tightly fitting lids, preferably in dark corners, where the stable refuse may be kept, until it can be removed. This should be done at least once a week, since under suitable conditions the larvæ reach full growth in about five days, and many of them wander to loose *débris* in the neighbourhood to pupate.

The possibility of flies breeding from manure spread over land is another important and practical point on which Howard (1911, p. 192) quotes some of Hine's unpublished observations. The latter found that flies came out in abundance from spread manure infested with larvæ, but that only one generation appeared, and that the spreading prevented the development of future generations in the same manure.

An example of the nuisance which may be created in the neighbourhood of large accumulations of rubbish has already been quoted (p. 75).

Masses of decaying vegetable refuse should not be tolerated, and it should be remembered that numerous flies are bred from badly kept rabbit hutches, etc.

Receptacles containing kitchen refuse should be kept closed to prevent flies laying their eggs in them. As previously pointed out, flies which happen to enter them, may be caught by employing suitable methods.

Newstead (1908) has pointed out that ash-pits may be so screened as to prevent the breeding of house-flies in them.

Earth closets and privies, which are not very carefully looked after, are prolific breeding places of flies. In towns they ought to be abolished, as far as possible, but where they must be retained they should be of the best type. Stiles (1910) has given much attention to this subject, and has published detailed instructions for building really sanitary privies, which are fly-proof, well ventilated, and have suitable receptacles, containing the necessary amount of water with a film of kerosene floating on it. The use of kerosene in privies, wherever possible, is to be strongly recommended, since it kills not only the eggs of parasitic intestinal worms, but fly larvæ of all kinds.

Permanent preventive measures, even though a staff of inspectors has to be employed, will always be less expensive in the end, and also very much more effective than the use of temporary methods in the form of insecticides, which must be applied repeatedly with continuous expenditure of time, labour and money. Temporary methods must, however, sometimes be employed, and various workers, mainly in America, have carried out extensive investigations on the use of insecticides for destroying larvæ in their breeding places.

Howard (1911, p. 194) found it to be "perfectly impracticable to use air-slaked lime, land plaster, or gas lime with good results. Few or no larvæ were killed by a thorough mixture of the manure with any of these substances. Chloride of lime, however, was found to be an excellent maggot killer," in the proportion of one pound to eight quarts of horse manure. Ninety per cent. of the larvæ were killed in less than twenty-four hours.

While kerosene gives good results in small experiments, "on a large scale this substance cannot be used with good effect," owing to the difficulty of obtaining thorough mixing.

Hermes found that fly larvæ in manure are very tenacious of life, and "that insecticides which will kill them must be strong, in fact from two to five times as strong as those which are useful against other insects."

Howard (1911, p. 197) quotes some unpublished experiments by Forbes, of Illinois, which show that "the breeding of the house-fly in manure can be controlled by the application of a solution of iron sulphate—two pounds in a gallon of water for each horse per day—or by the use of two and one-half pounds of dry sulphate per horse per day." It is stated also that iron sulphate has the advantage of completely deodorising the manure, and does not appear to injure it or the soil to which it is applied.

Any attempt to control the breeding places of flies in cities must be regulated to some extent by local bylaws, which might with advantage be based on the excellent regulations enforced in the District of Columbia. Much can also be done by suitable posters and leaflets, and by interesting the people and educating the children.

In camps and stations, where the night soil is buried in trenches, special care is necessary in making the trenches sufficiently deep, and in covering the excreta immediately after deposition in the trenches with a sufficient quantity of soil. The mere presence of dry earth over the excreta will not prevent the flies from emerging, if, owing to the neglect of suitable precautions, eggs have been deposited before the night soil is covered. If considered desirable, some material may be added to kill any larvæ which may be present. Much attention has already been paid to this subject, and the various methods which have been adopted or suggested need not be given in detail.

CHAPTER XXVIII

SUMMARY AND CONCLUSIONS

The subjects chiefly considered in each chapter, and the conclusions arrived at, are here briefly recapitulated.

The common-house-fly, *Musca domestica*, occurs in all parts of the world, and is the fly most commonly found in houses. In the height of the fly-season at least 90 % of the flies caught on sticky papers or in traps belong to this species. In the earlier months *F. canicularis* often predominates, but is displaced later by *M. domestica*. Many other species of non-biting flies, nearly all of which frequent putrefying substances and fæcal matter, are found in houses in small numbers. Owing to the numerous hairs scattered over their bodies and legs, most of these species are well adapted to carry bacteria from the substances they visit, and to distribute them on food materials within a few hours of contamination (Chapter II).

M. domestica breeds mainly in heaps of fermenting materials, especially piles of horse manure, but also breeds in refuse of all kinds and in human fæces. The females frequent these substances for the purpose of laying eggs, and at the same time walk over them and feed on them. The life-cycle from egg to sexual maturity is completed under favourable conditions in three to four weeks. The larvæ of the house-fly together with those of closely allied species, and members of the genus *Pycnosoma*, are found in trenches in which night soil is buried near camps and stations in the tropics (Chapter III).

In connection with the distribution of bacteria, the alimentary canal and its appendages constitute the most important system in the internal anatomy of the fly. The alimentary canal is long and complicated, consisting of the œsophagus, proventriculus, ventriculus, intestine and rectum. A branch of the œsophagus, the crop-duct, passes to the crop, a very distensible blind sac, situated in the anterior part of the abdomen. The salivary glands are greatly developed (Chapter IV).

The oral lobes situated at the end of the proboscis of the fly are provided with minute channels, the pseudo-tracheæ, into which liquid food is sucked through a form of grating, which prevents most particles of large size entering the œsophagus. Occasionally when feeding on fæcal material containing parasitic ova, to which flies are greatly attracted, great exertions may cause larger particles, such as ova, to enter the mouth direct, without the filtering action of the pseudo-tracheæ coming into action (Chapter V).

The crop acts as a reservoir into which fluid food is passed previous to its entering the intestine. The fluid in the crop is only passed into the intestine gradually through the proventriculus, which acts as a valve. When feeding on soluble substances this fluid in the crop, which is often highly contaminated with bacteria, is regurgitated through the proboscis in order to moisten and dissolve the food (Chapter VI).

Flies can travel for considerable distances, up to 1000 yards, at least in open districts, but probably do not often travel far in towns. In houses they walk over everything, including food, and deposit both fæcal material and 'vomit,' or fluid regurgitated from the crop, on every article over which they walk. After feeding they habitually regurgitate a portion of the crop contents, and other flies suck up the vomit, and infect themselves with any bacteria which may be present in it.

Flies defæcate very frequently, especially when well fed, many masses of fæces being deposited in the course of the day (Chapter VII).

Outside houses flies congregate on fermenting and decaying refuse of all sorts, carcases of animals and fæces.

If flies are provided with a sufficient quantity of liquid food they can be kept in captivity for two or three weeks or more in small glass cages in which their habits can be easily studied (Chapter VIII).

Infected flies not only carry bacteria on the surfaces of their bodies and limbs, and thereby contaminate substances over which they walk within a few hours of infection, but also distribute the bacteria they have ingested with their food by means of 'vomit' and fæcal deposits. Non-spore-bearing bacteria only survive a few hours, at most about twenty-four hours, on the limbs, but flies infect substances over which they walk with such organisms for several days. This infection is brought about by the flies constantly dabbing down their proboscides moistened with fluid regurgitated from the crop. Food, such as milk, syrup and sugar, may be infected in this way for several days. In the crop many of the ingested bacteria survive for several days, but no clear evidence of their multiplication in this situation or in the intestine has yet been obtained. The majority of the non-spore-bearing types pass through the intestine, and are present in a living condition in the fæcal deposits. Many of the experiments have been carried out with the easily recognizable non-spore-bearing *B. prodigiosus*, but other experiments indicate that several of the disease-producing species, such as *B. typhosus*, *B. enteritidis* (Gaertner), *B. tuberculosis*, and *B. anthracis* (non-sporing forms in blood) behave in the same way. Almost all the experiments have been carried out with *cultivated* strains, and it is possible that *uncultivated* strains, direct from naturally infected material, may be able to withstand competition with the other organisms which are present in the fly's intestine for even longer periods.

Spores, as ascertained by experiments with spore-bearing cultures of *B. anthracis*, may remain alive and virulent on the limbs and in the intestinal canal for at least three weeks. It is also important to note that in the case of flies, which become infected with anthrax spores, and die of empusa disease or cold, the spores remain alive and fully virulent in their bodies, if kept dry in bottles, for years. Such dead flies might easily be a source of infection.

Flies feeding on tubercular sputum suffer from diarrhœa, a

fact which may be of some importance in relation to their potentiality for spreading infection.

Flies do not appear to be affected by the presence in their alimentary tracts of bacteria pathogenic to man (Chapter IX).

City flies carry both in and on their bodies very large numbers of bacteria, many of which are of fæcal types, and are obtained from excrement. The bacteria are more numerous in flies obtained from congested and dirty areas. In cities flies do not migrate to any great extent from the neighbourhood of the area in which they are bred. In a few instances pathogenic species or allied types have been isolated from 'wild' city flies (Chapter X).

Certain types of bacilli, mostly belonging to the non-lactose fermenting group, are apparently so adapted to the conditions prevailing within the alimentary tract of the larva and adult, that, when ingested by the larva, they pass through the metamorphosis, and are present in the imagines, when they emerge from the pupæ. Of these the most interesting is Morgan's No. 1 bacillus, since it is often intimately associated with epidemic diarrhœa, and may have a causal relationship to the disease. *Cultivated* strains of *B. typhosus* and *B. enteritidis*, when fed to larvæ, do not survive, but experiments carried out by Faichnie indicate that *uncultivated* strains may be capable of surviving. The spores of *B. anthracis* can undoubtedly survive. Flies bred from larvæ living in material infected with anthrax spores are therefore capable of communicating the disease for some days after they emerge (Chapter XI).

The bacteriological evidence connecting 'wild' flies with the spread of specific diseases is at present very incomplete. Some of the evidence is old, and some too imperfectly recorded to be satisfactory. Careful and trustworthy bacteriological work is greatly needed, as the subject is beset with many difficulties. Bacteria of many kinds are present in great numbers in the intestines of flies, and several varieties closely resemble important disease-producing types, so that isolation and identification are matters requiring laborious and patient work, involving all the known means of diagnosis. Only a small proportion of the flies are likely to be infected with disease-producing types at any given time, and owing to the long incubation period of some of the diseases under consideration the infected flies may have disappeared before the disease is recognized and investigations started. Suitable opportunities for investigation must however occur from time to time, and if these are utilized definite and reliable information on the subject will be obtained.

Apart from definite bacteriological proofs, other evidence clearly points to flies being the carriers of infection in certain outbreaks, in which the other principal sources of infection have been carefully excluded (Chapter XII).

B. typhosus is said to have been isolated from 'wild' flies associated with outbreaks of typhoid fever on several occasions, and experimentally flies can carry and distribute this bacillus for several days. There is some evidence that flies are factors in causing the autumnal increase in the disease in this country, but it is unlikely that they play an important part in well-sewered towns. On the other hand, the evidence is very strong that they are the dominating factor in the dissemination of the disease in military and other camps, and in stations in the tropics. In such places infection is mainly acquired from the trenches in which night-soil is insufficiently buried, or from fæcal matter deposited in situations to which flies have access. The infected material is derived from 'carriers' or incipient or mild cases of the disease (Chapter XIII).

In temperate climates epidemic diarrhœa is the most important disease flies are supposed to transmit. It is undoubtedly true that unlimited opportunities are afforded to flies of conveying presumably infected material from the intestinal discharges of patients to the food of healthy infants, and also that there is a close relationship between the curves graphically illustrating the rise and fall of the annual outbreak of epidemic diarrhœa and the rise and fall of the annual prevalence of flies. In the hot summer of 1911 flies were numerous and epidemic diarrhœa very prevalent, but in the cold and wet summer of 1912 flies were few and epidemic diarrhœa uncommon. Evidence of this nature, whilst very suggestive, is not altogether conclusive. Unfortunately, though the disease is admitted to be infectious, the causative organism has not been identified with certainty. In some outbreaks Morgan's bacillus is very frequently present in the fæces of children suffering from the disease, and it is very significant, that while it has been found not uncommonly in the intestines of flies associated with such outbreaks, it seldom occurs in the intestines of flies from non-diarrhœa infected localities.

The annual mortality due to this disease is so great that a serious attempt to conclusively ascertain the part played by flies in its dissemination by exterminating them in some suitable areas, usually exhibiting a high mortality, though expensive, would be justified (Chapter XIV).

Most of the evidence relating to the spread of cholera by flies is somewhat old, but is so remarkable that careful investigation of this problem is highly desirable (Chapter XV).

Flies are greatly attracted to tuberculous sputum, and can carry and distribute *B. tuberculosis* contained in it for several days. Whether they are serious factors in the spread of the disease yet remains to be proved (Chapter XVI).

Flies feeding on blood containing non-spore-bearing anthrax bacilli can carry and distribute these bacilli in a virulent state for several days. Opportunities for infecting themselves from the bloody discharges of diseased animals probably often occur. Spores of *B. anthracis* can be carried for longer periods, and flies, which die while containing the spores, remain infective for long periods. Further spores ingested by the larvæ are present in the flies which develop from them. The part, if any, played by flies in the spread of this disease has not been ascertained.

Though evidence is lacking there can be little doubt that the spores of other pathogenic bacilli, such as *B. œdematis maligni* and *B. anthracis symptomatici*, behave in the same way as anthrax spores (Chapter XVII).

The organisms of other bacterial diseases, especially ophthalmia, may be distributed in the ways already mentioned, but little definite evidence on the subject is available (Chapter XVIII).

It is also possible that non-biting flies disseminate the virus of certain non-bacterial disease, more especially the *Spironema pertenuis* of Yaws (Chapter XIX).

Experimentally it has been shown that flies can carry and distribute the smaller ova of 'worms' parasitic in the human intestinal canal. Though they are very greatly attracted to such ova in fæcal deposits, the part they play in their dissemination under natural conditions has not been ascertained (Chapter XX).

The larvæ of some species of non-biting flies cause myiasis of various kinds in man. Some live in the tissues lining natural cavities or in wounds, causing serious loss of tissue, extensive wounds and even death. Others live under the skin, and are the cause of much irritation, and the larva of one species sucks blood from wounds which it produces. The larvæ of several species have been found in the intestinal tract, occasionally giving rise to uncomfortable sensations, or even serious inconvenience and ill-health, but often producing no symptoms (Chapter XXI).

In temperate climates adult flies appear to be subject only to one serious disease, that caused by the fungus, *Empusa muscæ*, which destroys large numbers in the late summer and early autumn. If some means could be devised of artificially infecting flies with this fungus, a ready means of controlling their numbers would be obtained (Chapter XXIII).

Externally various parasites, such as mites and false-scorpions, are often found on flies. These creatures, some of which live on various articles of human food, such as cheese, are undoubtedly transported to fresh feeding grounds by flies, but it is at present doubtful whether the majority of them feed on the flies. Internally various species of flies, especially in the tropics, are infested with flagellate protozoon parasites, and nematode worms.

Larvæ and pupæ are frequently destroyed by parasitic hymenoptera (Chapter XXIV).

The natural enemies of flies and their larvæ, such as spiders, wasps, ants, predaceous flies, lizards, toads and birds, probably destroy large numbers, but are incapable of effectually checking their multiplication (Chapter XXV).

Many species of flies breed in or visit human excrement. Of these the most important house-frequenting species are *M. domestica*, *F. canicularis* and *F. scalaris*, though several others are occasionally found in houses. In camps on the other hand many excrement frequenting species visit food, and under suitable conditions may distribute disease-producing bacteria (Chapter XXVI).

Flies which enter houses may be caught on papers or in traps, or may be destroyed by other means. In order to limit their numbers, however, the breeding places must be removed or rendered unsuitable. This can only be accomplished by educating the community, establishing inspectors, and enforcing bylaws framed to meet the needs of different localities (Chapter XXVII).

The filth-carrying capacity and foul associations of the house-fly have been clearly demonstrated, but prolonged and careful observations are yet required before we are in a position to understand its exact relationship to disease under varying conditions. For the elucidation of some of the problems, which have been indicated, expert knowledge is required, but accurate observations by workers without special scientific training would be of the greatest assistance. The writer hopes that those who are interested in public health matters, both at home and abroad, will be able to gather from these pages some information, which may be useful to them in planning investigations on the widely scattered problems opened up by the demonstration of the capacity of non-biting flies to disseminate disease-producing micro-organisms.

APPENDIX

Recent work on measurements of flies (p. 264), effects of different foods and duration of feeding during the larval stages (p. 266), range of flight (p. 273), changes of habits of flies (p. 276), colour preference (p. 282), hibernation (p. 282), survival in the adult fly of micro-organisms ingested by the larva (p. 284), typhoid fever (p. 284), dysentery (p. 285), summer diarrhœa (p. 287), cholera (p. 326), anthrax (p. 332), leprosy (p. 332), trypanosomiasis (p. 334), infection by non-biting flies of wounds caused by biting flies (p. 335), myiasis (p. 338), Empusa disease (p. 345), parasites of adult flies (p. 347), parasites of larvæ (p. 348), enemies of flies (p. 349), measures against adult flies (p. 350).

Measurements of flies (see p. 15).

Hermes (1907, 1911) carried out most interesting experiments relating to the effects of under- and over-feeding of the larvæ on the flies (*Lucilia* and *Sarcophaga*) subsequently produced from such larvæ. In the course of these investigations he weighed the larvæ at intervals, and in some cases weighed the adults which emerged before they had had any opportunity of feeding. He did not, however, distinguish between the sexes, nor did he measure the adults or attempt to breed from single females. He has published an excellent plate showing the sizes of the adults (*L. cæsar*) which emerged from larvæ fed for various times.

The writer has recently made somewhat similar observations and experiments on blow-flies (*C. erythrocephala*), which are easily handled in captivity. Not only were 'wild' specimens, caught in various localities, accurately measured, but adults bred from eggs deposited by single females were also measured. The larvæ from which these adults were bred were allowed to feed for various times on different foods. Until evidence to the contrary is forthcoming it may be justifiable to assume that conditions, similar to those which tend to produce individuals of different sizes amongst artificially bred flies, are responsible for the production of the variations in size noted amongst 'wild' flies. Hermes (1907) has shown that under natural conditions variations in the food supply of the larvæ often occur.

So far as the writer is aware these are the first experiments in which 'wild' flies, and those produced from larvæ reared artificially under varied conditions, have been accurately compared by measurement.

In order to estimate the variations in the sizes of 'wild' flies the author measured a number of blow-flies (*C. erythrocephala*) caught during the last few years in different localities. In carrying out such observations it is necessary to choose certain easily established fixed points, between which the measurements can be accurately made. In this set of experiments the length of the thorax from its anterior border to the tip of the scutellum[1] (Fig. 3), the length of the wing from the point where the costal vein joins the conjoined stem of the auxiliary and first and second longitudinal veins to the apex of the wing (Figs. 3 and 4), and the maximum breadth of the head (Fig. 1) were measured. These measurements were made under a low power of the microscope with the aid of an eye-piece micrometer. The degree of variation which occurs may be gauged from the fact that no two specimens of wild flies with similar measurements were discovered. Similar variations, the nature and extent of which are set out in Tables 32 and 33, occurred amongst bred examples, and consequently it seems unnecessary to give the measurements of all the wild flies examined in tabular form. The mean length of the thorax in wild males was 4·78 mm., in wild females 4·61 mm., the mean length of the wing in males 9·39 mm., in females 9·76 mm., and the mean breadth of the head in males 3·68 mm., and in females 3·74 mm. The largest male measured—thorax 5·22 mm., wing 9·31 mm., head 4·13 mm., and the smallest—thorax 4·46 mm., wing 8·93 mm., head 3·32 mm. The largest female measured—thorax 5·51 mm., wing 11·49 mm., head 4·60 mm.—and the smallest—thorax 3·99 mm., wing 8·83 mm., head 3·32 mm.

[1] As the tip of the scutellum is an easier point to determine than the base, the tip was taken as a fixed point after ascertaining, by a series of measurements, that the scutellum does not vary appreciably in length in relation to the rest of the thorax either in the male or the female.

The greatest length of thorax observed was 5·51 mm. and the smallest 3·99 mm., the greatest length of wing 11·49 mm. and the smallest 8·45 mm., the greatest breadth of head 4·60 mm. and the smallest 3·27 mm. An interesting point in relation to the sizes of the eyes in the two sexes may be noted. If males and females, possessing heads of the same breadth, be examined it will be seen that the space between the eyes in the female (mean 1·22 mm.) is nearly five times as great as the space (mean ·26 mm.) between the eyes in the male. The male eye (mean 1·63 mm.) is on the contrary, however, nearly one-third broader than the female eye (mean 1·16 mm.).

Experiments to determine the effects on the adult flies of different foods and the duration of feeding during the larval stages.

A number of experiments, of which three are quoted, were conducted in order to ascertain to what extent the flies which

Explanation of Plate XXV.

Blow-fly *A*, upper central figure, and some of the flies bred from eggs deposited by it (natural size).

Row 1.—Seven flies, four males and three females, bred from undisturbed larvæ fed on *fish*.

On the left is the largest male, then two of intermediate size, and the fourth specimen represents the smallest male. The three specimens on the right represent from left to right, the largest, an intermediate and the smallest females.

Row 2.—The three specimens on the left represent the flies, two males and one female, bred from larvæ allowed to feed on *fish* for seven days, and the four on the right the females bred from larvæ allowed to feed for six days.

The small object on the right in line with the puparia represents a larva which failed to pupate after five days' feeding.

Row 3.—Seven flies, three males and four females bred from undisturbed larvæ which fed on *meat* for 11 days. In each group the largest specimen is on the left and the smallest on the right.

Row 4.—From left to right the two males bred from larvæ allowed to feed on *meat* for 11 days, the two males from larvæ allowed to feed for 10 days, and the three flies, two males and one female, from larvæ allowed to feed for 9 days.

Row 5.—On the left two males, and on the right two females, in one of which the wings failed to expand, bred from larvæ allowed to feed on *meat* for 8 days.

Under each specimen is placed the pupa case from which it emerged.

Each fly shown in this plate is marked * in Table 32.

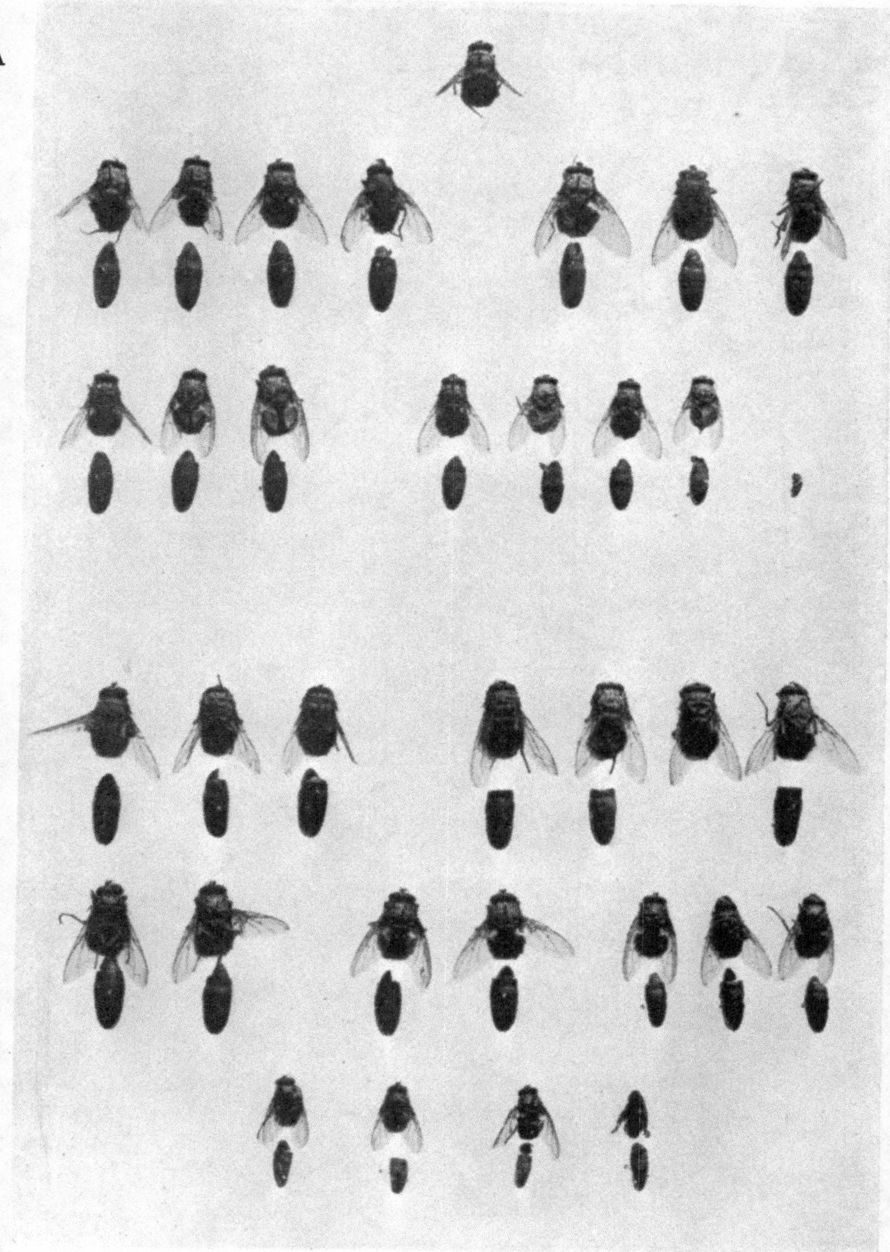

Flies bred from Blow-fly A.

emerge are effected by the conditions prevailing during the larval stage. Female blow-flies were captured, and each individual was induced to deposit her eggs in a separate cage. Some of the eggs obtained from each fly were transferred to cooked fish placed on earth, some to cooked fish without earth, some to cooked meat placed on earth, and some to cooked meat without earth. The larvæ, which developed from those placed on the cooked fish and meat resting on earth were not disturbed, and eventually went under ground and pupated. The flies which emerged were allowed to live for two or three days before being killed. Specimens of the larvæ, which were placed on fish and meat without earth, and therefore had no suitable substance into which to burrow and pupate, were removed after feeding for various times and placed on earth without food. The majority of these after wandering about for a short time disappeared under the earth and pupated.

While the fish and meat were renewed at frequent intervals it should be noted that while the cooked meat soon became very dry, the fish remained moist under the dried skin.

Experiment 1. A small female blow-fly, *A* (*C. erythrocephala*), giving the following measurements, thorax 4·46 mm., wing 8·74 mm., head 3·61 mm. deposited eggs on July 18th, and the larvæ hatched out next day. Some of the larvæ were transferred to cooked fish placed on earth and after feeding for eight days disappeared into the earth. From these twenty male and seventeen female flies emerged between the 34th and 36th days after the deposition of the eggs. The measurements of these flies, which exhibited considerable variation in size, are given in Table 32. It should be noticed, however, that all are larger than the parent in every measurement. The mean length of the male thorax was 4·95 mm., of the female thorax 5·07, of the male wing 9·59 mm., of the female 10·16 mm., the mean breadth of the male head 3·76 mm. of the female head 3·95 mm.

Three flies emerged from larvæ allowed to feed for seven days on fish and then placed on earth. In their thoracic measurements these are larger than the parent. Four flies emerged from larvæ allowed to feed on fish for six days, all of them smaller than the parent. These seven flies also emerged

Table 32 giving the measurements of flies bred from eggs deposited by Blow-fly A.

(Thorax 4·46 mm., wing 8·74 mm., head 3·61 mm.)

Larvæ fed on Fish.
Measurements of flies in mm.

Thorax	Wing	Head	♂	♀	
5·22	10·35	3·94	—	1	Flies emerging in 34–36 days after the deposition of the eggs from pupæ of undisturbed larvæ which fed for 8 days on fish placed on earth.
,,	10·21	,,	—	1*	
,,	9·64	3·80	1*	—	
5·17	10·35	4·03	—	1	
,,	10·07	3·94	—	1	
5·13	10·26	,,	—	1	
,,	10·16	3·99	—	2*	
,,	9·88	,,	—	1	
,,	,,	3·80	1	—	
,,	9·58	,,	1	—	
,,	9·50	,,	1	—	
5·03	10·40	3·99	—	1	
,,	10·26	3·89	—	1	
,,	10·11	3·99	—	1	
,,	10·07	3·94	—	1	
,,	9·73	3·80	1	—	
,,	9·69	3·75	1	—	
,,	9·64	,,	1	—	
,,	9·40	,,	1*	—	
4·98	10·16	3·99	—	1	
,,	9·97	3·89	—	1	
4·94	10·30	3·94	—	1	
,,	10·07	3·84	1	—	
,,	9·97	3·89	—	1	
,,	9·83	3·80	2	—	
,,	9·59	,,	1	—	
,,	9·54	3·75	1	—	
,,	9·50	3·70	1*	—	
4·89	10·07	3·94	—	1*	
4·84	9·59	3·65	1	—	
,,	9·50	3·75	1	—	
,,	,,	3·70	1	—	
4·79	9·54	3·70	1	—	
,,	9·50	,,	1	—	
4·60	8·78	3·80	1*	—	
4·75	9·92	3·75	—	1*	Larvæ allowed to feed on fish for 7 days
,,	9·02	3·51	1*	—	
4·56	8·64	3·42	1*	—	
4·27	8·59	3·27	—	1*	Larvæ allowed to feed on fish for 6 days
4·03	8·55	3·27	—	1*	
3·89	7·98	3·13	—	1*	
3·61	7·31	2·80	—	1*	

Larvæ fed on Meat.
Measurements of flies in mm.

Thorax	Wing	Head	♂	♀	
5·32	10·45	4·03	—	1	Flies emerging in 35–36 days after deposition of eggs from pupæ of undisturbed larvæ which fed for 11 days on meat placed on earth.
5·27	10·30	3·84	—	1*	
5·22	10·64	,,	—	1*	
,,	10·54	3·89	—	1	
,,	10·49	3·75	—	1	
,,	10·45	3·80	—	1	
,,	10·40	3·94	—	1*	
5·17	10·45	3·99	—	1*	
,,	10·02	3·80	1*	—	
5·13	9·97	3·46	1*	—	
4·98	9·59	3·51	1*	—	
4·94	9·40	,,	1	—	
4·79	10·30	3·56	—	1	
5·08	10·07	3·80	1*	—	Larvæ allowed to feed on meat for 11 days
,,	9·83	,,	1*	—	
4·79	9·50	3·61	1*	—	Larvæ allowed to feed on meat for 10 days
,,	9·45	,,	1*	—	
4·41	8·64	3·37	1*	—	Larvæ allowed to feed on meat for 9 days
4·18	8·78	3·32	—	1*	
4·13	8·21	3·18	1*	—	
3·56	7·69	2·80	—	1*	Larvæ allowed to feed on meat for 8 days
3·42	6·93	2·61	1*	—	
3·32	6·74	2·61	1*	—	
2·47	—	1·94	—	1*	

* Flies shown in Plate XXV.

between the 34th and 36th days. Larvæ allowed to feed for five and four days only failed to pupate.

A few larvæ transferred to cooked meat placed on earth fed for 11 days before burrowing. Four males and nine females emerged on the 35th and 36th days after the deposition of the eggs. Except in regard to their head measurements these flies were decidedly larger than those obtained from the fish-fed larvæ, the mean length of the thorax in males being 5·05 mm., in females 5·18 mm., the mean length of the wing in males 9·74 mm., in females 10·44 mm. and the mean breadth of the head in males 3·54 mm., in females 3·85 mm.

Two flies emerged from larvæ fed on meat for 11 days and then placed on earth, and two from larvæ fed for 10 days. All four surpassed the parent in size. Three flies, all smaller than the parent, emerged from larvæ fed for nine days, and four flies from larvæ fed for eight days. The latter were all very small individuals, and in one of them the wings failed to develop. These 11 flies also emerged on the 35th and 36th days.

The measurements of every fly which emerged from the eggs laid by blow-fly *A* are given in Table 32, and photographs of some of the more interesting examples are shown on Plate XXV.

Experiment 2. A large female blow-fly, *B* (thorax 5·22 mm., wing 10·64 mm., head 4·27 mm.) deposited eggs on July 17th, from which larvæ emerged on July 19th. A number of the larvæ were allowed to feed on fish placed on earth. These fed for eight days, and 29 males and 31 females emerged between the 35th and 37th days after the deposition of the eggs. All were considerably smaller than the parent in every measurement. The mean length of the thorax in males was 4·73 mm., in females 4·68 mm., of the wing in males 9·12 mm., in females 9·56 mm., and of the breadth of the head in males 3·48 mm., in females 3·58 mm.

Two flies emerged from larvæ allowed to feed on fish for eight days and then placed on earth, four from larvæ allowed to feed seven days and three from larvæ which fed for six days. The latter were very small. Larvæ allowed to feed for five and four days only failed to pupate. These nine flies also emerged between the 35th and 37th days.

On meat the undisturbed larvæ fed for 11 days, and the flies which emerged between the 39th and 41st days after the deposition of the eggs, were smaller than the majority of specimens, which developed from fish-fed larvæ.

Two larvæ were kept for 12 days on meat before being placed on earth. Both pupated, but while one fly failed to extricate itself from the pupa case, the other emerged. Two flies, which emerged from larvæ allowed to feed for 11 days, were rather small, three flies from larvæ which fed for ten days were still smaller, and a fly which emerged from a larva, allowed to feed for nine days only, was, though perfect, very small.

The smallest fly emerged on the 35th day, but the other six between the 39th and 41st day.

The measurements of every fly which emerged from the eggs laid by blow-fly *B* are given in Table 33 and photographs

Explanation of Plate XXVI.

Blow-fly *B*, upper central figure, and below it four rows of flies bred from eggs deposited by it (natural size).

Row 1.—Six flies, three males and three females, bred from undisturbed larvæ fed on *fish*. In each group the largest specimen is on the left, the smallest on the right.

Row 2.—On the left a male and a female bred from larvæ allowed to feed on *fish* for 8 days; in the centre two males and one female bred from larvæ allowed to feed for 7 days; on the right one male and two females bred from larvæ allowed to feed for 6 days.

The small object on the right below the line of puparia represents a larva which failed to pupate after 5 days' feeding.

Row 3.—Two males and one female bred from undisturbed larvæ, which fed on *meat* for 11 days.

Row 4.—On the left one male bred from a larva allowed to feed on *meat* for 12 days; then a male and a female bred from larvæ allowed to feed for 11 days; next two males and a female bred from larvæ allowed to feed for 10 days; on the right a male bred from a larva allowed to feed for 9 days.

The two small objects on the right represent larvæ, allowed to feed on meat for 8 days, which failed to pupate.

The pupa case from which the fly emerged is placed either below or at the side of each specimen. Each fly shown is marked * in Table 33.

The lower central figure represents blow-fly *C*.

Row 5.—Four males and two females bred from the eggs deposited by *C* on a small piece of meat (see Table 34).

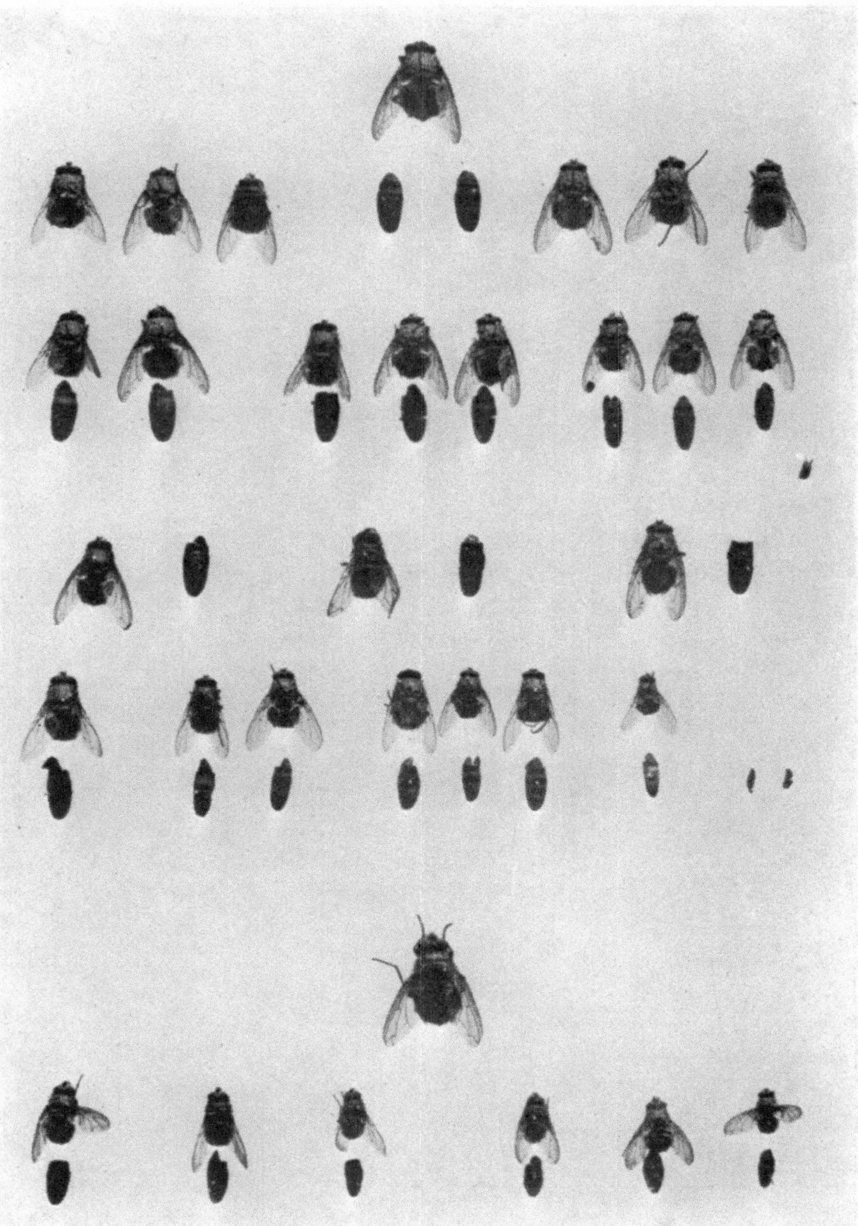

Flies bred from Blow-flies B and C.

Table 33 *gives the measurements of flies bred from eggs deposited by Blow-fly B.*

(Thorax 5·22 mm., wing 10·64 mm., head 4·27 mm.)

Larvæ fed on Fish.

Thorax	Wing	Head	♂	♀	
Measurements of flies in mm.					
4·94	9·12	3·61	1*	—	Flies emerging in 35–37 days after the deposition of the eggs from pupæ of undisturbed larvæ which fed for 8 days on fish placed on earth.
4·89	9·39	3·65	1	—	
4·84	9·88	3·70	—	1	
"	"	3·65	—	1	
"	"	3·61	—	1*	
"	9·73	3·61	—	1	
"	9·40	3·56	1	—	
"	9·31	3·51	1	—	
"	9·26	"	1	—	
"	"	3·32	1	—	
"	9·12	3·56	1	—	
"	9·07	"	1	—	
"	"	3·42	1	—	
"	9·02	3·51	1	—	
"	"	3·46	1	—	
4·79	9·88	3·70	—	1	
"	9·54	3·56	—	1	
"	9·21	3·46	1	—	
4·75	9·83	3·61	—	1	
"	9·75	3·65	—	1	
"	9·69	3·56	—	1*	
"	9·59	3·61	—	1	
"	9·50	3·70	—	1	
"	"	3·61	—	2	
"	9·35	3·56	—	1	
"	9·31	3·61	1	—	
"	9·16	3·51	1*	—	
"	"	3·32	1	—	
"	9·12	3·46	2	—	
"	9·07	3·56	1	—	
"	9·02	3·42	2	—	
"	8·93	3·46	1	—	
4·70	9·64	3·56	—	1	
"	9·50	3·65	—	1	
"	"	3·46	—	1	
"	9·45	3·61	—	1	
4·65	9·69	"	—	1	
"	9·54	3·51	—	1	
"	9·40	3·61	—	1	
"	9·31	3·51	1	—	
"	9·21	3·56	1	—	
"	9·02	3·42	1	—	
"	8·83	3·46	—	1	
4·60	9·59	3·61	—	1	
"	9·35	"	—	1	
4·56	9·59	3·56	—	1	
"	9·40	"	—	1	
"	"	3·37	—	1	
"	9·12	3·51	1	—	
4·46	9·69	"	—	1	
"	9·54	3·56	—	1	
"	9·45	3·51	—	1	
"	9·26	3·46	—	1*	
"	9·07	3·51	1	—	
"	"	3·46	1	—	
"	8·93	3·42	1*	—	
"	8·64	3·27	1	—	

Thorax	Wing	Head	♂	♀	
Measurements of flies in mm.					
4·65	9·35	3·56	1*	—	Larvæ allowed to feed on fish for 8 days
4·56	9·88	3·70	—	1*	
4·65	8·93	3·46	1*	—	Larvæ allowed to feed on fish for 7 days
4·56	"	3·37	1	—	
4·46	9·40	3·56	—	1*	
4·37	8·88	3·32	1*	—	
4·08	8·12	3·08	—	1*	Larvæ allowed to feed on fish for 6 days
3·99	8·26	3·08	—	1*	
3·89	7·88	2·95	1*	—	
Larvæ fed on Meat.					
4·65	9·02	3·42	1*	—	Undisturbed larvæ which fed 11 days. Flies emerging in 39–41 days.
"	8·83	"	1*	—	
4·60	9·50	3·61	—	1*	
4·65	8·78	3·46	1*	—	Larvæ allowed to feed on meat for 12 days
4·18	7·98	3·04	1*	—	Larvæ allowed to feed on meat for 11 days
4·08	8·36	3·04	—	1*	
4·37	8·40	3·27	1*	—	Larvæ allowed to feed on meat for 10 days
4·08	"	3·08	—	1*	
3·32	7·03	2·61	1*	—	
2·99	6·08	2·28	1*	—	Larvæ allowed to feed on meat for 9 days

* Flies shown in Plate XXVI.

of some of the more interesting examples are shown on Plate XXVI.

Though the experiments quoted were few in number they were conducted with the greatest care, and the measurements made with as much accuracy as possible, consequently it may perhaps be permissible to offer the following tentative conclusions: that the size of the fly depends on the quality and quantity of the food of the larva, and the time during which it feeds. On moist food the larvæ become full fed more rapidly. On dry food though the larvæ take longer to mature the flies which emerge may be of large size. The smallest individuals seem to be produced by relatively short periods of feeding on dry food. In 'wild' flies variations very similar to those observed in bred flies are met with, and are due probably to similar causes.

Griffith (1908) has shown that when the larvæ are kept cool the flies which emerge are small, and incapable of reproduction. Possibly the small specimens produced in these experiments were sterile.

The effects on the pupa cases are very marked. Undisturbed meat-fed larvæ produce strong dark coloured puparia, while those of the fish-fed larvæ are lighter in colour. The puparia of larvæ allowed to feed for short periods are very pale and fragile.

In the situation in which these experiments were conducted the mean daily maximum temperature over the whole period was 76° F. and the mean daily minimum 52° F.

Experiment 3. A very large female blow-fly, *C* (thorax 5·60 mm., wing 11·21 mm., head 4·32 mm.) deposited eggs on a small piece of meat. In five days the meat had become very hard and covered with moulds. No other food was supplied to the larvæ. Only six of the larvæ pupated, and from these six very small flies emerged on the 41st day. Their measurements are given in the following table.

The parent fly together with the six flies mentioned are shown in Plate XXVI.

Table 34 *showing the measurements of flies bred from eggs deposited by Blow-fly C.*

Thorax	Wing	Head	♂	♀
3·99	7·88	2·99	1	—
3·80	7·69	2·89	1	—
3·37	7·41	2·75	—	1
3·23	6·55	2·42	1	—
3·13	6·50	2·42	1	—
2·89	6·27	2·28	—	1

Range of flight (see p. 74).

In the months of July, August and the first week of September, 1912 Hindle and Merriman (1913) conducted a series of experiments on the range of flight of *Musca domestica* in the town of Cambridge. In the course of these experiments upwards of 25,000 flies were liberated under very variable meteorological conditions, and 191 were recovered at one or other of the 50 observation stations employed for their recovery. Before liberation the flies were thoroughly dusted with coloured chalks (see p. 76).

When the flies were liberated in the morning the traps and fly papers were examined in the afternoon of the same day. Subsequently, however, the observation stations were visited every morning, and therefore, any flies then recovered would have been exposed to the winds of the preceding day. This point should be remembered in examining the results shown on their charts, for in some cases the flies seem to have travelled with the wind owing to its change of direction on the day of recovery. Eleven experiments were made and the authors describe each in detail with the assistance of charts and full meteorological data. To illustrate the method employed experiment 6 is quoted.

Experiment 6. 6th—12th August, 1912. "2400 red coloured flies were liberated from the ground at 11.30 a.m. on August 6th. A strong wind (11 miles per hour) was blowing at the time of liberation, and several showers fell during the day, but nevertheless, no less than 34 flies were recovered at distances ranging up to 325 yards from the point of liberation. It will be noticed that most of the 15 flies, which travelled a distance of more than 150 yards, had flown either across, or in the teeth of, the wind prevailing on the day previous to their recovery. In this case, a number of flies were recovered from rooms at an altitude of 30 feet, and in many cases the insects must have flown over buildings at least 50 feet high."

In the following chart five flies recovered on August 6th are indicated by the letter *a*, those caught on August 7th by the letter *b*, and so on. The distance traversed is also indicated in each case.

Unfortunately the experiments were seriously handicapped by the difficulty of obtaining flies in sufficient numbers and the adverse meteorological conditions. Nevertheless some interesting conclusions could be drawn from these observations, the most unexpected being that flies tend to travel either directly against the wind or across it. "The main exceptions to this rule were those recovered within a radius of about 150 to 200 yards from the point of liberation, and probably these flies were individuals that had merely selected the first shelter they could find." The writers consider that two explanations of this phenomenon are possible: "(1) the flies may tend to fly against any current of air to which they are subjected. This property is known as positive anemotropism, and is possessed by some other insects and birds." (2) "The flies may travel against the wind, being attracted by any odours it may convey from a source of food."

These experiments further indicate that (*a*) the chief conditions favouring the dispersal of flies in a town are fine weather and a warm temperature; (*b*) the height at which the flies are liberated, and also the time of day influence their dispersal. When set free in the afternoon they do not scatter so well as when liberated in the morning; (*c*) the maximum flight in thickly housed localities is about a quarter of a mile.

A different aspect of the problem relating to the flight of flies has been recently investigated by Hodge (1913). Plagues of flies were reported from the cribs of the water-works, situated a mile and a quarter, five miles and six miles out in Lake Erie from Cleveland. On investigation it was found that there was nothing to attract flies to these places, or materials of any kind

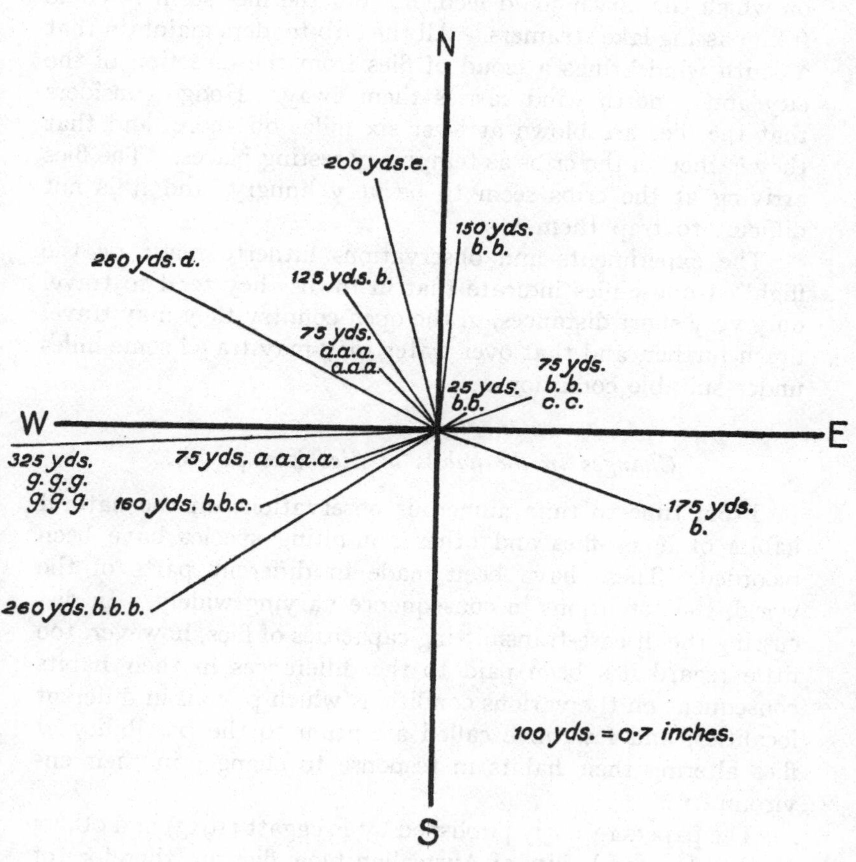

Chart 5.

	Date		Direction of wind	Velocity of wind in miles per hour	Thermometer Max.	Thermometer Min.	Rainfall in inches
(*a*)	August	6th	S.E.	11	68	56	0·1
(*b*)	,,	7th	W.S.W.	10	65	53	0·2
(*c*)	,,	8th	W.	8	66	52	0·16
(*d*)	,,	9th	W.	6	67	54	0·04
(*e*)	,,	10th	S.	5	67	52	0·0
(*f*)	,,	11th	W.	6	66	49	0·08
(*g*)	,,	12th	E.	4	64	49	0·03

on which the larvæ could feed, nor did the flies seem to come from passing lake steamers. All the crib-tenders maintain that a south wind brings a cloud of flies from the direction of the city and a north wind carries them away. Hodge considers that the flies are blown at least six miles off shore, and that they gather on the cribs as temporary resting places. The flies arriving at the cribs seem to be very hungry, and it is not difficult to trap them.

The experiments and observations hitherto made on the flight of house-flies indicate that in towns they tend to travel only very short distances, in the open country they may travel much further, and that over water they may travel some miles under suitable conditions.

Changes in the habits of flies (see p. 78).

From time to time numerous observations on the natural habits of house-flies and other non-biting species have been recorded. These have been made in different parts of the world, the conditions in consequence varying widely. In discussing the disease-transmitting capacities of flies, however, too little regard has been paid to the differences in their habits consequent on the various conditions which prevail in different localities, and few have called attention to the possibility of flies altering their habits in response to changes in their environment.

The papers recently published by Froggatt (1913) and others on the changed habits of Australian blow-flies are therefore of peculiar interest in calling attention to two important facts—that in different parts of the world different species of flies may be responsible for similar diseases, and that great changes may take place in the habits of certain species within comparatively short periods of time.

Froggatt's paper mainly refers to that form of myiasis in sheep known as 'blown wool,' of which he gives the following description. "Usually, the flies lay their eggs upon the wool of the rump near the tail, but should the wool be accidentally soiled on the flank they may be deposited there. When the sheep is caught, it will be noticed that the wool is discoloured or dark on the surface, and quite hot to the hand, resulting from the decomposition, inflammation, and moisture caused by the swarms of maggots beneath. Opened out with a pair of sheep shears, a putrid, vile-smelling mass of wool is found beneath ; if in an advanced stage, the maggots extend right down to the skin which is red and inflamed. The whole mass of squirming maggots is in all stages of development, from great big fat creatures to some just hatched ; for when once a sheep is blown and smelly, other flies are attracted, and these drop their eggs or living larvæ in clusters of a dozen or fifty, gummed together with a secretion that also glues them to the wool as they pass from the retractile slender ovipositor of the fly."

At present this disease appears to exist in certain parts of the world only, Great Britain, Australia, New Zealand and Hawaii.

It " has been known from a very early date in Great Britain," where, though occasionally caused by the larvæ of *Lucilia cæsar* or *Calliphora erythrocephala*, it is due usually to those of *L. sericata*. In New Zealand also it is due to the larvæ of *L. sericata* (Gilruth, 1908).

In Australia on the other hand though *L. sericata* is common its larvæ have never been found in blown wool, and the disease is caused mainly by the larvæ of *Calliphora oceaniæ* and *C. villosa*, and occasionally by those of *C. rufifacies*. In Hawaii the disease has made its appearance only recently, and is there due to the larvæ of *Calliphora dux*, an insect long established in the Islands, but which has only recently shown a partiality for live wool.

Though the disease has been known in Great Britain for many years it seems to have spread recently into districts previously unaffected. " A distinctly important point brought out in the inquiry relates not only to the wide-spreadness of maggot and its increasing frequency, but to its spread to high-lying hill pastures, where, until recently in many places, the attack seems to have been almost unknown" (MacDougall, 1909).

This author quotes a large number of reports from sheep-owners in various parts of Scotland. All are agreed that the trouble became serious between 1899 and 1904. Extracts from two of these reports may be of interest. "Till 1893 or 1894 we had no trouble with the maggots, unless in sheltered, woody or low ground. About this time the fly began attacking ewes grazing on the low hills; they have been getting worse every year, and now I am fully of opinion that sheep grazing at 1900 to 2300 feet above the sea level are just as likely to be attacked as sheep grazing in sheltered, woody, or low ground pastures. Even on the low ground in the last few years there has been a steady increase year by year" (D. R. Ballater). "In this district (Breadalbane) the fly is rapidly extending its area, and many high-lying farms, where up to quite recently maggots were unknown, are now badly infested." Carpenter (1902) speaking of 'maggot' in Ireland makes the following statement. "It seems that, over a limited area, one of two kinds of flesh flies, have forsaken the usual habit of their family, so that the maggots have become parasites instead of scavengers. There can be no doubt that this change of habit has been induced by the domestication of sheep by man. We have taken an originally alpine race of animals, crowded them on the plains, and by artificial selection increased the qualities—such as fat and thick wool—that tend to attract the fly."

"Blow-flies are indigenous to Australia; specimens were collected by the naturalists who visited our shores in exploring expeditions as far back as the early part of last century, before there could be any chance of their being introduced by man from other countries.

Now, under natural conditions, blow-flies confined their attention to decaying animal and vegetable matter festering around camps. When settlers came into the country, they were, at the worst, what we might call 'casual domestic pests,' attracted into the house and larder by their keen sense of smell to food upon which they deposited their eggs. Sometimes, it happened that they obtained access to a neglected wound on a farm animal, and it became maggoty."

Froggatt is exceptionally qualified to speak on the changes which have taken place in the habits of blow-flies in Australia.

He has resided in the country while the change has been taking place, and though now Government Entomologist, New South Wales, was at one time interested in sheep. His experiences and observations may therefore be quoted at length.

"Thirty years ago, when the writer was personally interested in sheep on the Murray frontages, one could mark lambs at any time of the year and not even worry to dag the ewes, unless they were in a particularly bad state from too much young grass in a good season; one seldom found maggots in the lambs, and never in the wool. The only maggots one dealt with in sheep were in the heads of rams, where they had injured their hard heads fighting, so that the broken skin had become blown."

Rabbits at that time were uncommon in this district, and though there were some severe droughts, "and dead sheep were scattered all over the plains and ranges, yet the flies had not forsaken their natural rôle as scavengers, and become parasitic upon live sheep." "In the bush, away from the waste and rubbish about town and homestead, blow-flies were not constant attendants to one riding or walking through the timber or scrub, as they are at the present day." Blow-flies were first observed in abnormal numbers by Froggatt during the drought of 1890—1.

"During the last six months of 1910, while making visits to the west and south of New South Wales, the writer found the open forest, and the flats along the creeks and billabongs, swarming with blow-flies, while, about any homestead, they simply clustered, like swarms of bees, round the wire doors—particularly those near the kitchen."

"Though blown wool may have been common before, in some holdings, it was not until 1903 that the writer had any record of it doing any noticeable damage to the wool or sheep. In the following year, it was recorded from a number of widely separated districts as a very serious trouble to the sheep-owners; and, in the last five years, it has become one of the most serious problems to fight and to control, in the working of sheep. At the present time, there is hardly a district in which sheep are running where blown wool is not found; and, though perhaps the trouble is most intense in the south, west, north-west and Riverina districts of New South Wales, it has been found close to Sydney and all down the south coast. The trouble is still spreading, so that practically the whole of New South Wales is infested. Recent reports show that the trouble is spreading through Queensland; and, as the blow-flies are not much affected by cold, it will probably be found before long, infesting Victorian flocks in a similar manner."

That the blown wool disease has become serious only in recent years is admitted by several writers, who attribute the change in habits of the flies to different causes.

Froggatt considers that the destruction of birds and other insect-destroying animals by wholesale poisoning, adopted to get rid of the rabbits, and other means has allowed the flies to increase abnormally. The clearing of the forest lands has had a similar effect. Finally, he attributes their change in habits to the last great drought. "This drought was remarkable for the fact that, unlike many of the previous and more local ones, it was felt over the greater part of the pastoral country in Australia. Then, flocks had to be shifted all over the country, leaving in their wake thousands of dead sheep clothed with wool that was not worth collecting. The scavenger or blow-flies deposited their eggs among this wool, and thus apparently acquired the habit of detecting foul wool. This sharpened sense, which we might say is now inherited, has become intensified, so that it requires very little moisture, mucus or blood upon the wool to attract the flies; thus, wool, under these conditions, has become a regular food supply to large numbers of these fly maggots."

Woodburn (1913) thinks the fly trouble has been consequent upon the destruction of rabbits.

Whatever the cause may be the fact appears to be clearly established that two species of indigenous blow-fly in Australia and another species of indigenous blow-fly in Hawaii have developed parasitic habits within recent years.

In this connection the researches of Hermes (1907) on the sarcophagid flies at Cedar Point beach near Sandusky, Ohio, are of considerable interest. On this narrow strip of sand the fish cast up by surf-producing storms are the sole food of these flies and their larvæ. "The surf-producing storms occur at comparatively regular intervals, a low surf taking place about every three days, a heavier surf every six or seven days, and a still heavier surf every 14 or 15 days. Now the very fact that the life histories of *Compsomyia macellaria*, *Sarcophaga assuida*, *Lucilia cæsar* and *Sarcophaga sarraceniæ* cover, respectively, a period of 8 or 9 days, 12 or 13 days, 14 or 15 days and 18 or 19 days, seems to indicate a peculiar coincidence, if nothing more. The factor 3 plays an important rôle, viz. 3 × 3, 3 × 4, 3 × 5 and 3 × 6, which corresponds in general to the occurrence of the surf. Were adults to emerge from their pupa cases at a time when no fish or very few fish were present on the beach the probabilities are that such individuals would suffer starvation. If this were often repeated the tendency would be to impair the vigor of the species, especially by interfering with the normal egg-laying habit. This latter would certainly be the case if the usual number of adults were to emerge with an under supply of food present upon which the eggs could be deposited. The large number of larvæ for the short supply of food would result in producing smaller individuals, which has been proven by experiments. That the sarcophagids given in the list are normal, as compared with individuals of the same species breeding elsewhere, is evident to the most superficial observer, and they are certainly not less numerous.

"Considering the above facts and also bearing in mind that the food supply is influenced by the comparative regularity of the surfs, there seems then to have been somewhere in the past an adaptation to surf-producing storms. When the adult fly emerges from the pupa case it is likely to find available food on the beach, or has but a very short time to wait for it. Then, since egg deposition and food supply are so intimately connected, eggs are deposited and the cycle begins anew."

"It would be useless to speak of a correlation to surf-producing storms if the life histories of the species studied here corresponded to the life histories of the same species in localities remote from a beach."

Enough has been said to show that sarcophagid flies at any rate are capable to some extent of changing their habits to suit their environment, and it is highly probable that other flies, both biting and non-biting, are capable of doing so. In many parts of the world the sanitary conditions are being rapidly altered and improved, and in consequence the usual breeding grounds of the house-flies are being rendered less suitable. It seems not impossible that their habits may become materially altered, at least in some localities, in such a manner that the larval stages may be passed in materials at present regarded as unsuitable.

Indoor Habits (see p. 83).

Colour preference.

If it could be shown that flies are averse to alighting on objects or walls of certain colours the fact might be used in protecting houses, stables, and milk sheds from invasion. Up to the present only three investigators have devoted any attention to this subject.

Fé noticed that flies did not rest upon walls covered with blue paper. He therefore blue-washed the walls of his milk-sheds, and thought that insects did not visit them so frequently. Galli-Valerio (1910) and Hindle (1913), who have carried out elaborate experiments, have however been unable to detect any colour preference or colour aversion. It seems unlikely therefore that the adoption of any particular colour for the walls of houses and stables will have any effect on the numbers of flies entering them.

Hibernation (see p. 85).

There has been much speculation as to the stage in which house-flies pass the winter months. In warmed houses, kitchens and bake-houses, where the temperature is relatively high, adults may be found in an active condition throughout the winter, and in the presence of sufficient food material may even continue to breed, but little is known as to their mode of passing the winter under natural conditions. Most observers, however, seem to think that the winter is passed in the adult condition.

The most recent and extensive attempt to solve this problem has been made by Copeman (1913).

He quotes an interesting communication made to him by Dr Laver, of Colchester, on the hibernation of flies. This observer "had come to the conclusion that, in addition to the more or less active individuals which are usually to be found throughout the winter months in bake-houses and other warm situations, considerable numbers of flies in the adult stage hibernate *outside* dwellings, in various sheltered situations; the under-surface of the thatch of farmyard stacks having been found by him to constitute specially-favoured winter quarters." In a later communication Dr Laver stated that the flies were most usually to be met with on the north sides of hay stacks.

Copeman acting on Dr Laver's observations obtained on two separate occasions large numbers of flies in a dormant condition from a large attic of the rectory house, Ingoldisthorpe, near King's Lynn. Flies were also obtained in March, 1913, from the thatch of an old disused hen-house and in May from the attic of a farm house. Austen, who examined the specimens, was unable to find a single example of *M. domestica*. The flies mostly belonged to the genera *Pollenia*, *Pyrellia* and *Fannia*.

Twenty-five corn and hay stacks were also carefully examined. In the corn stacks no hibernating flies were found. In the hay stacks, although flies of other species were present, no specimens of the house-fly were obtained.

Skinner (1913) considers that house-flies pass the winter as pupæ, since specimens caught early in the year are fresh, and in many cases the ptilinum has not completely retracted.

The writer has had little experience with house-flies, but observed numerous blow-flies on sunny days at the end of February, 1914, in sheltered gravel pits, situated at considerable distances from houses. Males and females, both large and small, were seen, which seemed to have emerged recently from pupæ, as they were in perfect condition, and their chitin was relatively soft. Moreover, he has obtained in March, 1914, pupæ of different species from the earth in the neighbourhood of manure heaps, and has hatched the flies from them (see p. 297).

The Survival in the Adult Fly of Micro-organisms ingested by the Larva. (See Chapter XI, p. 114.)

More than ten years ago Daniels (1904) made experiments in order to ascertain whether organisms ingested by the larva survived in the adult. The details of his experiments were apparently not published, and his conclusions are stated in the following words. " In some of the Chinese houses, *Musca domestica,* and several species of Lucilia and Sarcophagi are abundant. The Chinese method of disposal of excreta is probably ultimately destructive to pathogenic organisms, but in the early stages of the process before this destruction has taken place these flies may convey disease.

There is no evidence that the *larvæ* of these flies bred in the excreta harbour as *imagines* the human intestinal bacteria. As far as experimental work has gone even *B. coli communis* does not seem to be carried in this manner."

Krontowski (1913) infected larvæ of *S. carnaria* and *mortuorum, L. cæsar* and *M. domestica* with *B. typhosus* and *B. dysenteriæ.* He was unable to find these organisms in the fæces of the adults, which emerged, or to infect milk by allowing them to feed on it.

Typhoid Fever. Experimental Evidence (See p. 129.)

Thomson (1912) carried out some very interesting investigations in 1907, but only published them in 1912. His observations in India on the habits of flies in relation to the disposal of night soil in trenches are specially interesting. " As soon as the trench was filled in, the flies laid their eggs on it. No eggs were visible on the surface, since the flies burrowed down into the crevices, but on turning over the small lumps of earth, little masses of eggs, like snow, were found over the whole trench. In a few days the eggs were hatched, and the larvæ straightway burrowed down to the layer of excrement. So numerous were they at Meerut in the beginning of April, that on digging down about six inches, a distinct layer of larvæ was found, feeding on filth."

Experimentally he found *B. typhosus* in 30 per cent. of artificially infected flies 24 hours after feeding, but never found this organism in the flies 48 hours after feeding. It was present in 50 per cent. of the samples of fly fæces he examined passed up to 6 hours after infection, but was never found in fæces passed after 24 hours. *B. typhosus* was found in flies fed on the urine of a carrier for 24 hours. He further states that he frequently found in the intestines of flies typhoid-like, but non-agglutinable, bacilli.

Dysentery. (See p. 146.)

The writer greatly regrets that the important work of Bahr (1912), who made a very careful study of dysentery in Fiji, was overlooked in the first edition. Bahr makes the following remarks on the prevalence of flies in that region. "House-flies (*Musca domestica*) constitute a great plague in Fiji. They swarm during the hot weather (November to April) in Suva; in the sugar districts they are prevalent throughout the year, finding suitable breeding-places in the decomposing vegetation necessarily connected with this industry. In many of the islands the traveller becomes covered from head to foot with these insects immediately he ventures out of his lodging. In the sugar districts life is made endurable only by the provision of fly-proof netting over the doors and windows. In these districts nearly every house is provided with at least one fly-proof room. Flies are especially numerous in the Fijian villages, where they find abundant congenial breeding-places in the refuse heaps.

"I need hardly point out that in consequence of this great profusion of flies every article of food is liable to gross contamination by these insects; and it is my suggestion that the fly season in Suva corresponds exactly with the annual epidemic of dysentery. After the great hurricane in March, 1910, there was a sudden and large increase in the number of cases of dysentery concurrently with a vast increase in the number of flies, which found in the rotting vegetation resulting from the hurricane favourable breeding-grounds.

"In the sugar districts there appears to be no definite dysentery season, and there apparently is no seasonal variation in the number of flies.

"The infection of patients, who are in hospital suffering from other complaints, with dysentery can best be explained by the agency of flies."

The methods of disposing of the excreta in the Colonial Hospital, Suva, afford very easy opportunities for flies to infect themselves from fresh excreta.

"The phenomenal preponderance of flies in Fiji, the great frequency of dysentery there, the concurrence of the fly season with the dysentery season, the many opportunities supplied by the insanitary conditions obtaining in the villages, plantations and public institutions for contamination of food by infected flies, are distinctly in favour of regarding Fijian epidemic dysentery as a fly-borne disease."

Bahr produces further evidence in support of this hypothesis from his observations and experiments.

He isolated Shiga's bacillus, identified by culture and agglutination tests, from the intestines of flies caught on dysentery patients, and was able to isolate the same organism from artificially infected flies up to the fourth day. It is interesting to note that some of the bacilli recovered from the flies, though agglutinated "by anti-serum in a dilution of 1 : 200," gave slightly different sugar reactions. Besides dysentery bacilli he also isolated other non-lactose fermenting bacilli, which could be differentiated from dysentery bacilli by their failure to agglutinate with a polyvalent anti-dysenteric serum.

Bahr (1914) later conducted other experiments on the transmission of the dysentery bacilli, Shiga-Kruse and Y-types, through the intestinal tracts of house-flies, kept in a glass house "in which the temperature approached that of the tropics, reaching as high as 91° F. in the daytime." He was unable to recover the organisms from the intestines of the flies after the fifth day, and observed no evidence of multiplication of these bacilli in the flies.

Krontowski (1913) only found dysentery bacilli, Shiga-Kruse type, in artificially infected flies up to the third day.

Ebeling (1913) considered that an outbreak of dysentery, which occurred amongst the cavalry attached to the tenth German Army Corps during the 1911 manœuvres, was due to fly infection, but produced very little evidence in support of his views.

Summer diarrhœa. (*a*) *Epidemiological evidence.* (See p. 150.)

Reflections on the manner in which flies possibly pass the winter and on the influences which induce the appearance of large numbers of them in certain years, caused the writer to study closely the known facts which have led certain observers to think that flies are the main disseminators of the virus of epidemic diarrhœa in the late summer. These studies have led to the evolution of hypotheses regarding certain habits of flies, and regarding their connection with diarrhœa. Whether further research will prove their truth or not the writer hopes that some of those who read these pages and carefully consider the charts, which illustrate them, will be sufficiently interested to investigate the problem more closely than has hitherto been done. The considerations, which have mainly influenced the writer in arriving at his conclusions, are set forth in the order in which they occurred.

It has been pointed out by a number of observers that the curve for the 4 foot underground temperature corresponds more closely to the curve for diarrhœa deaths than any other varying seasonal fact. The remarkable correspondence of these two curves is illustrated in Chart 6 which gives the mean earth temperature at 3 ft. 2 inches in depth during the third quarter for each year at Greenwich from 1870 to 1913, and the curves for diarrhœa deaths in England and Wales since 1870, in Cambridge since 1882, in Birmingham since 1887 and in Manchester since 1891. It will be seen that during the last

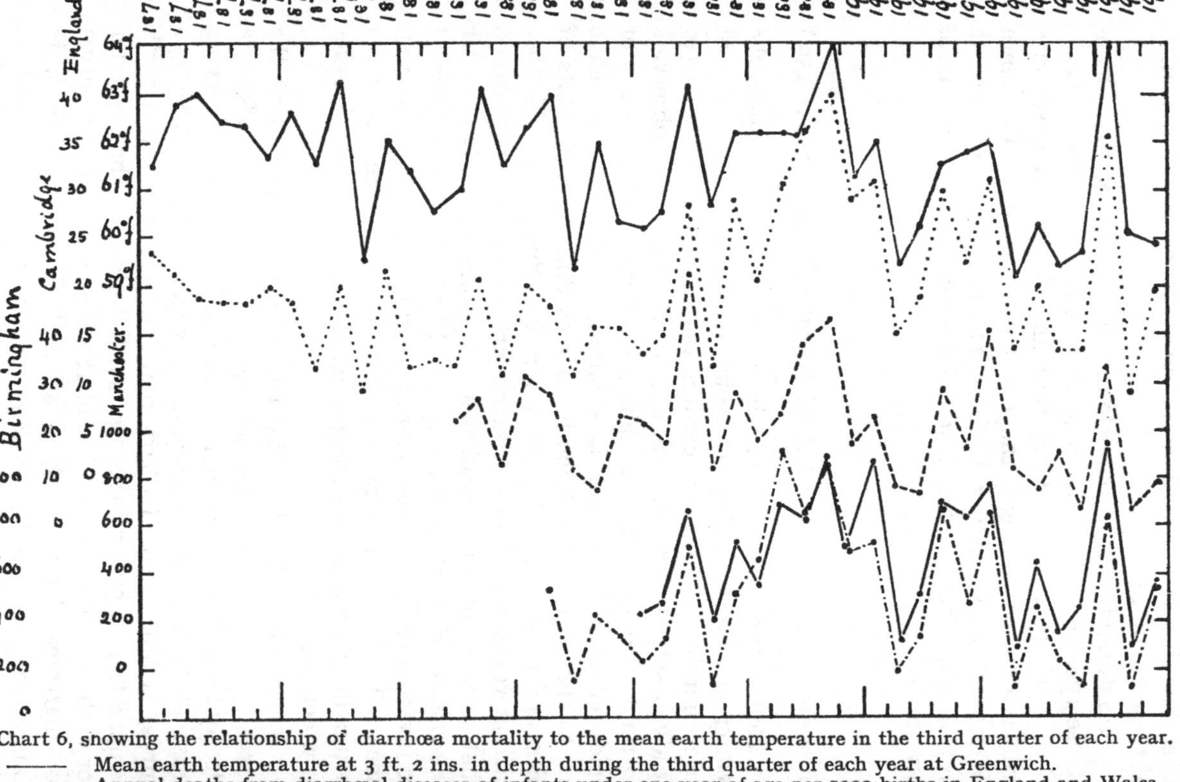

Chart 6, showing the relationship of diarrhœa mortality to the mean earth temperature in the third quarter of each year.

——— Mean earth temperature at 3 ft. 2 ins. in depth during the third quarter of each year at Greenwich.

.... Annual deaths from diarrhœal diseases of infants under one year of age per 1000 births in England and Wales.

– – – Annual deaths from diarrhœa in Cambridge.

·——· Deaths from epidemic diarrhœa during the third quarter of each year in Manchester.

–·–·– Deaths from epidemic diarrhœa and enteritis during the third quarter of each year in Birmingham.

30 years the curve for the *annual* deaths from diarrhœal diseases of infants under one year per 1000 births in England and Wales has shown fluctuations corresponding to those of the earth temperature curve except in 1887, 1890, 1896, 1897, 1898, 1905, and 1913[1].

The conditions in different places vary so greatly that it could be scarcely possible to take into account the factors, which have caused the irregularities just mentioned. The writer, therefore, influenced at first mainly by reflections on the activities and breeding habits of flies, determined to study closely the conditions which prevailed during the last *ten* years in Cambridge, Manchester and Birmingham. These three places were selected because the writer is well acquainted with the meteorological conditions of Cambridge, and epidemic diarrhœa is uncommon there; he studied the bacteria present in flies collected during two years in Birmingham, and Niven has published a very careful account of his highly suggestive observations in Manchester.

In Cambridge the *annual* deaths from diarrhœa in infants have been taken in preparing the curve in Chart 6. The numbers are very small, but the curve, except in the years 1905, 1908, 1909, 1910 and 1913, follows that illustrating the earth temperature. In Manchester the number of deaths, which is considerable, during the *third quarter* of each year has been taken. Here the two curves closely correspond, except in the year 1913. In Birmingham, where the number of deaths during the *third quarter* has been selected, the curves correspond except in the years 1905, 1910, and 1913. In both these cities, however, the curves for the diarrhœa deaths in no way correspond to the earth temperature curve in the years 1895, 1896, 1897 and 1898, and therefore the conditions prevailing during these years have also been studied in detail.

The evidence brought forward by Niven and others in support of the hypothesis that the annual epidemic of diarrhœa

[1] The data on which the curves for the mean earth temperature at Greenwich and the deaths from diarrhœa in England and Wales have been constructed have been obtained from the Registrar-General's Report for 1911. The figures for 1912 and 1913 have been kindly supplied by the Meteorological Office and by the Registrar-General.

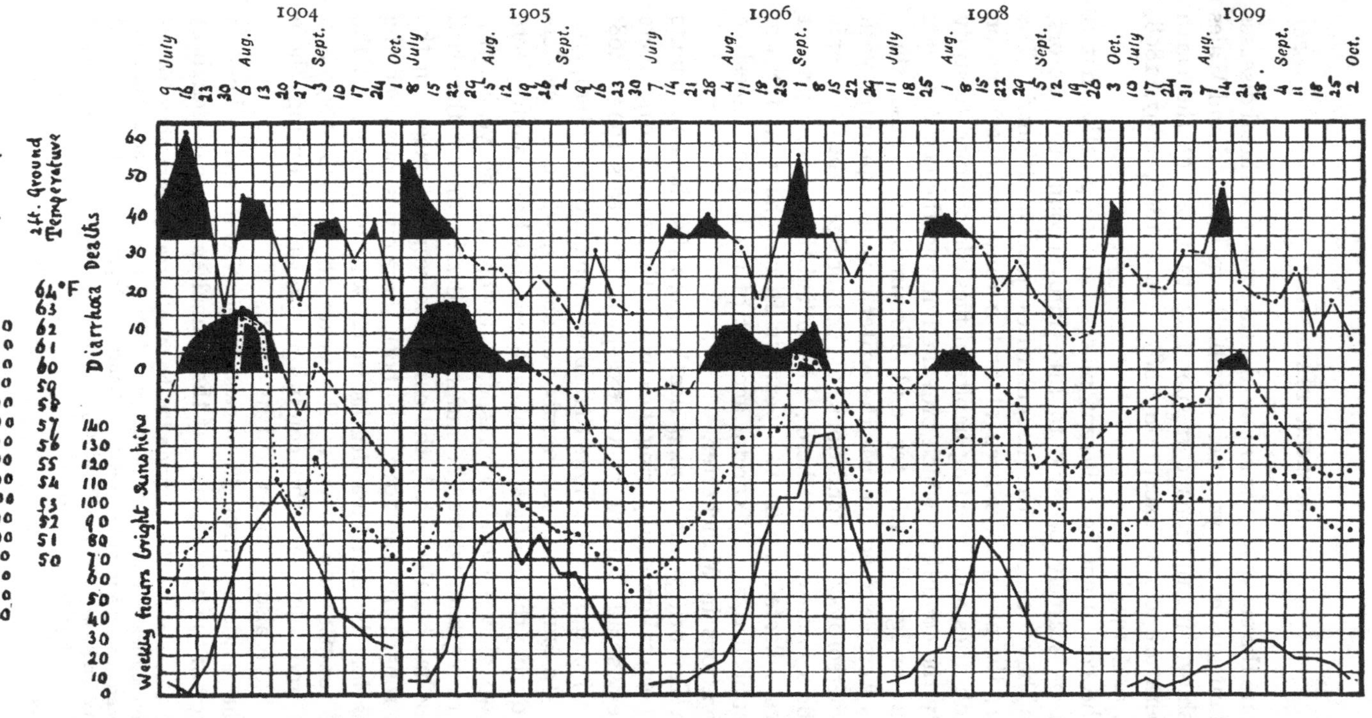

Chart 7, showing the weekly hours of bright sunshine, the mean weekly ground temperatures at 2 ft., the weekly numbers of flies caught per trap, and the weekly diarrhœa deaths during the third quarters of **1904, 1905, 1906, 1908 and 1909** in Manchester.

•——• Hours of bright sunshine, –·–·–· 2 ft. ground temperature, •······• Flies per trap, —— Diarrhœa deaths.

is due mainly to fly infection has been discussed already in considerable detail (p. 150), but in considering the influences which are likely to affect the numbers of flies and the deaths from diarrhœa it is necessary to consider some of the points more fully.

The most complete data at present available in regard to the numbers of flies present in houses in infected areas are those compiled by Niven for the city of Manchester during the years 1904, 1905, 1906, 1908 and 1909. Chart 7 illustrates by means of curves the weekly deaths from diarrhœa in Manchester, the numbers of flies caught per trap, the mean weekly ground temperature at a depth of two feet, and the weekly hours of bright sunshine during the third quarter of each year. It is evident that the numbers of flies can be gauged only very roughly by the method employed of counting the numbers caught in bell-traps (see p. 152). Further it should be pointed out that in 1909 bell-traps were not employed but sticky papers, so that the numbers are not strictly comparable with those obtained for the other years. In spite of the admitted crudeness of the method employed in estimating the numbers of flies a study of the chart reveals an extraordinary resemblance between the curves representing the numbers of flies and those indicating the diarrhœa deaths. The latter curve moreover lags about a week behind the fly curve. Again, except in the year 1906, the 2 ft. ground temperature curve very closely resembles the curve indicating the number of flies.

Though the similarity in the curves is highly remarkable it may be contended that the conditions prevailing in the ground at 2 ft. affect flies and the virus of epidemic diarrhœa independently, since as yet insufficient direct evidence exists, mainly owing to our lack of knowledge of the virus of diarrhœa, in support of the view that flies are the chief distributors of the disease.

The mortality due to this disease is so great that any evidence bearing on this important problem ought to receive careful consideration.

Attention may be directed first to the influence of the 2 ft. ground temperature on the numbers of flies. Clearly the adult flies cannot be affected. Niven thinks the larvæ in the breeding-grounds are influenced, considering that when the air temperature is rising the conditions for the fly larvæ are becoming favourable, and after the external temperature has fallen the heat of the soil continues to favour the larvæ so that a high mean temperature for the third quarter of the year indicates favourable conditions for the continuous production of flies. The larvæ, however, generally breed in fermenting materials, in which a high temperature, not greatly influenced by slight changes in external conditions, is maintained, and therefore it seems to the writer that the ground temperature exerts its influence mainly in some other way. Moreover Niven's hypothesis does not explain the somewhat sudden increase in the number of flies, which occurs when the 2 ft. ground temperature reaches a certain level, which we may call the 'critical point.' To account for this the writer is inclined to the hypothesis that the influence is exerted on the pupæ from which the flies only emerge when the temperature conditions become favourable, rather than on the larvæ.

House-flies generally appear first on warm sunny days in the early summer, the latter part of May and June, and the larvæ, which develop from these eggs, seek when full fed suitable positions in which to pupate. They may select the upper and cooler portions of manure heaps (Griffith, 1908) or their dry fringes or more often they wander off, sometimes for several feet or even yards, in search of dry and sheltered spots, where they secrete themselves in cracks or holes, or even burrow in the soil or pupate under piles of rubbish. Little seems to be known as to the wanderings of house-fly larvæ[1],

[1] Since the above was written an interesting paper by Hutchinson (1914) on the "migratory habit of house-fly larvæ" has appeared. In manure heaps in the open he often noticed "a tendency to congregate" at the edges of the heaps near the ground. On examining a place where a heap had been he found some pupæ buried half an inch or more in the soil close to the edges. In one instance numerous larvæ were noticed near the top of a heap. Eight days later the pile was examined. No pupæ were found near the top but 9000 were collected in the lowest layers, and 100 in the soil. In the examination of 50 heaps pupæ were found in masses at the edges, as many as 30,000 being found in some heaps. Hutchinson also carried out experiments with the following apparatus:

"A large galvanized iron pan, measuring 5 by 3 feet, with side 4 inches or of the situations selected for pupation, except in highly artificial breeding-grounds such as dust bins (p. 45). In high, was made. In this stood a container on legs 8 inches high. This container measured 4 by 2 by 2 feet. The sides and bottom were of heavy wire, ¼-inch mesh, supported by a light wooden framework. Twelve cubic feet of manure well infested with eggs and larvæ were placed in this container and sprinkled with water. Water was also poured into the pan below to a depth of about 1 inch. Surrounding and covering both pan and container was a fly tight enclosure made of a large cage 6 by 6 by 6 feet. This prevented further infestation of the manure, and an arrangement of traps at the top of the cage made it possible to capture and keep a record of any flies that might emerge. At the time for the emergence of flies the sides of the cage were darkened with a black cloth in order to drive the flies into the traps at the top. Each day the larvæ were collected from the pan and counted, and each day the manure in the container was sprinkled thoroughly with water and the pan was washed out and again partly filled with water to drown the larvæ which fell into it. The records of Experiment No. 1 are summed up briefly" below.

Date 1913	Larvæ collected from pan	Flies from trap	Date 1913	Larvæ collected from pan	Flies from trap
Aug. 27	337	—	Sept. 5	304	22
28	715	—	6	—	88
29	1550	—	7	—	102
30	10,000	—	8	—	23
31	8000	—	9	—	19
Sept. 1	2160	—	10	—	9
2	670	3	12	—	5
3	263	18	15	—	6
4	—	8			
				23,999	303

"A few flies at the time of emergence fell into the water of the pan and were drowned. Allowing for these and for the few which may have escaped from the cage during the opening and shutting of the door, the total number of flies may be placed at 350. It will be seen from these figures that out of a possible total of 24,350, 24,000, or a little more than 98 per cent., were destroyed through the catching of the larvæ in the manner described."

In other somewhat similar experiments, about 99 per cent. of the larvæ were destroyed. From his observations and experiments Hutchinson concludes that "it is quite certain that the migratory habit is deeply ingrained and highly characteristic of house-fly larvæ."

He is of opinion that exposed manure piles do not become reinfested and that "even under the most favorable conditions maggots will rarely be found in a given lot of manure after 10 or 12 days exposure."

Finally he suggests that traps of the nature described should be used in stables, and other places where fresh manure has to be dealt with.

Levy and Tuck (1913) who also made a number of observations on this subject make the following statement. "We therefore announce the biological fact that the house-fly does not pupate in manure if the full-grown larvæ can find any means of reaching and entering the earth."

middensteads the full-fed larvæ crawl to the sides or to the top of the framework, or locate themselves in dry spots, often getting as far as they can from the moist situations in which the growing larvæ flourish (p. 45).

Records of their habits under more natural conditions are scarce. Smith (1907), however, records some careful and most interesting observations on the habits of the larvæ of a very closely allied species, *M. enteniata*[1], in India.

"On turning over a three days' old deposit of fæces, a mass of maggots was disclosed beneath. The disturbed maggots at once began to make for cracks in the earth or to go down dung beetle holes or worm holes. Meanwhile ants attacked them and carried some off. While ants had already begun to weaken the defensive wall of fæces by eating it away. The fæcal covering was replaced, but on the following day nothing remained but dry, hard fæces, no longer adherent to the ground. The fæcal mass crumbled up and in a few days all trace of it had gone. Where were the maggots?

"Diggings into the soil below a fæcal deposit four days old brought to light many maggots at a depth of 5 to 6 inches. Larvæ and the earth, in which they had been found, were placed in a jar under a net. Fourteen days from the estimated hour of their birth as larvæ flies appeared, and proved to be *M. enteniata*. A good many similar observations have been made, and always in the main with like result, but often with much fewer flies and sometimes with different species of flies.

"Sometimes the digging below a dried deposit did not bring to light any maggots, though plenty had been present in the same fæces before it became dry. This was the case with a deposit on some hard, dry soil in a flower pot—sections of the earth were made in vain—nevertheless, from this soil under a net, flies appeared on the 14th and 15th days."

A deposit of cow dung "was noted to cover hundreds of maggots; next day none were found. Digging in the ground beneath and around brought to light a few maggots widely dispersed and at 2 or 3 inches in depth. From these and from the soil in which they were found, as well as from similar deposits, the following flies amongst others were obtained, *M. domestica* and *M. enteniata*."

Straton (1907) states that "in the laboratory flies have emerged from specimens of night soil covered with six inches of well powdered earth" and Aldridge (1904) that "in about one pint of soil taken from a (night soil) trench, 520 pupæ were counted, and from these 329 flies were hatched." In a later paper Aldridge (1907) relates that "from one-sixth of a cubic foot of soil taken from a trench at Meerut and placed in a cage, 4042 flies were hatched." Dwyer collected 500 from a cage covering three square feet of a trench at Mhow. According to Aldridge (1904) "by turning up the soil of trenches at different ages, the stages of development can easily be followed."

[1] In dealing with all but the most recent observations, especially in tropical climates, it should be remembered that great advances have recently been made in the identification of species, superficially resembling one another, but

The observations, which have just been quoted, show that the full-fed larvæ often bury themselves, if the breeding-grounds afford suitable opportunities for so doing, and one at least of Smith's observations indicate that they may migrate.

If, in the absence of conclusive information in regard to house-fly larvæ, arguments derived from the habits of allied larvæ are permissible, very considerable migrations possibly occur, especially at night[1], when the breeding-grounds are so situated that migration is possible. Hermes' (1911) interesting observations on the habits of the larvæ of *L. cæsar*, which migrate during the night and burrow before pupating, have been quoted already (p. 25).

When bred in captivity in jars half filled with earth or sand the larvæ of *M. domestica*, *C. erythrocephala* and *L. cæsar* all burrow to near the bottom before pupating.

Up to the present the effects of temperature on pupæ have been little studied. It is well known, however, from the researches of Newstead, Griffith and others, that while under favourable temperature (65° F. to 75° F.) and food conditions, the pupal stage lasts five to seven days, under less suitable conditions it may last 14 to 28 days, or even considerably longer. Griffith (1908) showed that at 65° F. to 75° F. "the whole process from egg to fly was completed by the eighth or ninth day," but that when the larvæ and pupæ were kept cold 57 days might elapse before the emergence of the flies. He also found that "when the larvæ were kept in proper warmth until they formed pupæ, the flies came out even in a rather cold temperature, and quickly in the warm." On the other hand "when the larvæ were kept cool and the pupæ warm, some flies came out but all were small; it has been a regular occurrence that cold surroundings and plenty of food have produced small flies, if

differing in habits, and that too much reliance should not be placed on the older identifications of species.

Patton and Cragg (*Text-book of Medical Entomology*, 1913, p. 335) can find no reliable distinguishing characters between *M. enteniata* and *M. nebulo*, and state that it is very difficult to distinguish the female of *M. domestica* from the female of *M. nebulo*.

[1] Hutchinson (1914) says that he has frequently seen house-fly larvæ migrating by night from his experimental cages.

any." Such small flies are, according to Griffith, incapable of reproduction.

From the limited experimental data at present available it seems very probable that larvæ, developing under favourable conditions from eggs laid in fermenting materials by flies which have appeared early in the summer, may give rise to pupæ, the majority of which remain in sheltered and relatively cold situations till the surrounding temperature conditions become suitable. In this way an accumulation of numerous pupæ, from which flies are ready to emerge, may be formed. The advent of suitable temperature conditions would then result in large numbers of freshly emerged flies.

The thermometers which record the earth temperatures are usually placed in exposed positions and record the underground temperatures in situations, which in the height of summer, must be warm. Probably the temperatures recorded in such situations are higher than those which prevail at the same depth in dry and shady places or in damp places protected from the direct rays of the sun[1]. The pupæ are found in the latter situations and, though it is hardly likely that the larvæ ever burrow to a depth of two feet, are probably exposed to temperature conditions corresponding to those recorded by thermometers buried to a depth of one to two feet in the open.

A glance at Chart 7 will show that the curve for the numbers of flies and that for the 2 ft. ground temperature correspond in a remarkable way. If the larvæ were influenced the fly curve would follow and not correspond with the 2 ft. curve, since some time must be allowed for the larvæ to become full-fed, the pupæ to form, and the flies to emerge. On the other hand, if the hidden pupæ from which the flies are ready to emerge are affected by the temperature changes, an increase

[1] The writer being unable to find any information relating to this point has recently placed standard earth thermometers short distances apart in exposed and shady situations. The observations hitherto recorded tend to show (1) that on warm sunny days the soil at depths of one and two feet is several degrees warmer in exposed than in sheltered situations, and (2) that the temperatures recorded are influenced to some extent by the character of the soil.

in flies would correspond with a rise of the ground temperature to the critical point.

If this explanation of the source of the swarms of flies in the middle of the third quarter of the year is correct the condition of the weather in the last two weeks in May and in June ought to have a great influence on the numbers which eventually appear, since unsuitable weather at that time would result in a dearth of flies which lay the eggs from which the earlier swarms of late summer mainly arise.

This question involves a consideration of the source from which the early summer flies are derived. The evidence at present available (p. 282) seems to indicate that few house-flies hibernate as adults, and from observations on other species of flies, the writer is inclined to think that the winter is passed in the pupal stage.

In the autumn of 1912 three samples of dog fæces were collected and placed in separate jars half filled with earth. The tops of the jars were closed with gauze, and the jars were left outside in a sheltered position during the winter. On 25th March, 1913, the jars were examined. The first contained 110 pupæ, the second 215 and the third 245, or 570 in all, of which 133 were large, 427 small and 10 of the *Fannia* type. These pupæ were kept in a warm room, and from the large specimens flesh-flies (*Sarcophaga*) emerged in April and May, and from the smaller three species of anthomyid flies during the first three weeks of April.

Thinking that pupæ might be found in sheltered situations in the neighbourhood of manure heaps, the writer examined the soil near heaps in March, 1914. In the *damp* soil under a hedge near one heap at a depth of about six inches several large muscid pupæ, amongst others, were found. From these, when kept in a warm room, blow-flies, *C. erythrocephala*, emerged in the beginning of April. In the soil close to the second heap, which was situated in an open field, a number of smaller pupæ were found. From these anthomyid flies emerged.

Unfortunately little time has been available for prosecuting this line of research, and only a few hours have been devoted to it, nevertheless it has been demonstrated that blow-flies, flesh-flies and anthomyid flies pass the winter as pupæ. Three points of special interest were noticed, namely that worm or beetle holes were not numerous where the pupæ were found, that the pupæ were often located in masses of damp earth, and that they were extremely local. In fact near both heaps the majority of the pupæ were close together, and there was no evident reason why one situation more than another was chosen for pupation.

As already stated (p. 283) the writer has observed blow-flies, in quite perfect condition and apparently freshly emerged, in the end of February. The fact that some of these were very small is of interest.

It is true that the pupæ of *M. domestica* have not been found, but opportunities for making observations have been so limited that it may be permissible to argue from the habits of allied genera. If *M. domestica* passes the winter in the pupal stage, from such of the pupæ as are located in situations easily influenced by the air temperature flies will emerge on warm days in early summer. Moreover it is not impossible that the winter pupæ behave differently from summer pupæ in response to temperature conditions. Griffith (1908) noticed " that flies were found earliest, and sometimes in great numbers, at a certain large refuse heap, where they appeared and disappeared according to the weather, long before there were any in the town, except in bake-houses and restaurant kitchens."

After discussing the conditions which are likely to influence the emergence of the flies from the pupæ it may be as well to consider those which are likely to influence their breeding habits, and activities, including the capacity of the adults for distributing disease-producing bacteria.

The flies, which appear in the early part of summer, have either hibernated as adults or emerged from pupæ. Though little information has been obtained in regard to this point up to the present it is possible that the former may be ready to lay eggs within a few days, but the latter, which probably compose the great majority, will require a fortnight of suitable weather to acquire sexual maturity. It is unknown whether the development of sexual maturity is markedly retarded by cold weather or not, but that it is retarded is exceedingly probable, judging by what is known in regard to the relationship of insects to temperature conditions.

It is on the other hand a well established fact that bright sunshine has the greatest effect on the activities of flies. They are active in bright sunshine even when the air temperature is relatively low, and even more active when bright sunshine is combined with a high air temperature. It would seem therefore that a spell of bright weather in early summer lasting about three weeks is required for the flies to reach sexual maturity and lay eggs in large numbers. The majority of the flies, which develop from these eggs, will emerge when the ground temperature conditions become suitable, usually in the third quarter of the year. The flies, which occur later, depend on good breeding conditions in the third quarter.

At this stage it seems desirable to consider in some detail the probable effects of the meteorological conditions, which appear to be the main factors in influencing the breeding habits and activities of the flies which appear in the late summer, namely (A) bright sunshine in the early summer, (B) the ground temperature in the third quarter and (C) bright sunshine in the third quarter of the year. At the same time, assuming that flies are the chief disseminators of the virus of epidemic diarrhœa, we may consider the probable effects of these factors on the annual epidemic.

(A). *Bright sunshine in early summer.*

Since the house-flies which have survived the winter rarely appear before the middle of May bright sunshine before that period of the year will have no effect on them. On the other hand, bright sunshine in the latter half of the second quarter and during the third quarter will have very marked, though somewhat different, effects. The effect of bright sunshine during the second half of the second quarter may be considered first. In this period of the year it will influence the breeding capacity of the few adults, which are about, but will have no effect except indirectly on the annual diarrhœa epidemic.

(1) If during the early summer the weather is dull, *i.e.* without two or more consecutive weeks during which more than 35 hours[1] of bright sunshine per week are recorded, the few flies which appear will be inactive, possibly fail to acquire sexual maturity, and will deposit few eggs. As a consequence the number of flies which emerge when the ground temperature reaches the critical point in the third quarter will be too small to produce an extensive epidemic (see Charts 11, 13, 16[2]).

(2) If during two or more consecutive weeks more than 35 hours per week of bright sunshine are recorded in the early summer the flies will be active, and lay eggs. In consequence numerous flies will emerge from the buried pupæ if the ground temperature reaches the critical point, and an outbreak of diarrhœa will follow. The numbers likely to emerge depend on the duration and period of the early bright weather.

(*a*) If an interval of dull weather, as often happens, intervenes between the sunny period and the rise of the ground temperature to the critical point flies will emerge from the majority of buried pupæ at one time, and the consequent diarrhœa epidemic curve will rise rapidly, but in the absence of other favourable conditions, the epidemic will be of short duration (Chart 12).

(*b*) If on the other hand the bright weather is of long duration and especially if it extends up to the time when the ground temperature reaches the critical point larvæ and pupæ in all stages will be present, and flies will continue emerging in large numbers for some weeks. The curve of the consequent diarrhœa epidemic ought therefore to rise sharply and continue at a high level for some weeks (Charts 9, 15).

(B). *The effects of ground temperature.*

If pupæ are present in the soil flies will emerge when the temperature of the soil as recorded by the 2 ft. earth thermometer

[1] This figure has been selected as the result of the study of Charts 8—19.

[2] That part of the chart which refers to the conditions in Manchester is referred to in each case. When the conditions in Birmingham are specially referred to the letter B is placed after the chart number.

in the open approaches the critical temperature. This critical temperature appears to be about 60° F. in Manchester and 56° F. in Birmingham. The critical temperature may be really different in these two cities or the apparent difference may be due to the varying conditions under which the flies breed or under which the temperatures are recorded[1]. In this connection it may be mentioned that during the last ten years the mean temperature in the shade during the third quarter of the year in Manchester has been 59·0° F. and in Birmingham 57·6° F. and it is not impossible that flies in Birmingham respond to lower temperatures than those in Manchester, since allied species have been known to change their habits (p. 276) and adapt themselves to their environment (p. 282).

Even though the pupæ are present few flies will emerge if the ground temperature never rises within 2° F. or more of the critical point (Chart 11 B). A slow rise in the ground temperature when near the critical point will result in the gradual emergence of flies from the more favourably situated pupæ, and a correspondingly slow rise in the diarrhœa curve (Chart 17 B).

If pupæ are present in the soil in small numbers only few flies will emerge, even though the ground temperature is favourable, and the annual epidemic will not occur (Chart 16).

As has been pointed out previously the presence or relative absence of the pupæ in the soil depends on the sunshine in early summer.

As the ground temperature falls towards and then below the critical point the emergence of flies will gradually diminish and eventually almost cease when the temperature reaches a point 2° or 3° F. below the critical point.

(C). *Bright sunshine in the third quarter of the year.*

During the third quarter the occurrence of bright sunshine influences flies in two ways. The flies are more active in breeding, and owing to the favourable emerging conditions produced by the coincident high ground temperature the

[1] See footnote p. 296.

generations succeed each other with great rapidity, only three or four weeks elapsing between the deposition of the eggs and the emergence of the adults. Apart from breeding the flies are more active in their movements, and more hungry, and therefore more liable to carry infection.

(1) If the early summer has been dull and bright sunshine small in amount in the third quarter flies will be few, and epidemic diarrhœa uncommon, whether the ground temperature reaches the critical point or not (Charts 11, 16).

(2) If the early summer has been dull, and in the third quarter a spell of bright sunshine occurs after the ground temperature has reached the critical point, flies will appear in large numbers about three or four weeks after the commencement of the bright spell, and they will be very active. Consequently a severe diarrhœa outbreak may be expected within a week of their appearance (Chart 19).

(3) If the early summer has been bright and flies are emerging, a spell of bright sunshine will increase the activities of the flies, and the diarrhœa curve which has already ascended may be expected to rise rapidly to a higher level (Chart 10).

(4) Owing to the decreased activities of flies the death curve may be expected to decline about a fortnight after dull weather commences, and, if the dull spell is of sufficient duration, two or three weeks, the decline may be expected to continue, more particularly if the ground temperature has fallen, since very few flies are likely to emerge to take the place of those which have died. On the other hand, if the dull spell is of short duration the recurrence of bright weather may lead to a temporary recrudescence of the epidemic. Continued bright weather in the early autumn may cause the epidemic to continue in the fourth quarter of the year.

It is possible to summarize these deductions briefly in the following way :

Dull early summer and third quarter, flies few, little diarrhœa.

Dull early summer, and bright third quarter, late but sharp epidemic, its length depending on the continuance of bright weather.

Bright early summer, and dull third quarter, early and usually short epidemic.

Bright early summer and bright third quarter, early and considerable epidemic, its duration depending on the continuance of bright weather.

The value of these deductions, based on a consideration of the habits of flies, may now be tested by reference to the known facts in respect to meteorological conditions and epidemic diarrhœa.

In regard to the city of Manchester it is possible during the years 1904, 1905, 1906, 1908 and 1909 to study the weekly prevalence of flies in conjunction with the meteorological conditions. The data relating to the third quarters of these years are given in Chart 7 and the meteorological conditions prevailing during the second quarters may be ascertained from Charts 8, 9, 10, 12, 13. In consideration of the fact that the writer's views have just been given in detail it is unnecessary to do more than mention the chief points of interest in each year.

In 1904 bright weather prevailed in June and the early part of July, and the ground temperature reached the critical point about July 16th, and, as we should expect, large numbers of flies were caught in traps during the next fortnight. During the first fortnight of August the weather was very bright, breeding conditions at their best and the flies very active, and in consequence very large numbers were caught in traps. Subsequently a fortnight of dull weather occurred, and fewer flies were caught, but the numbers were considerable as good emerging conditions still prevailed. The curve for diarrhœa deaths follows the main lines of the fly curve, rising abruptly because the ground temperature reached the critical point rapidly, and dropping rapidly owing to the dull fortnight at the end of August.

In 1905 a long period of bright sunshine prevailed throughout June and July, and the ground temperature remained above the critical point for some weeks from July 8th to August 19th. The third quarter was dull, and as might be expected, an epidemic of some weeks duration with a sharp initial rise, declining when the weather became very dull in the beginning of September, occurred.

In 1906 the bright sunshine in June though fairly plentiful was irregular, and moderately bright weather prevailed in July. The ground temperature, after remaining a little below the critical point for some weeks, reached this level about July 28th, and remained above it till September 15th. As we might expect, owing to the early good breeding conditions and the slow rise of the ground temperature, the fly curve rose steadily, and flies were numerous during the eight weeks mentioned. A period of bright weather at the beginning of September, leading to increased activity of the flies, caused still greater numbers to be caught in traps. The diarrhœa death curve in this year follows the fly curve in a very remarkable manner.

In 1908 very bright weather prevailed at the end of May and at the end of June. Flies in large numbers might therefore be expected when the ground temperature reached the critical point at the beginning of August. In this year the period of fly activity was short, the ground temperature being above the critical point for four weeks only and during this period the weather was bright. Later it was dull. A short but sharp epidemic occurred.

In 1909, except during one week in the early part of August, the weather was dull, and the ground temperature only remained above the critical point for a fortnight in August. Fly[1] conditions were poor and the epidemic small.

These are the only years in which it is possible to compare fly counts with diarrhœa deaths and meteorological conditions, but through the kindness of Dr J. Niven of Manchester, Dr J. Robertson of Birmingham and Dr A. J. Laird of Cambridge, the writer has been able to prepare charts showing the meteorological conditions and the diarrhœa deaths in those areas for the last ten years.

If flies are responsible for the annual epidemic the diarrhœa mortality should reflect the meteorological conditions which mainly influence flies. For the purpose of determining the

[1] See p. 291.

effects of the meteorological conditions on the diarrhœa mortality in Birmingham, Manchester and Cambridge charts showing the mean weekly maximum temperature, the mean weekly shade temperatures, the mean weekly earth temperatures at 1, 2 and 4 ft., the weekly hours of bright sunshine and the weekly rainfall from May to September during the years 1904–13 were prepared and studied. Little evidence was obtained suggesting that the air temperatures or rainfall have any specially marked influence, and the 2 ft. ground temperature was found to be the one which corresponded most closely with the diarrhœa death curve. The mean weekly maximum air temperature is related to some extent to the sunshine curve, though the peaks of these curves, especially in early summer, often do not coincide. It is not suggested that warmth apart from sunshine has no influence, but that its influence is much less marked than that of sunshine. The curve of the mean shade temperature coincides less frequently with the sunshine curve. The influence of warmth is dealt with later (p. 323).

For the sake of simplicity it has been considered sufficient, therefore, to reproduce only the curves representing the weekly hours of bright sunshine, the mean weekly 2 ft. temperature, and the diarrhœa deaths.

In studying these charts it becomes clearly evident that in the three selected areas the curves representing the 2 ft. ground temperatures in any year are very similar in shape, but vary considerably in regard to the actual temperatures recorded. The mean for the third quarters from 1907 to 1913 in Cambridge is 1·7° F. higher than the mean for Manchester, and the mean for Manchester is 4·2° F. higher than the mean for Birmingham. The ground temperature records are probably influenced by the nature of the soil, the positions in which the thermometers are placed and other local conditions. In Cambridge the earth thermometers are sunk in gravel in a very open but low position. In Manchester they are sunk in loam in a fairly large yard surrounded by buildings. In Birmingham they are placed in a fairly open position in an urban district, the geological formation being soft sandstone, and the elevation 500 ft.

If epidemic diarrhœa was entirely dependent on the ground temperature or on conditions which influence flies Cambridge ought to show a high mortality, but this is so far from being the case that Cambridge has proportionately many times fewer deaths than Manchester or Birmingham.

Except in the year 1911[1], when exceptionally favourable fly conditions prevailed, the deaths in Cambridge during the last seven years have been very few. The Cambridge charts have been introduced to bring this fact into prominence. In large cities such as Birmingham and Manchester diarrhœa prevails to some extent throughout the year and cases of the disease and infected carriers are always sufficiently numerous to afford ample opportunities for flies to infect themselves, whereas in Cambridge winter cases are rare and carriers probably uncommon. In the present state of our knowledge it seems reasonable to assume that in Cambridge epidemic diarrhœa is uncommon because flies have few opportunities of infecting themselves and distributing the virus.

We may now consider the charts relating to Birmingham and Manchester. The diarrhœa death curves are in many years very similar though, as has been pointed out, the Birmingham 2 ft. ground temperature never reaches the same level as that of Manchester, the critical point in Manchester being apparently about 60° F. and in Birmingham about 56° F.

In 1904 the early summer was moderately bright and the pupæ in the soil at the beginning of the third quarter probably plentiful. The ground temperature reached the critical point about July 16th, and with numerous flies ready to emerge and the conditions favourable for the continuance of emergence a considerable epidemic with a sharp initial rise might be expected. This occurred in both cities, but the diarrhœa death curve reached a higher level in Birmingham, where the weather was very bright in the early part of August. The peaks of the diarrhœa curves correspond to the sunshine peaks in the beginning of August. While the Manchester curve drops rapidly owing to the dull fortnight at the end of August, there is a slight secondary rise in the Birmingham curve corresponding

[1] The Cambridge ground temperatures have been recorded since 1907.

to the sunny period in the beginning of September after a relatively dull week.

In 1905 the conditions in Manchester (see p. 303) were favourable for a continued epidemic with a moderately sharp rise, since favourable egg laying conditions only commenced on June 10th, three weeks before the ground temperature somewhat rapidly rose to the critical point. In Birmingham the ground temperature remained near the critical point for two weeks before rising above it, favouring a less rapid rise in the death curve.

The conditions in 1906 were similar in both cities, and they have been considered previously (p. 304). It may be noted that the highest peaks of the diarrhœa curves correspond with the sunshine peaks in the early part of September.

In 1907 bright sunshine was moderate in amount in Birmingham throughout the summer, but in Manchester was much below the average. In neither city did the ground temperature reach the critical point, and there was little diarrhœa in either. It is interesting to note that Griffith (1908) observed "a large proportion of small flies" in this year.

In 1908 similar conditions prevailed in both cities. These have been considered previously (p. 304).

In 1909 the early summer was unfavourable for flies, and in Manchester, except in the second week in August, remained unfavourable. Here there was a slight rise in the diarrhœa death curve following this week, but the epidemic was slight. In Birmingham a favourable period for egg laying occurred between July 17th and August 21st, but the ground temperature remained above the critical point for a fortnight only (August 14th–21st). The latter part of the third quarter was unfavourable. The curve for diarrhœa deaths has a small peak corresponding to the favourable period of much sunshine and high ground temperature in the early part of August.

The chart for 1910 to some extent resembles that for 1909 and need not be discussed in detail. The highest peak of the Birmingham death curve corresponds with the favourable fly period when 43 hours of bright sunshine were recorded in the week in which the ground temperature reached its highest level.

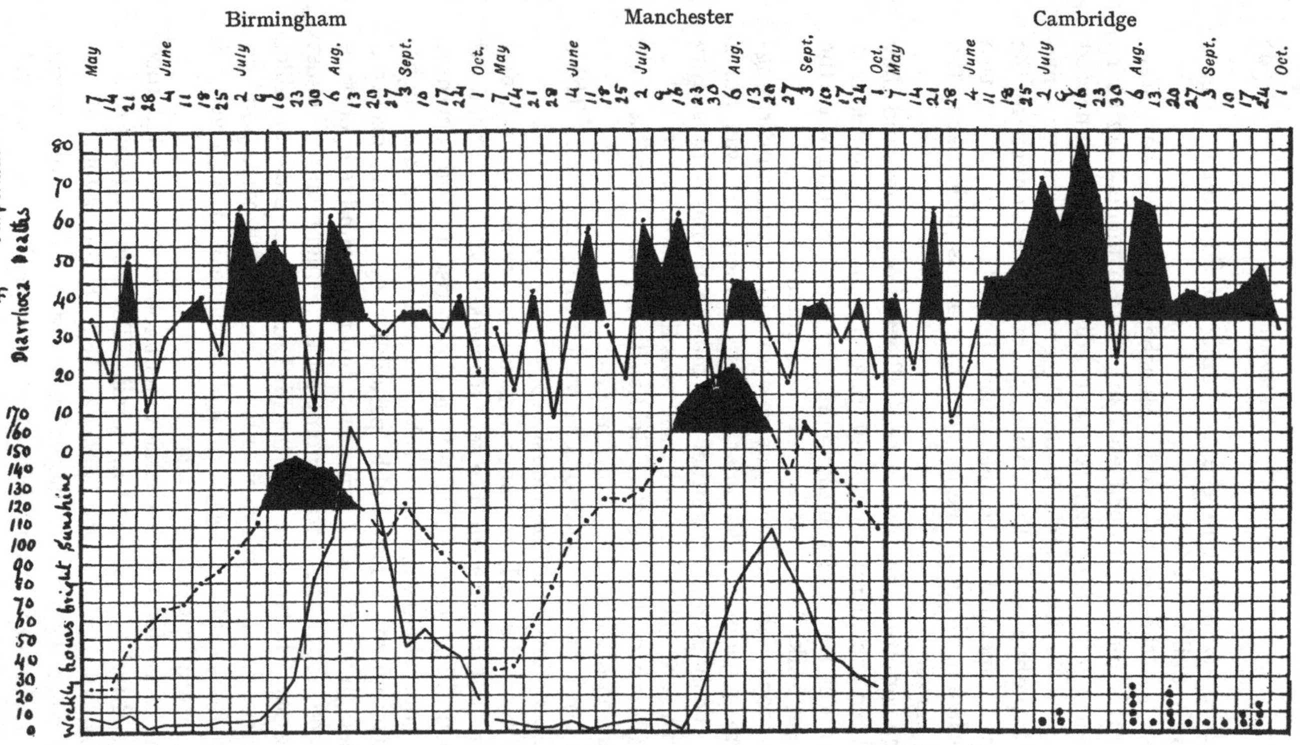

Chart 8, showing the weekly hours of bright sunshine, the mean weekly soil temperatures at 2 ft in depth, and the deaths from epidemic diarrhœa from May to September in **1904**.

Explanation of Charts 8—19: ·—· Weekly hours of bright sunshine. ·–––·–––. 2 ft. ground temperature. —— Diarrhœa deaths. In Cambridge · signifies one death. Here the temperatures have been recorded only since 1907.

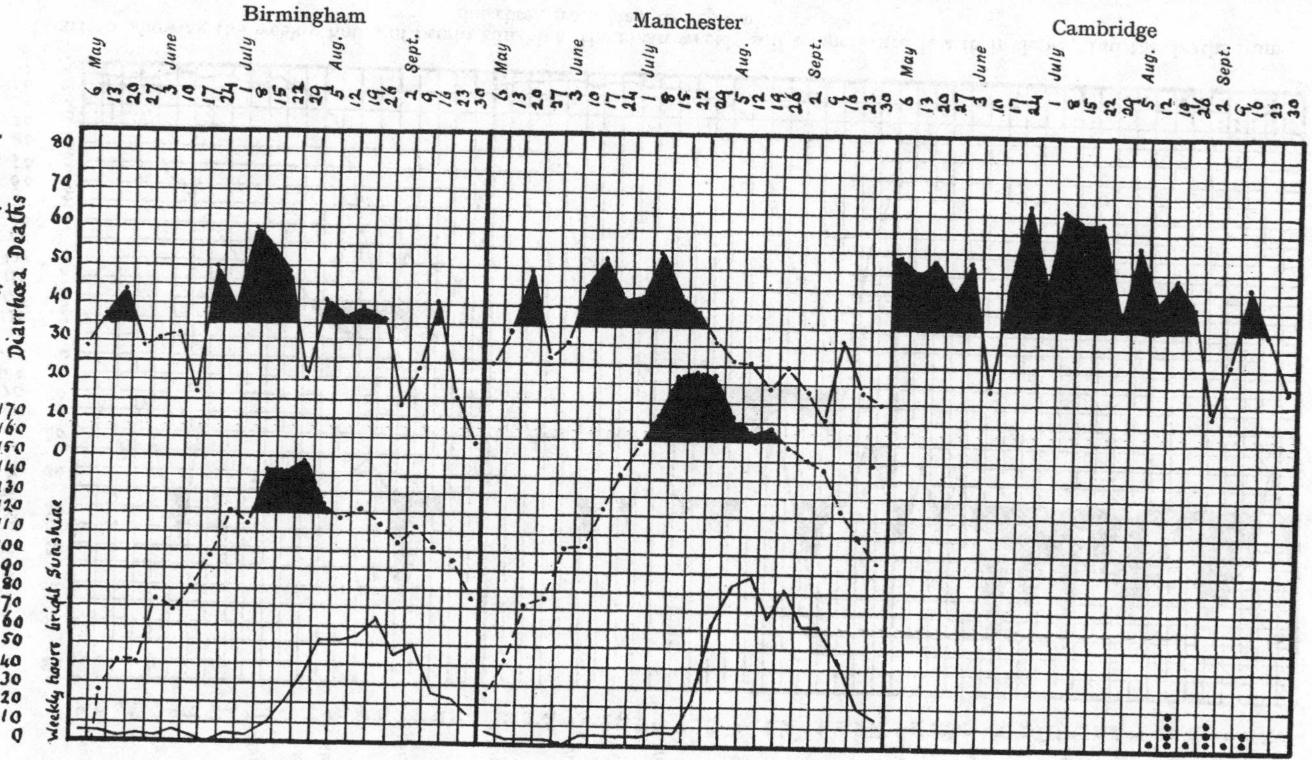

Chart 9, showing the weekly hours of bright sunshine, the mean weekly soil temperature at 2 ft. in depth, and the deaths from epidemic diarrhœa from May to September in 1905.

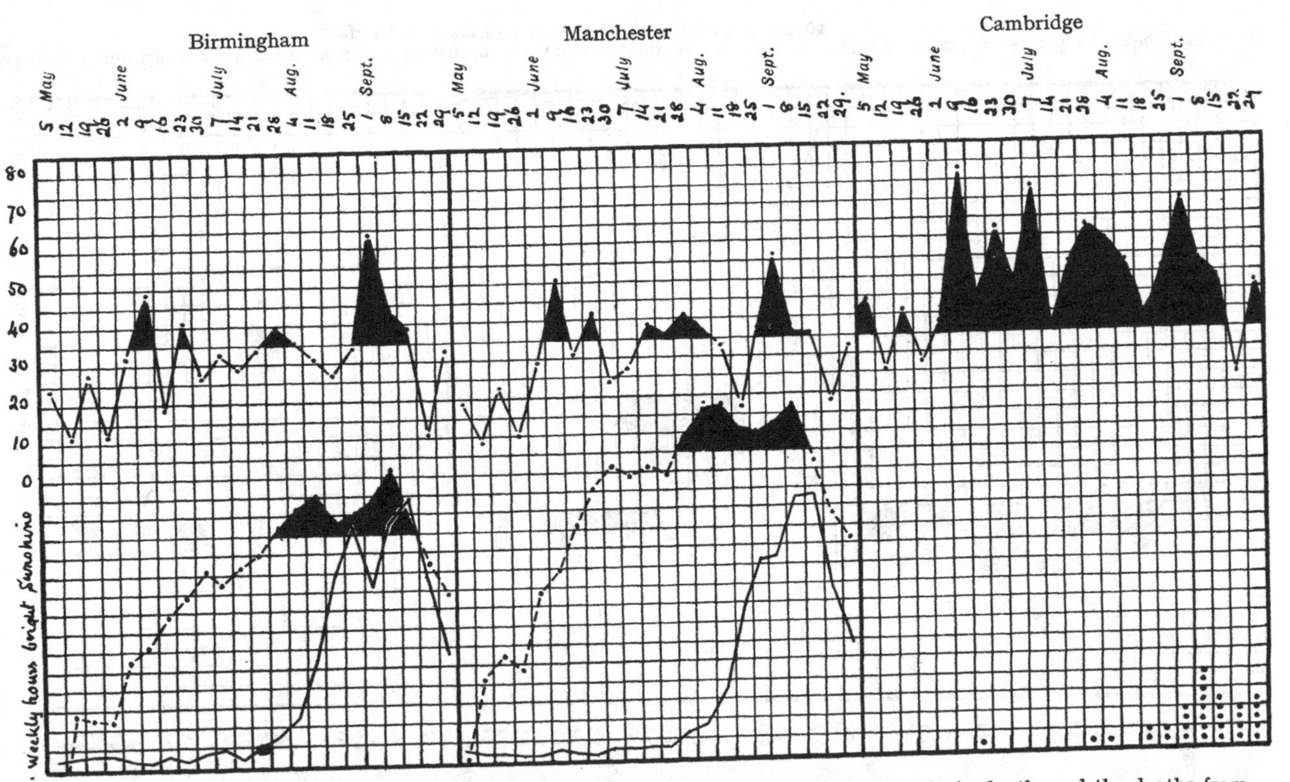

Chart 10, showing the weekly hours of bright sunshine, the mean weekly soil temperature at 2 ft. in depth, and the deaths from diarrhœa from May to September in 1906.

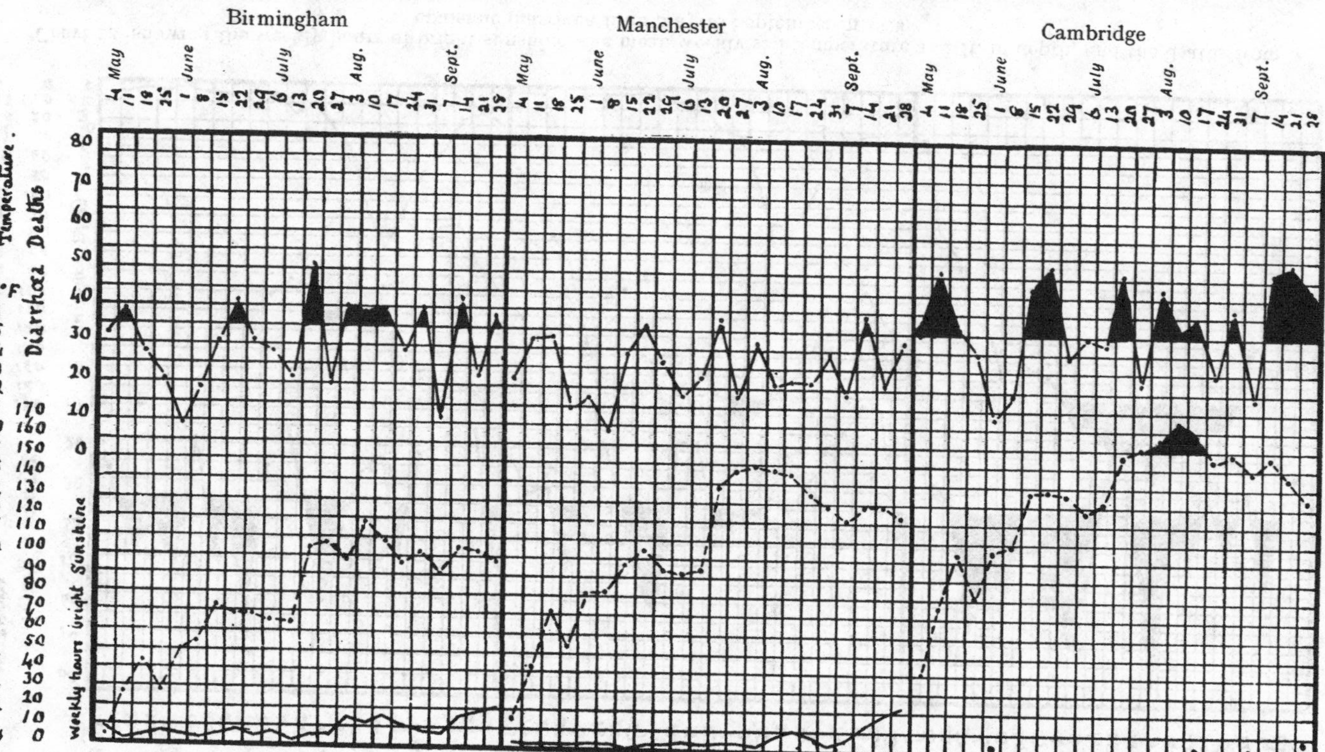

Chart 11, showing the weekly hours of bright sunshine, the mean weekly soil temperature at 2 ft. in depth and the deaths from epidemic diarrhœa from May to September in 1907.

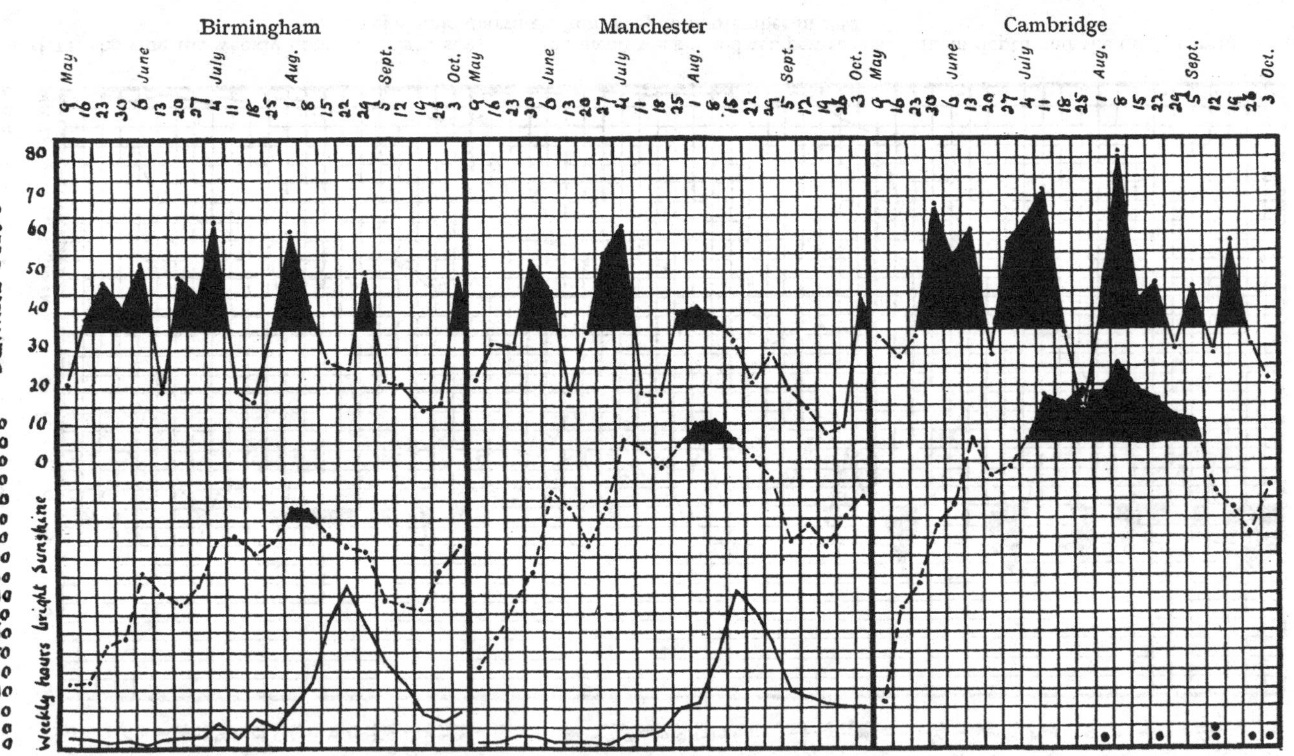

Chart 12, showing the weekly hours of bright sunshine, the mean weekly soil temperature at 2 ft. in depth, and the deaths from epidemic diarrhœa from May to September in 1908.

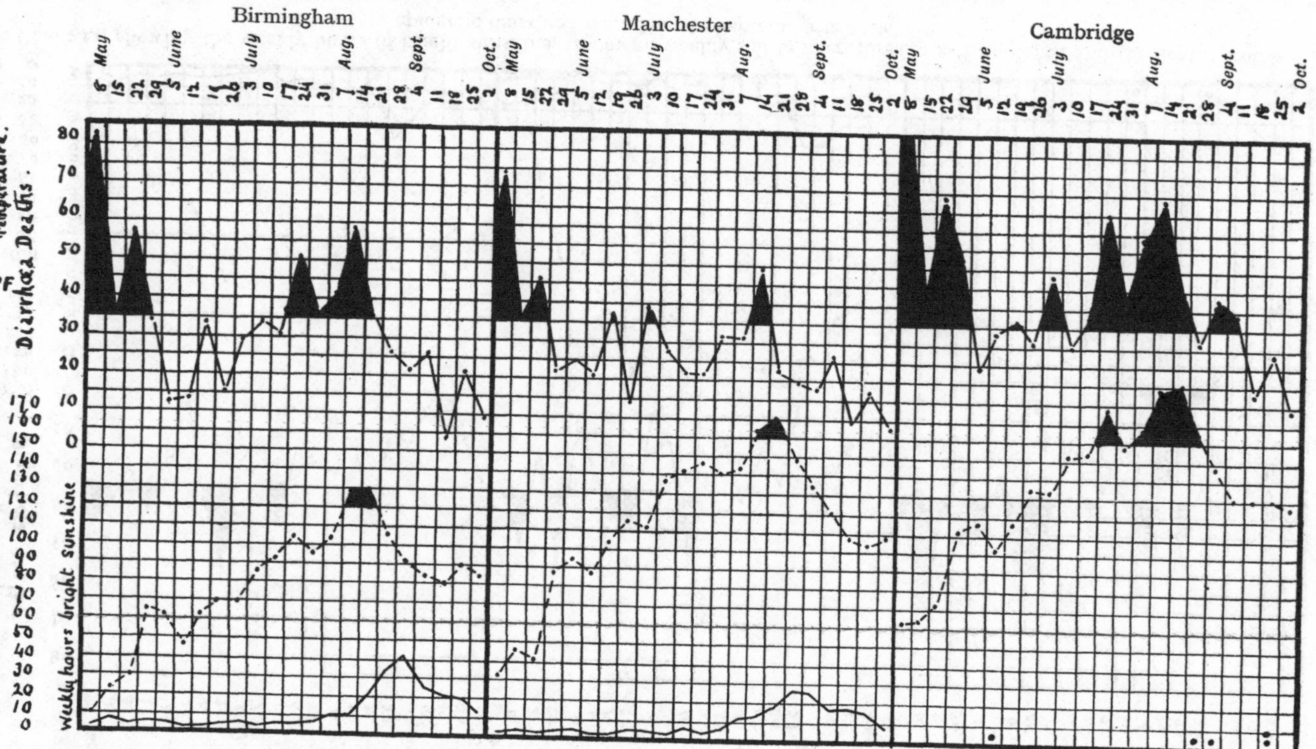

Chart 13, showing the weekly hours of bright sunshine, the mean weekly soil temperature at 2 ft. in depth, and the deaths from epidemic diarrhœa from May to September in **1909**.

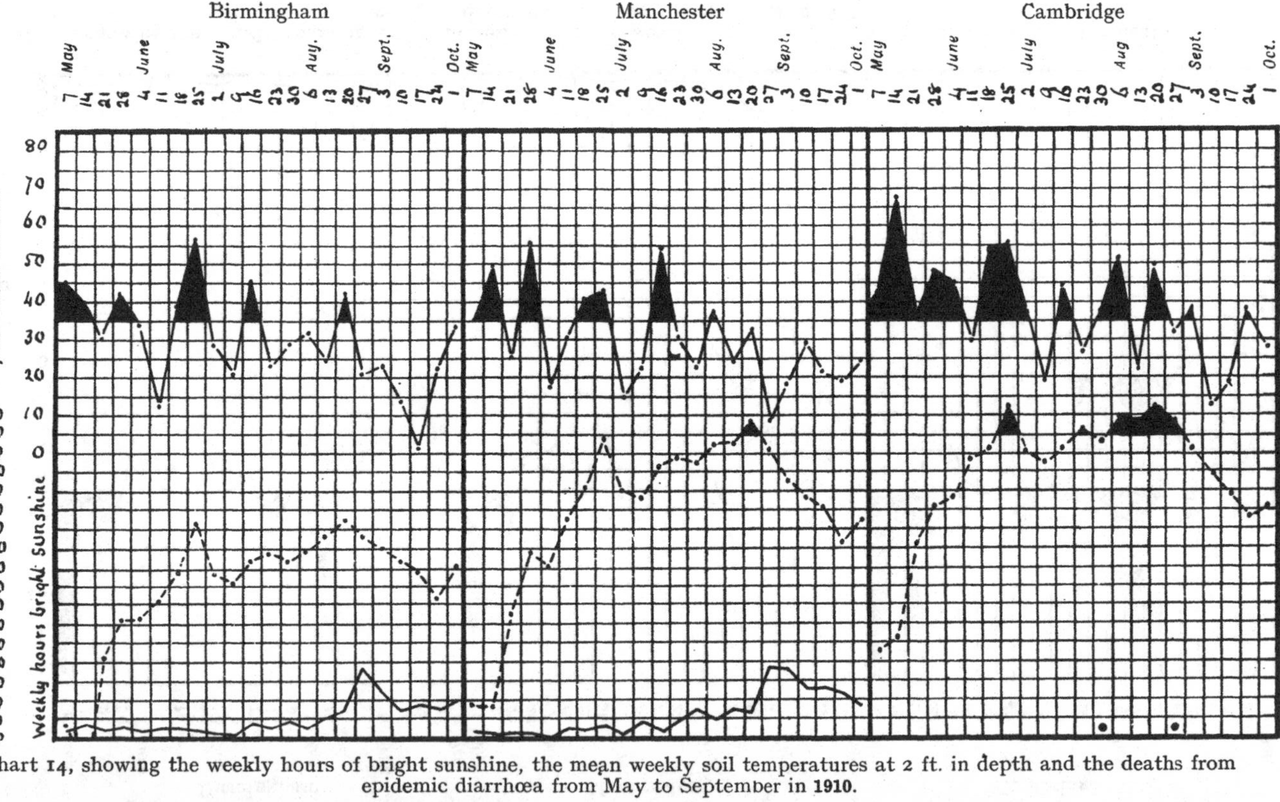

Chart 14, showing the weekly hours of bright sunshine, the mean weekly soil temperatures at 2 ft. in depth and the deaths from epidemic diarrhœa from May to September in 1910.

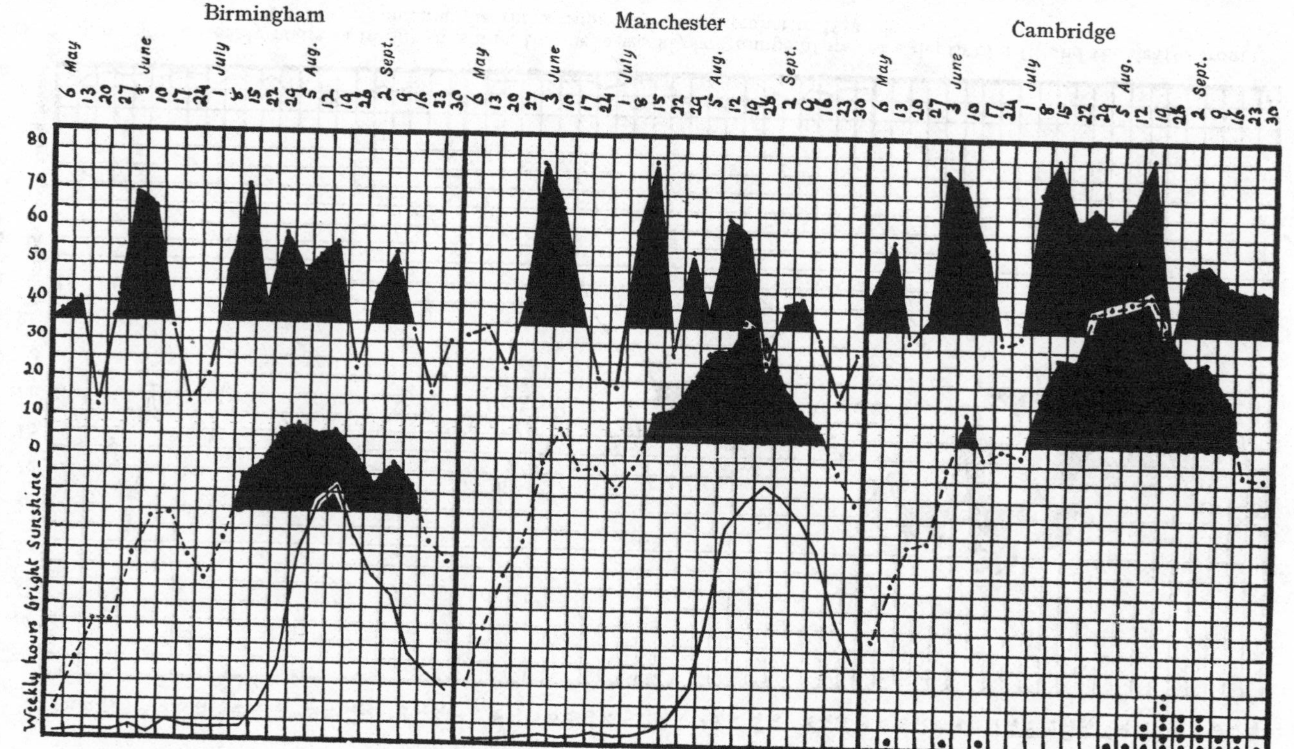

Chart 15, showing the weekly hours of bright sunshine, the mean weekly soil temperatures at a depth of 2 ft. and the deaths from epidemic diarrhœa from May to September in 1911.

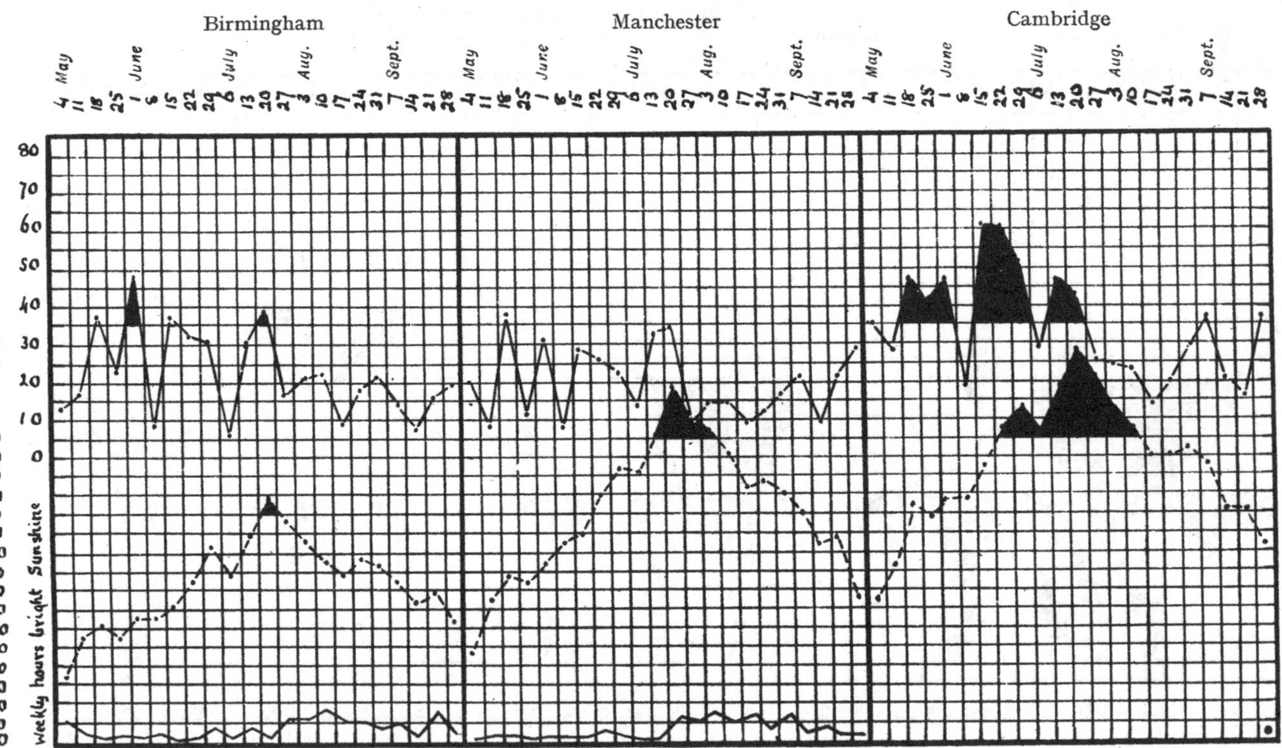

Chart 16, showing the weekly hours of bright sunshine, the mean weekly soil temperatures at a depth of 2 ft. and the deaths from epidemic diarrhœa from May to September in 1912.

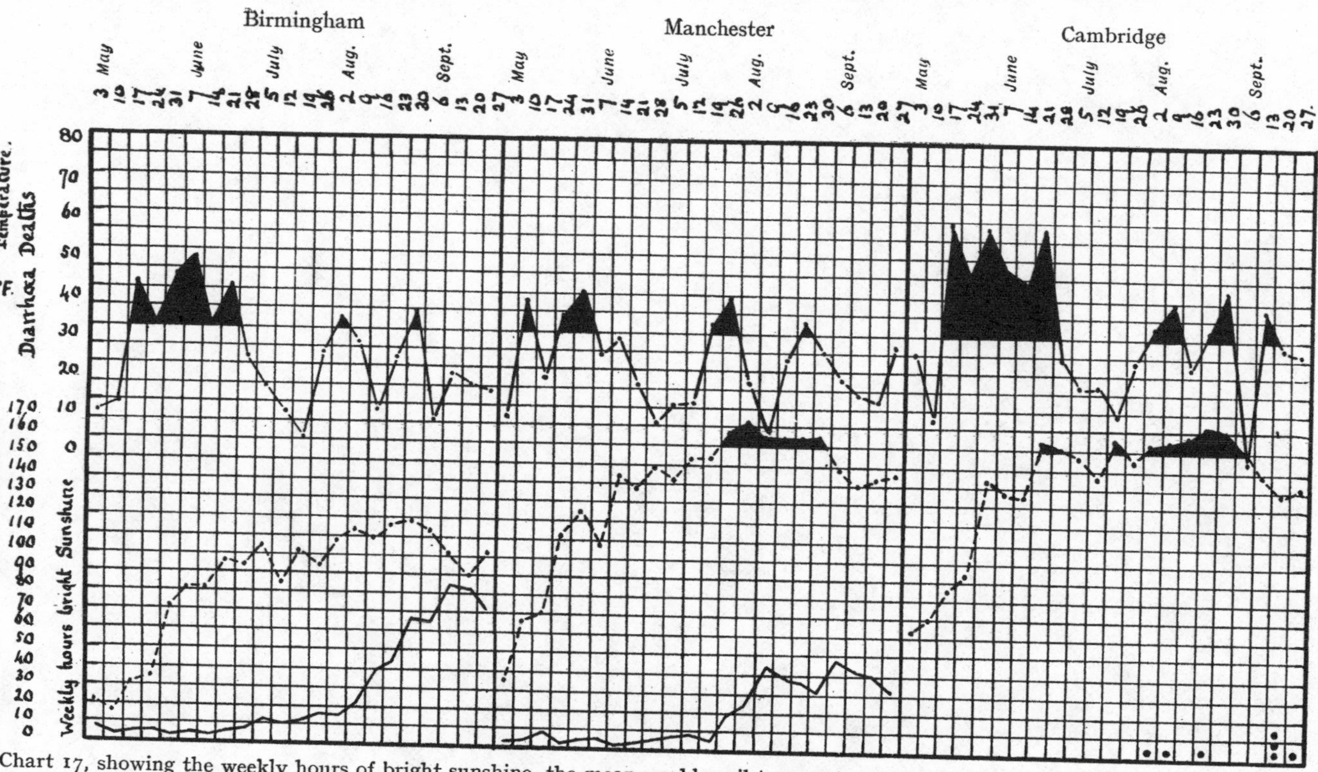

Chart 17, showing the weekly hours of bright sunshine, the mean weekly soil temperatures at a depth of 2 ft. and the deaths from epidemic diarrhœa from May to September in 1913.

the third quarter. In the Manchester death curve the two peaks corresponding with the sunshine peaks are interesting.

It may be stated, therefore, that in Birmingham and Manchester, at least in each of the ten years under consideration, the diarrhœa epidemic seems to depend on such weather conditions as are most likely to influence the numbers of flies and their activities in the late summer, and that the mortality from this disease and its time incidence may be approximately calculated in each year by studying in detail the curves recording the weekly hours of bright sunshine between the middle of May and the end of September, and the 2 ft. ground temperature during the third quarter.

On the other hand the following table shows that comparatively little information can be gained from the mean records of the meteorological conditions prevailing during the third quarter of the year.

Table 35 *showing the mean maximum and mean shade air temperatures and* 2 *ft. ground temperatures for the third quarter, the mean hours of bright sunshine from the middle of May to the end of the third quarter, and the deaths from diarrhœa during the third quarter in Birmingham and Manchester in* 1904–1913.

	Birmingham					Manchester				
	Max. air temp.	Mean air temp.	2 ft. earth temp.	Hours of bright sunshine	Deaths	Max. air temp.	Mean air temp.	2 ft. earth temp.	Hours of bright sunshine	Deaths
1904 ...	66·7	58·8	55·5	38·8	845	67·3	60·1	59·6	36·5	626
1905 ...	65·4	58·4	55·5	34·1	442	65·0	58·8	59·6	32·6	615
1906 ...	69·1	60·7	56·1	32·8	833	67·6	60·4	59·9	32·5	780
1907 ...	64·9	57·4	53·7	30·1	135	64·5	58·0	57·0	24·7	92
1908 ...	64·1	57·8	54·2	35·7	436	64·6	58·6	58·1	31·5	427
1909 ...	64·3	57·3	53·0	29·9	218	63·3	57·7	57·5	25·2	171
1910 ...	63·8	55·3	53·5	28·9	179	64·3	58·0	57·7	28·4	236
1911 ...	72·9	63·3	57·9	41·9	808	71·1	63·0	61·8	42·9	956
1912 ...	61·4	55·6	53·3	22·9	113	62·5	56·8	57·6	20·5	103
1913 ...	65·4	51·3	54·4	28·9	534	65·9	59·3	59·5	22·6	378

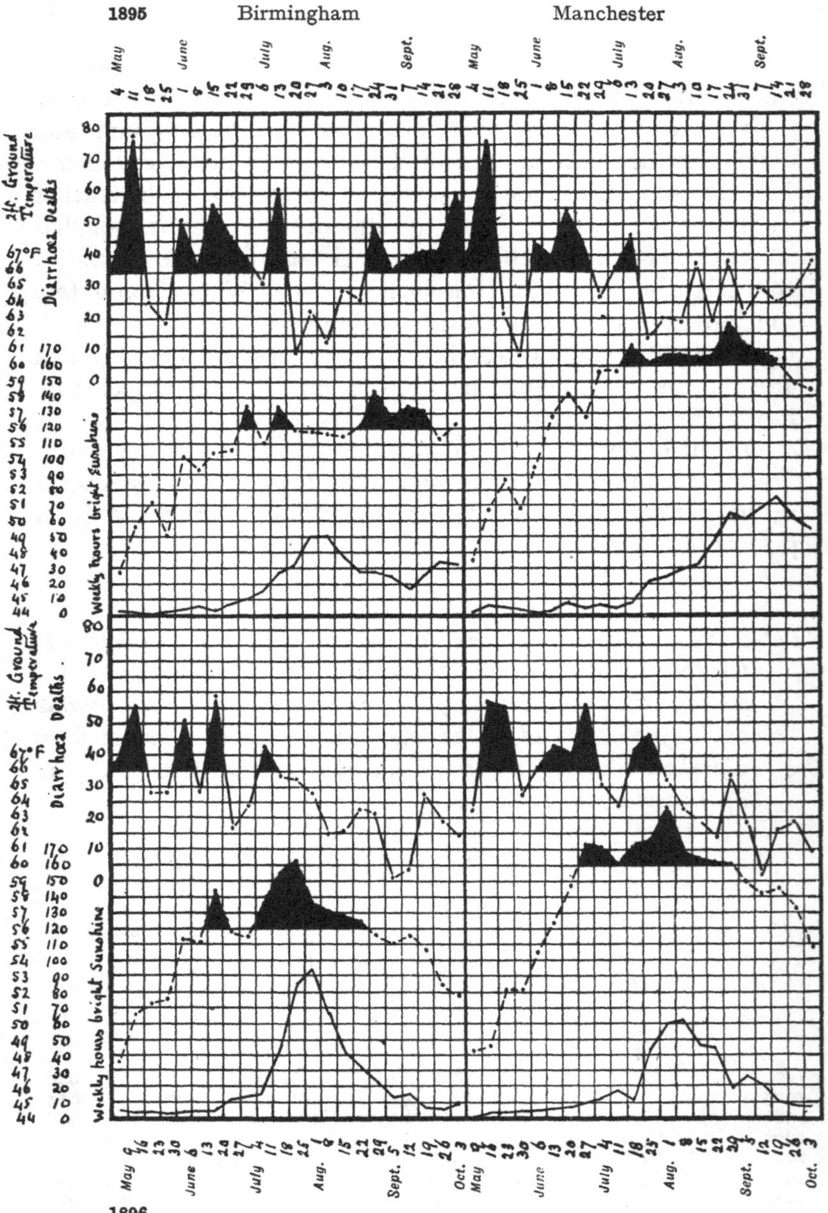

Chart 18, showing the weekly hours of bright sunshine, the mean weekly soil temperatures at a depth of 2 ft. and the deaths from epidemic diarrhœa from May to September in 1895 and 1896.

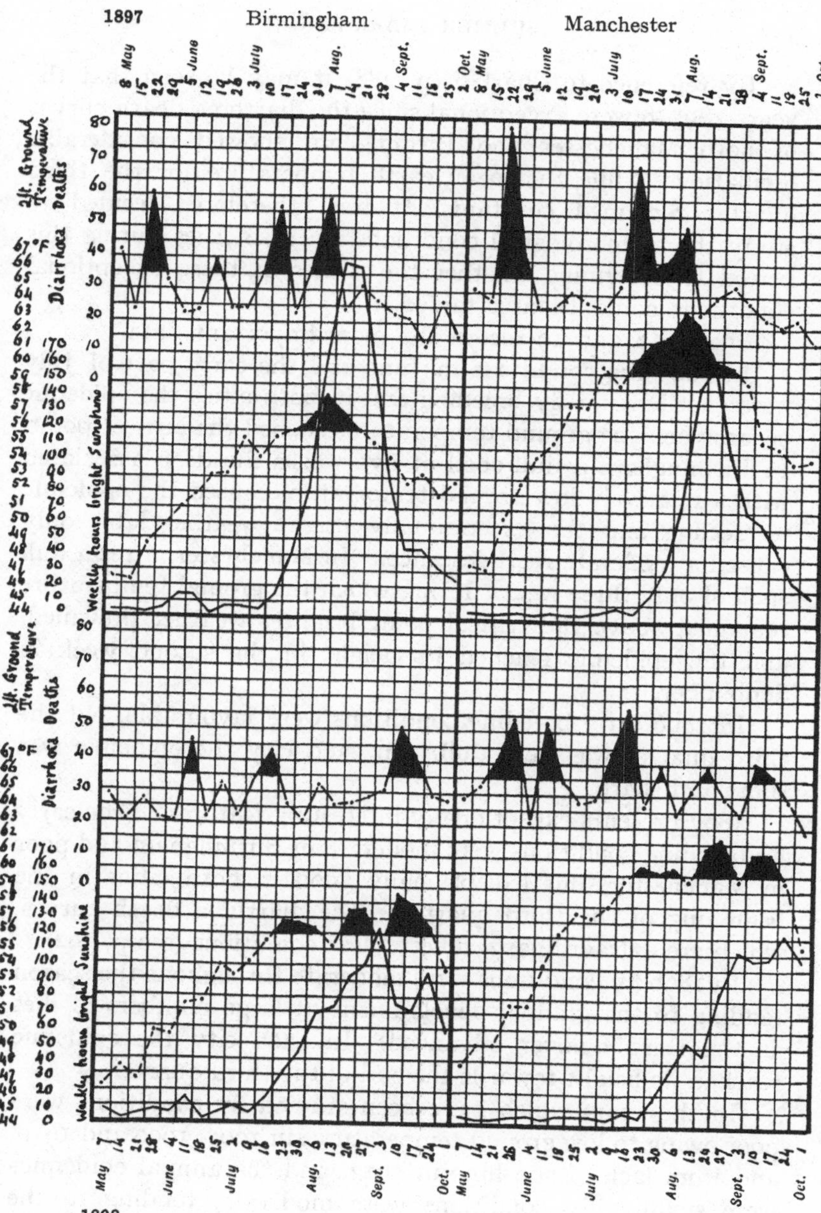

Chart 19, showing the weekly hours of bright sunshine, the mean weekly soil temperatures at a depth of 2 ft. and the deaths from epidemic diarrhœa from May to September in **1897** and **1898**.

By reference to Chart 6 (p. 288) it may be seen that the years 1895–8 were exceptional since the diarrhœa death curves in both Manchester and Birmingham showed considerable oscillations, while the mean earth temperature for the third quarter remained constant. It was, therefore, decided to study the meteorological conditions in these cities during this period to determine whether the causes of these exceptional conditions could be ascertained.

Charts 18 and 19 record the more important data.

In 1895 the conditions in June and the early part of July were excellent for fly breeding and in both cities the epidemic began when the ground temperature reached the critical point. In Birmingham a dull spell of five weeks duration associated with a relatively low ground temperature caused the epidemic to decline and the exceptionally bright weather later only caused a moderate recrudescence. In Manchester, after a dull spell of only three weeks during which the ground temperature remained above the critical point brighter weather prevailed, and the epidemic reached its height in the second week in September.

In 1896 early breeding conditions were favourable, but the third quarter was very dull. In each city the epidemic was short and sharp.

1897 presents exceptionally interesting features. The early fly breeding conditions were moderate in Birmingham and poor in Manchester, but exceptionally good in both cities in the beginning of the third quarter. The diarrhœa death curves, which are extraordinary, reflect these conditions (see p. 302).

In 1898 fly conditions were moderate throughout the season tending to the gradual development of large numbers of flies as the third quarter advanced. In each city the epidemic reached its height towards the end of the third quarter.

In the years which have been studied fly conditions were poor owing to low ground temperatures in 1907, 1909 and 1910, and from lack of sunshine in 1912, and the annual epidemics were small. Fly conditions were moderate, tending to the presence of large numbers at the end of the third quarter in 1895, 1898, 1906 and 1913, and late epidemics occurred. Owing to long bright periods in the early parts of the third quarters, excellent fly conditions, usually of short duration, prevailed in 1896, 1897, 1904, 1905, 1908 and 1911, and sharp epidemics occurred.

The apparent correlation of the diarrhœa death curve to the prevalence of bright sunshine, which adversely affects all disease-producing organisms at present known but increases the activities of flies, is a significant point, in favour of the fly-borne as against all other hypotheses relating to diarrhœa dissemination.

Epidemic diarrhœa seems to be a food infection, and if its virus responds to temperature in the same manner as other known disease-producing organisms which multiply in food, the air temperature ought to have a marked influence on the incidence and severity of the disease, since such organisms multiply more rapidly as the temperature of the medium in which they are living rises, causing the consumer to receive a larger dose. Before the air temperature can have this effect, however, infection of the food must have occurred.

In this secondary manner no doubt a high air temperature is an important factor in each annual epidemic, and possibly by aiding personal infection is responsible for the slight rise in the death curve, which takes place even in poor fly years during the third quarter, since conditions for bacterial multiplication are always more favourable owing to the higher mean temperature at this time of year.

That in years of considerable epidemics the occurrence of the disease is not directly related to high air temperatures is shown in several ways. The death curve bears no resemblance to the mean weekly maximum air temperature curve, and lags several weeks behind it. In years with poor early fly breeding conditions, but good breeding conditions in the third quarter, the diarrhœa death curve only rises when sufficient time has elapsed for flies to emerge and by this time the air temperature curve has often fallen (1905). No doubt when a high air temperature coincides with a period when flies are numerous and active, as in 1897 and 1906, it has a profound influence on the incidence of the disease.

The writer is well aware of the danger of basing conclusions on purely epidemiological data, and puts forward his hypotheses with some hesitation. The evidence in support of them is acknowledged to be scanty, but in view of the importance and obscurity of the problems a detailed consideration of any hypothesis, which may throw some light on the subject, is justified, if it attracts the attention of those who are in a position to investigate such matters, and directs research into channels hitherto little explored.

Finally, it may be pointed out that these hypotheses only apply to temperate climates. In the East excessive heat, dryness, and sunshine are inimical to both flies and pupæ, and it seems probable that, in India at any rate, the conditions become favourable when the soil temperature is falling, the humidity of the air is increasing and the ground has been moistened by rain.

In the first edition it was pointed out (p. 6) that an attempt ought to be made to prove the connection of flies with epidemic diarrhœa, by reducing their numbers in selected areas, where the disease was usually prevalent. Armstrong (1914), who has recently done this, gives an account of his work " in the borough of Bronx, New York City, in a neighbourhood inhabited solely by Italians, and presenting the typical conditions associated with overcrowding, filthy streets, refuse-littered vacant lots, waste-strewn roadways, insanitary stables, etc.—one area, inhabited by 311 families or 1725 individuals, and containing a population of 362 children under the age of 5, was selected, and within this area every effort was made to eliminate the housefly and to break the contact which the insect was supposed to make between filth and food. Another area, containing the same number of families, was permitted to pursue its usual insanitary course. Through nurses supplied by the Bureau of Public Health and Hygiene and by the New York Health Department, careful records of all the facts of morbidity and mortality in the two areas were taken weekly for a period of eight weeks from July 21 to September 13. These findings were later compared and it is on the most significant of them—namely, those dealing with diarrheal diseases of infants—that the greatest emphasis should be placed."

"The methods of opposing the activity of the house-fly may be briefly outlined. First, an educational campaign was carried on by nurses among the mothers in the first area selected. The oral injunctions of the nurses were supplemented by the distribution at frequent intervals of literature in Italian and English, describing and depicting the house-fly dangers. Free tickets were distributed in the Park admitting the people to a moving picture theater near by, where an arrangement was made by which there was displayed for a week the anti-fly picture films. The seventeen hundred doors and windows in the area were carefully screened. Under the auspices of the local Boy Scout organization, large fly-traps were constructed and placed in the court ways, yards and stables."

"In so small a number of children the mortality figures will be too few to be of any significance. On the other hand, the results of the work from the standpoint of diarrheal morbidity are striking and significant. It was found, for instance, that there were in the protected area twenty cases of severe diarrheal disturbances in infants under five years of age, while among the 'outside' infants, in the same age-group, there were fifty-seven similar cases. The ratio here is nearly one to three."

So similar were the two areas selected for comparison "that of the infants in the protected area 88 were breast-fed and 14 bottle-fed, while among the infants 'outside' 85 were breast-fed and 15 bottle-fed."

"Practical results of the investigation indicate the possibility of immensely improving the sanitary condition of a community by the simple procedure of enforcing those sanitary regulations which have to do with fly-breeding nuisances. The statistical results justify the placing of a greater emphasis on educational work among mothers regarding the dangers of the house-fly in the lives of infants. This element should become a more important factor in infant-welfare work."

(*b*) *Bacteriological investigations* (see pp. 159–172).

As pointed out in the first edition (p. 172) all organisms giving the cultural reactions of Morgan's bacillus do not necessarily belong to one species. Lewis (1912, p. 276), who first demonstrated that bacilli of this type may be separated into groups by agglutination tests, has continued his work on this subject. His most recent investigations (1913) show that agglutination reactions serve to discriminate in a striking fashion between cultures of Morgan's bacillus, which by cultural and chemical tests are indistinguishable. The groups into which cultures of Morgan's bacillus can be divided by their agglutination reactions are distinct, and a serum prepared with any one member of a group will agglutinate all other members of that group. Members of these groups were isolated from various sources, normal children, milk, mice and diarrhœa cases, but it is unfortunate that "no line of demarcation can be drawn by agglutination reactions between strains of Morgan's No. 1 Bacillus which by their source might be supposed to be pathogenic or non-pathogenic respectively."

Alexander (1913) has also published further investigations carried on during the year 1912, from which he concludes that the lactose fermenting bacilli found in the fæces are of little importance in the production of intestinal disturbances. During the two years 1911 and 1912 he isolated Morgan's bacillus from the fæces of 4 % of healthy children, and from 13·4 % of diarrhœa cases.

Cholera (see p. 173).

The recent investigations of Greig on the occurrence of the cholera vibrio in the urine (VII, 1913, *d*), its presence in the gall-bladder (VII, 1913, *c*) and on its persistence in the stools of convalescent patients and contacts (VII, 1913, *b*), together with his observations on the epidemic of cholera at Puri in 1912, have materially added to our knowledge regarding the spread of the disease.

Hitherto it has been generally considered that in regard to

its distribution in the tissues of man the cholera vibrio is limited to the alimentary tract and that "the absence of infection of the gall-bladder and bile ducts by the comma bacillus places the disease in quite a different position from typhoid in this respect." (Rogers, 1911, p. 65.)

Greig, however, who has had exceptional opportunities for study, has demonstrated that the cholera vibrio is sometimes excreted in the urine (in 8 out of 55 cases examined), and that it is not infrequently present in the gall bladder, occurring not only on the surface of the mucous membrane, but also, deeper in the submucous tissue. His investigations on 271 fatal cases showed it to be present in the bile of 80.

These observations are of great importance since they show that conditions suitable for the prolonged life of the organism in the body not infrequently occur, and that, besides acute or temporary carriers, permanent chronic cholera carriers, like typhoid carriers, may exist, capable, when the circumstances are favourable, of disseminating the disease over long periods. The influence of typhoid carriers has already been discussed (p. 127), and it seems reasonable to suppose that cholera carriers convey disease in the same manner.

Greig has not only shown the possibility of the existence of cholera carriers, but has actually demonstrated that they do occur, and has moreover investigated an epidemic caused by one of them.

Persons, who have recovered from cholera, are usually discharged from hospital as soon as possible, and, in India at any rate, it is seldom possible to trace their movements. Greig found that about 36 per cent. were discharged in an infective condition, with cholera vibrios in their stools. In order to gain some information as to the proportion of these infected persons who become chronic carriers Greig (VII, 1913, *b*) made daily examinations over prolonged periods of the stools of eleven prisoners convalescent from cholera. In the majority of cases the vibrios ceased to be excreted very shortly after the acute attack, but in a small proportion (3 out of the 11 examined) the vibrios were "at intervals in the stools for longer periods." In two cases in which the prolonged excretion of the cholera vibrio was noted, there were long intervals, as in enteric fever, in which the stools remained free from cholera vibrios."

As an example of this condition Greig's observations on one of these cases is quoted in detail.

Name—Babaji Mahapatra, Hindu, Male. Age 27.
Date of attack—31st July 1912.

Date of examination of stools	Widal reaction cholera vibrio	Presence or absence of cholera vibrio in stools	Date of examination of stools	Widal reaction cholera vibrio	Presence or absence of cholera vibrio in stools
July 21 ..	..	–	Sept. 1 ..	..	–
Aug. 1 ..	..	+	,, 2 ..	..	Non-Agglutinating vibrios.
,, 3 ..	..	+			
,, 4 ..	..	–			
,, 5 ..	..	–	,, 3 ..	..	–
,, 6 ..	..	–	,, 4 ..	..	–
,, 11 ..	..	–	,, 6 ..	..	–
,, 12 ..	..	–	,, 7 ..	+(60)	–
,, 18 ..	..	–	,, 8 ..	..	–
,, 19 ..	..	–	,, 9 ..	..	–
,, 20 ..	..	–	,, 10 ..	..	–
,, 21 ..	..	–	,, 11 ..	..	–
,, 22 ..	..	–	,, 12 ..	+(60)	+ +
,, 23 ..	..	–	,, 13 ..	..	+ +
,, 24 ..	..	+ +	,, 14 ..	..	–
,, 25 ..	..	+ +	,, 15 ..	+(60)	–
,, 26 ..	..	–	,, 16 ..	..	–
,, 27 ..	..	–	,, 17 ..	..	–
,, 28 ..	..	–	,, 18 ..	+(100)	–
,, 29 ..	..	–	,, 19 ..	..	–
,, 30 ..	..	–	,, 20 ..	..	–
,, 31 ..	..	–			

.. = not tested; Widal + (60) = agglutinated in dilution of 1 in 60; vibrio – = not found; + = present; + + = present in large numbers.

"*Remarks.* This is an important case. The cholera vibrios were recovered from his stools 6 weeks after the attack. The discharge of the vibrios was markedly intermittent as in the case of *B. typhosus*. It is interesting to note that cholera-like vibrios occurred in the stool of this man on one occasion, but they did not react with a high titre agglutination serum. His blood also contained cholera agglutinins."

Other recent investigators have recorded similar results. Devecchi and Randone (1911, p. 347) state that the vibrios may be found in the stools up to the 35th day, and in the report of the International Sanitary Conference in Paris (1911) it is recorded that exceptionally it may be excreted for 12 months.

Greig (VII, 1913, *b*) also "examined 27 persons presenting no signs of disease and found six persons excreting the cholera vibrios in the stools. As these persons were attached to the cholera hospital as temporary staff they formed more suitable material for observations than a constantly moving population."

Cholera in Puri.

Greig carried out the researches, which have been quoted, during an epidemic which occurred in Puri, and also investigated a small outbreak, which occurred in the jail. Owing to the fact that about 300,000 pilgrims assembled in Puri in July 1912 the annual epidemic was larger than in previous years, and afforded valuable material for studying various problems connected with cholera.

During the epidemic in July and August, 1912, "flies were extremely abundant amounting almost to a plague ; an interesting point in this relation was that the appearance and disappearance of the flies synchronised with the arrival and departure of the great mass of the pilgrims: consequently temporary breeding places must have existed in Puri. Bacteriological examinations of the flies caught in the neighbourhood of collections of cholera cases at Puri showed the cholera vibrio was present on the external appendages, and, also, in the contents of the alimentary tract of the flies, demonstrating that the fly was a channel by which the virus was being conveyed from the infected to the uninfected individuals at Puri. Water I think could be excluded" (1, 1913). Encouraged by the results in the jail outbreak, about to be quoted, Greig extended the plan of disinfecting the fresh night soil to the town of Puri itself, using fresh chlorinated lime.

"The difficulties in carrying out the systematic disinfection of the fresh night soil in the town were very great owing to the extremely defective state of the private latrines and the absence of proper access to them. But in spite of these difficulties it was followed by a marked drop in the number of attacks and deaths from cholera. On 20th August, four days after it was begun, the deaths were 18. On 24th August, four deaths ; and by the end of August the epidemic ceased."

Outbreak of Cholera in Puri Jail.

Greig further had the opportunity of making a very careful investigation of an outbreak of cholera in Puri jail. " The epidemic was brought about in the following manner :—A patient, who had been attacked by cholera on the 6th July, 1912, was discharged from Puri Cholera Hospital. He wandered about until July 23rd, 1912, when he was arrested and sent to jail." A careful examination of the stools of this man on 28th July showed that he was excreting cholera vibrios in large numbers. It is of interest to note that he continued to excrete large numbers till he was released on 4th August.

A few days after his admission to the jail cases of cholera commenced to occur in the undertrial ward where he was. At that time there were 222 persons in the jail. " Including warders 17 cases of cholera with 5 deaths took place in the jail as the result of the introduction of the cholera virus by this carrier. The carrier was at once segregated, but before this was done he had had an opportunity of infecting latrines and flies ; the latter were very numerous in the jail and elsewhere in Puri at that time."

Greig, considering that water and other means of conveying infection could be excluded, and believing from his experience in the city that flies were the disseminating agents, decided to disinfect the fresh night soil of all the inmates of the jail. " Each person in the jail passed his night soil into a receptacle filled with a solution of cyllin of suitable strength, in this way the stool was rapidly disinfected and the access of flies during the process of disinfection was prevented, the fæces being submerged in the solution. Cases of cholera were occurring in the jail, but four days after the commencement of the systematic cyllination of the fresh night soil, the outbreak ceased."

Greig (1, 1913) concludes from his observations at Puri that " healthy ' carriers ' and flies were the main channels by which the infection of cholera was transmitted to the uninfected at Puri."

Chart 20 showing in graphic form the course of the epidemic in Puri jail, following the admission of the carrier, and the effect of the complete cyllination of all fresh night soil in the jail.

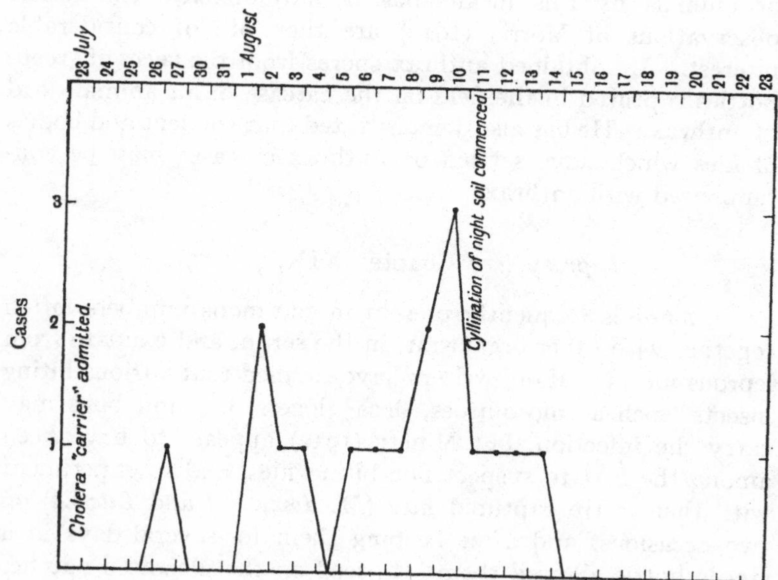

Seicluna (1912) thought that flies were partly responsible for the spread of cholera in Malta during the outbreak of 1911.

Alessandrini and Sampietro (1912) fed flies on materials containing cholera vibrios and found these organisms on the surfaces and in the fæces of these flies for 24–36 hours—vibrios were found only rarely in small numbers in larvae fed on such materials, but were never found in the pupæ. These observers also bred flies from larvæ, which had been kept in fæces swarming with cholera vibrios, but never found the vibrios either on them or in their intestinal contents. Moreover, though they investigated flies caught in surroundings in which natural infection might have occurred they never found any specimens carrying the vibrios.

Anthrax (see p. 180).

Although it has been demonstrated most conclusively that under experimental conditions flies can distribute both anthrax bacilli and their spores no evidence of infection in either man or animals by this means has been obtained. The recent observations of Morris (1912) are therefore of considerable interest. He obtained anthrax spores from the fæces of green-bottles captured in the field on the carcase of an animal dead of anthrax. He has also demonstrated that the feet and bodies of flies which have settled on anthrax carcases may be contaminated with anthrax.

Leprosy (see Chapter XIX, p. 189).

B. lepræ is frequently present in enormous numbers, often together with other organisms, in the serum and exudate from leprous ulcers. Many writers have claimed that various biting insects, such as mosquitoes, fleas, jiggers, lice and bugs may carry the infection, but Minett (1912) appears to have been among the first to suspect non-biting flies, and to experiment with them. He captured flies (*M. domestica* and *Lucilia*) on two occasions, and after keeping them for several days in a sterile bottle allowed them "to feed on the ulcerated patches present on several lepers for a short time before returning them to the sterile bottle. They were then kept for a period of three days before examination." The method of examination adopted was as follows:

"The flies were first killed with chloroform vapour; each fly was then placed in a thin sterile test-tube containing 4 c.cms. of sterile saline solution. They were allowed to soak in this for 48 hours, with frequent shakings, care being taken not to detach legs or wings. At the end of this period the fly was removed and the saline was placed for 5 minutes in a high speed electric centrifuge. The supernatant fluid was carefully drawn off with a pipette, and the deposit placed on a sterile glass slide and allowed to evaporate in the air, covered by a watch glass. This was then stained with Zeihl-Neelsen's differential stain, and examined for the presence of the bacilli. In this manner thirty flies were examined, and in one instance leprosy bacilli were detected.

"The same flies were then placed in fresh sterile test-tubes and their intestines teased out by means of sterile platinum needles, care being taken to break up the intestine itself and to express the fæces. Four c.cms. of sterile saline solution was then added to each tube, which was allowed to stand for 24 hours with frequent shakings. At the end of this period the fragments of the fly were removed by means of platinum loops, the fluid centrifugalised, and the deposit stained and examined as before. Of thirty specimens examined in this manner, four specimens contained well-formed leprosy bacilli, and one specimen showed their presence in a very degenerated form."

From his experiments Minett concludes "that flies must certainly be reckoned as possible factors in the dissemination of leprosy, if only as mechanical carriers; for it would be extremely easy for a fly, having previously fed on a leprous ulcer, to convey infection to others, either by way of cuts and abrasions on the skin, or possibly by the mucous membrane of the nasal cavity.

"Also the fact that undegenerated leprosy bacilli showing no plasmolysis, or other evidence of destruction, were detected in the fly's intestine after a period of three days, would seem to point to the conclusion that the waxy coating present on these bacilli is extremely resistant to the gastric juices, and that the organisms are presumably capable of carrying infection to a healthy person, if planted on a suitable medium, such as serum present on a cut or ulcer."

In other experiments Minett kept thirty flies in "sterile glass roll culture tubes" for 48 hours without food and "then fed them on serum known to be rich in bacilli, exuded from a freshly cut leprous nodule. This was effected by making a fairly deep cut in a suitable nodule, scraping the sides, and then placing the mouth of the tube containing the flies over the same. It was found that the flies fed on the serum and blood readily. They were allowed to feed in this manner twice daily for seven consecutive days. At the end of this period the flies were killed with chloroform vapour and shaken out of the tubes. 10 c.c. of sterile 0·75 per cent. saline solution was placed in each tube, and the fæces thoroughly shaken up, and allowed to remain for 24 hours to soak; then shaken up again, the saline centrifugalised in sterile tubes, and the deposit collected on slides, dried and stained as before. In order to concentrate the deposit, the saline obtained from five flies was mixed, making a total of six slides.

" On examination the results were as follows :

Two slides showed many typical bacilli present ;

Two slides showed many typical bacilli ; also a large number of bacilli showing well-marked granular degeneration ;

One slide showed well marked granules, but no typical bacilli ;

One slide was negative."

For obvious reasons it is impossible to attempt to prove this hypothesis of transmission from man to man by direct experiment.

Lebœuf (1912, 1913), who has spent some years in attempting to ascertain the part played by insects in the spread of leprosy, has also pointed out in a number of papers the possibility of this disease being transmitted by non-biting flies. He noticed that house-flies frequently settled on exposed leprous ulcers. Out of 23 flies which had settled on leprous ulcers known to contain many bacilli, 19 contained *B. lepræ*. In many the bacilli were present in large numbers. Fæces deposited within two days after feeding on ulcers contained some bacilli, showing no signs of degeneration. He observed leprosy bacilli in flies caught in the rooms of leprosy patients with ulcers, but not in 29 flies caught in the room of patients with non-ulcerating forms of leprosy. The bacilli were not found in flies caught elsewhere.

Lebœuf considers that flies may transmit the disease by depositing fæces on the nasal mucous membrane or on wounds, especially during sleep.

Noc (1912) also states that he has frequently found *B. lepræ* in the intestines of flies caught in the neighbourhood of patients suffering from leprous ulcers.

Trypanosomiasis (see p. 191).

Darling (1913) records the infection of a mule with a strain of *Trypanosoma hippicum* which had been maintained in guinea-pigs " by means of *Musca domestica*."

Infection by non-biting flies of the wounds caused by biting flies (p. 209).

Patton's interesting observations on the habits of *M. pattoni* have been quoted already. Patton and Cragg (1913) in a series of papers record further observation on this subject. "It is of peculiar interest to find that in the genus *Musca,* in which the proboscis is of the type from which the muscid biting flies have evolved, there are certain flies, which habitually feed on blood. Though they are confirmed blood suckers, and have no other food, the proboscis is not adapted for piercing, and presents no notable deviations from the type of the genus."

The great interest and importance of this group of flies lies in the remarkable manner in which they obtain their food. "Totally unable to penetrate the skin of the host themselves, they rely on other and better equipped flies to do it for them, and feed on the blood and serum which exudes from their bites. For this purpose they associate themselves with the biting Muscids, such as *Stomoxys*, *Bdellolarynx*, *Philæmatomyia* and *Lyperosia*, and with the *Tabanidæ*. An observer unacquainted with this group would remark on the large number of what appear to be ordinary house-flies on the cattle and horses in places where any of the above are numerous. Closer examination, however, reveals the fact that extremely few, if any, of the species present are really those which are habitually found in houses, but are flies which are seldom found away from cattle. We have frequently confirmed this by the examination of large numbers of flies brought from the neighbouring bazaar, and by the capture of flies from cattle.

"The behaviour of these flies is extremely interesting to watch. On approaching a biting fly in the act of feeding, the *Musca* will endeavour to thrust its proboscis into the wound, and to oust the rightful occupant ; often several will beset the same biter, and when they succeed in dislodging it, or when it has completed its meal, will thrust down their proboscides to suck up the blood which exudes from the wound. When a single individual succeeds in placing itself in position over the wound its attitude is exactly that assumed by the true biting muscids, such as *Philæmatomyia* and *Stomoxys*, for it crouches down and remains motionless while its abdomen can be seen to distend. Like the true biting flies also, they will gorge themselves with blood from one feed, and fly away to rest afterwards ; more frequently, however, the conditions are not sufficiently favourable, or the competition for food too great among themselves, to permit of this, and they will feed again on another animal after having exhausted or been dislodged from one source of supply. We have frequently seen as many as six individuals of *Musca pattoni*, a large fly, assembled around a single small *Philæmatomyia insignis*, waiting for it to withdraw its proboscis. The larger Tabanids, such as *Tabanus albimedius* and *T. striatus*, which make a deep and bleeding wound, provide a frequent supply of food.

" These flies are not entirely dependent on other biting flies for their food, for they will readily suck up the moisture which exudes from sores on the skin. That their food is blood and serum can be readily shown by dissection."

Patton and Cragg (1913 A) describe with beautiful illustrations *Musca gibsoni*, a fly which is common in September in the Pulney Hills, South India, at a height of 6000 feet, but is never seen in the plains, *Musca pattoni*, Austen, which is abundant in Madras throughout the year, *Musca convexifrons*, Thomson, which occurs in China, and is common in Madras throughout the year, and *Musca bezzii*, which is abundant during the middle of the year in the Nilgiri Hills, but is never seen in the plains of India. All these flies feed in the manner described.

In another paper on the interesting genus *Philæmatomyia* Patton and Cragg (1913, B) describe and illustrate *Philæmatomyia lineata*, which occurs in the cold weather in Madras and in the hot weather in the Pulney Hills. They have studied its habits carefully, " and now can say with certainty that it is not able to make a wound for itself, but that, like certain species of *Musca*, it relies on other flies to puncture the skin for it." On the other hand *Philæmatomyia gurnei*, Patton and Cragg, and *P. insignis*, Austen, are capable of making wounds for themselves.

Patton and Cragg's statements have been confirmed independently by Mitzmain (1913) in the Philippines, who describes his observations in the following words :

"A peculiar feeding relation has been observed to exist between *Stomoxys* and certain non-biting flies. I was curious to learn why such large numbers of non-biting flies were generally found in collecting insects from domesticated animals. Moreover, in an examination of extensive collections made with a net swung over the backs of the animals, the majority of the non-biting flies were found to have blood-engorged abdomens. When these were dissected and examined microscopically, mammalian blood was found to be the principal food constituent.

"A quiet bullock was selected for closer observation. On this animal 150 to 200 flies, mostly muscids, were seen. Many hundred dung flies, including house-flies, were scattered about on the floor of the stall, and occasionally one of these joined the blood-sucking flies on the body of the bullock.

"My attention was attracted by the peculiar grouping of the ecto-parasites ; groups of two to five predominated. On closer inspection the group was found to consist almost invariably of more than one species, a *Stomoxys* usually being the central figure. Where a *Stomoxys* was lacking, it was found that the group fed from a common area with the heads of the individuals in close contact. The food of these flies was found to be a droplet of freshly exuded blood, and among the blood imbibers often not an individual belonged to a species with a piercing mouth ; they consisted principally of house-flies. Other groups of flies surrounding a *Stomoxys* attracted attention by the fact that while it was feeding the rest waited. The latter gave evidence of great impatience and eagerness in the movements of nudging one another and colliding with the *Stomoxys*, apparently making efforts to dislodge it. The *Stomoxys* having been satisfied, the other flies pounced upon the feeding spot where trickled a well-rounded blood drop. These flies collected round the puncture, and lapped the blood as it oozed from the wound. In a moment the group disbanded with abdomens more or less reddened and distended, the individuals either flying off the host to rest or to join another biting *Stomoxys*. In many instances the *Stomoxys* was accompanied by a single fly which hovered above it until the *Stomoxys* was fully engorged and left the exuding blood to the disposal of the second passive parasite."

Mitzmain does not appear to have attempted to determine accurately the species of non-biting flies attending on the *Stomoxys*, and it is not unlikely that he was dealing with cattle-frequenting muscids or with species of the genus *Philæmatomyia*. "It is extremely probable that this genus is a large and widely distributed one, which has escaped the attention of entomologists on account of its close resemblance to non-biting muscids."

The practical importance of these observations lies in the probable capacity of this group of flies to transmit disease from one animal to another. The flies are necessarily to a large extent intermittent feeders, passing from place to place on the same animal, and from one animal to another, in the search for food, and always inserting their proboscides, perhaps bearing on their surfaces infective matter, into or near a wound or broken surface. "True biting flies, on the other hand, habitually take a full meal from one wound, and allow an interval of from one to three days to elapse before feeding again, in order to digest the meal. It is only when they happen to be disturbed while feeding that they will fly off to another animal, and in the majority of cases we must assume, if 'accidental infection' is to occur in a state of nature, that the infective organism is capable of living for at least twenty-four hours exposed to the external air. In cases where such a method of infection is suspected, the non-biting but hæmatophagous flies deserve at least as much attention as the true biters." Indeed Darling (1912) has shown already that non-blood-sucking flies can convey trypanosomiasis, a blood disease, from mule to mule (p. 191).

Myiasis (p. 211).

Human myiasis is so seldom observed in temperate climates that it has not been considered necessary to discuss in great detail the various conditions produced by the presence of dipterous larvæ in the living body. Some larvæ, which produce myiasis, are responsible for several conditions, while some invariably produce similar lesions; some attack men only, some attack animals, and a few are parasitic on both; some are habitually parasitic, others occasionally, and a few may be accidental parasites; some are wide-spread, others extremely local. The subject, in consequence of the diversity of habits displayed by the various larvæ and their wide-spread distribution, is so complex that a volume would be required to deal adequately with its various aspects.

In spite of the interest attaching to it myiasis has been little studied hitherto by medical men, except in the tropics, and hardly recognized by the public. In Chapter XXII, an attempt was made to arouse the interest of English readers by summarizing the more important investigations relating to flies, which cause myiasis in man, and giving in detail the cases which have been recorded in England.

Since the first edition was written in the early part of 1912 a number of interesting and important papers relating to myiasis have been published. With the exception of Froggatt's work dealing with the changes in the habits of flies producing myiasis in Australian sheep, which has been cited already (p. 276), the more important contributions published during 1913 are considered in the following pages.

A. *Blood-sucking larvæ* (p. 212).

Rodhain, Pons, Vandenbranden and Bequaert (1913) have shown that *A. luteola* is oviparous. The eggs are laid in damp soil, or possibly on ground inside or near huts contaminated with fæcal matter or urine. The larva which emerges is very active, and avoids the light, escaping in a very short time into the dust or earth. In the soil of different villages they found numerous larvæ, in different stages of development, and pupæ. Rodhain and Bequaert (1913) consider that the fly is distributed in the egg or larval stage in the dirty mats which the natives take about with them.

Roubaud (1913) has published a most interesting study of the four allied species, *A. luteola*, *A. prægrandis*, *Chæromyia chærophaga* and *C. boueti*, which are confined to tropical and subtropical Africa. According to Roubaud *A. luteola* is constantly associated with man, and lives more or less exclusively in his dwellings. It feeds on blood and also on fallen fruit and dejecta, and seems to be very sensitive to heat, dying rapidly if exposed to the sun or a temperature of 45° C. The female, which exhibits two definite periods of oviposition, and is capable of laying about 80 eggs, seems to deposit one egg at a time in holes in the soil or dust. The eggs are never laid on the bodies or clothes of sleeping persons. Roubaud says that the larvæ can always be found in large numbers by digging in the floors of native huts, if the sleeping mats are placed on the ground or very close to it. According to his experiments under the best conditions of food and temperature the larval life lasts 15 days, during which two moults occur. On the other hand under adverse conditions the larval stage may last as long as 76 days before pupation. Experimentally the larvæ exhibit very remarkable powers of resistance to starvation, being able to keep alive without food for three weeks after emerging from the eggs. Older larvæ can remain alive for a month without food. Roubaud has further observed that starving larvæ when buried in the soil are very sensitive to heat, becoming active and moving towards the source of heat, so long as the temperature is not above 38° C. On the other hand fed larvæ do not exhibit this sensibility to heat, and Roubaud thinks that it is by means of this thermotropism that the larvæ in the soil are guided to their host. *C. chærophaga* and *C. boueti*, on the other hand, are not dependent upon man, and live in the burrows of the wart-hog and ant-bear, emerging only at night.

B. *Larvæ deposited in natural cavities of the body* (p. 217).

Kimball (1893) in America reported the following very interesting cases of myiasis of the nose: "Case I. Private J. J. S., 18th Infantry; complained of pain in the forehead and orbits, anoexia and fever. His temperature taken under the tongue was 102·4° F. He was admitted to the hospital, and given the usual treatment for fever patients, but the following morning he was much worse. During the night he had been delirious and sleepless at times, constantly tossing about and trying to get out of bed. He complained of intense throbbing pain at the root of the nose and over the frontal region. The nose and lower eyelids were red and swollen. There was a discharge of bloody serum from the left nostril with an offensive odor. Chloroform was given by inhalation, and all the larvæ that could be seen, about 15 to 20 of them, were removed with a slender forceps, and then one drachm of carbolized oil was injected into the nostrils. The patient expressed great relief, but from time to time maggots were ejected in the act of sneezing or in blowing the nose. On September 21st the condition of the patient was worse than ever. Both eyes were closed by the swelling. Unremitting pain and sleeplessness were most distressing. Maggots escaped not only from the nose, but from the mouth as well when in the act of coughing. The fetor of the breath was extremely offensive. The velum palatinum was swollen to such an extent that deglutition was prevented. An injection was given of two drachms of chloroform (pure). The pain produced by the injection was allayed by injecting carbolized oil, and the nostrils were washed out by means of a post-pharyngeal syringe with a 10 volume solution of hydrogen dioxide. The effect was immediate and encouraging. Not less than a 100 dead larvæ were expelled, partly by syringing, partly by sneezing, by forcibly blowing the nose, and by coughing out those which came down through the posterior nares on to the pharynx. On September 23rd live maggots were again seen on looking into the left nostril, and the injection of chloroform was repeated for the third and last time. A score or more of dead larvæ were gotten rid of on this occasion. In all not less than 300 maggots were ejected.

"History. The patient said he had had a catarrh since last winter, and that for several months past the discharge had been offensive. The history he gave of the present illness was that in the afternoon of September 16th, about 36 hours before he had applied for medical aid, while asleep on a bench in the barracks he was awakened by a tickling sensation in the nose, which he thought was produced by a comrade with a straw. This, in all probability, was the time when the eggs or the larvæ were deposited by a fly within his nostril. The infection in this case was proved to be caused by the sarcophaga."

Kimball gathered on reliable information records of seven other cases of myiasis of the nose in the neighbourhood of Fort Clark. All but one of these proved fatal.

Wohl (1913) has collected the published reports of myiasis due to sarcophagid larvæ. Unfortunately in many of these cases very meagre details are given. Schnee (1853) extracted these maggots from an abscess of the nose, Kuznezo (1893) found them in the nose of a patient, who complained of itching and pain, du Salle (1857) extracted them through the nose from the frontal sinuses of a child, and Grube (1853) records destruction of the eye by these maggots in two boys.

Rieley and Howlett (1914) describe a form of nasal myiasis in Behar apparently due to the larvæ of a fly, which they describe under the name of *Pycnosoma flaviceps*. The larvæ are deposited on the mucous membrane of the nose, and burrow through it, feeding on the underlying structures and causing great destruction of the tissues, accompanied by severe constitutional symptoms. There is œdema of the upper part of the face, intense pain in the affected parts, severe frontal headache, and a rise of temperature up to 103° F. The mucous membrane of the nose is congested, swollen and ulcerated, and from the ulcers deep sinuses lead into the tissues. A blood-stained foul smelling nasal discharge is usually present. The larvæ may find their way into the frontal sinuses, and occasionally penetrate into the skull. Sometimes they emerge through the conjunctiva. Wohl (1913) cites cases in which the larvæ of *Sarcophaga* were found by Taschenberg (1870), Blake (1872) and Johnson (1892) in the middle ear, causing considerable destruction of tissue.

The Sergents (1913) report that on the Ahaggar Mountains, in Central Sahara, *Oestrus ovis* deposits eggs on the conjunctiva and the nasal mucous membrane of human beings, as it does in Algeria. Portchinsky (1913) also records some cases of human conjunctival infection with the larvæ of this fly.

C. *Larvæ deposited in wounds.*

de Moura (1913) has described a case of myiasis due to the larvæ of *M. putrida*, L. in an ulcerating cancer of the breast, and Neiva and de Faria (1913) in Brazil found the larvæ of *Sarcophaga pyophila* n. sp. in a suppurating wound of the parietal region.

D. *Subcutaneous myiasis.*

Tumbu-fly disease (p. 219).

Rodhain, Pons, Vandenbranden and Bequaert (1913) have shown by experiment that the larvæ of *Cordylobia anthropophaga*, immediately after emerging from the eggs, can penetrate the skin by the aid of their buccal hooks. In one experiment a larva took six hours to pass completely under the skin, the penetration being accompanied by slight pricking and itching sensations. Experiments on dogs and monkeys resulted in infection. The authors are of opinion, however, that the flies rarely lay their eggs directly on the skin, but usually deposit them on fæcal material on the ground, and the larvæ reach the parts which come into direct contact with the ground. Occasionally the eggs may be laid on clothing, which exhales the odour of sweat. Besides human beings, goats, rabbits, dogs and cats may be attacked, and in these animals the larvæ show a marked preference for the skin of the scrotum.

Heckenroth and Blanchard (1913) record four cases of cutaneous myiasis in French Equatorial Africa probably due to the larvæ of *Cordylobia rodhaini*, Gedoelst.

Dermatobia cyaniventris.

Surcouf (1913) has recently published one of the most interesting and important papers relating to the subject of myiasis. After pointing out that we are still ignorant as to how the larvæ of *Dermatobia cyaniventris* reach the host, he describes some interesting observations made by a number of different observers. As far back as 1900 Blanchard noticed packets of eggs attached to the abdomens of mosquitoes. Morales (1910) of Costa Rica believed that *D. cyaniventris* laid its eggs directly on the abdomens of mosquitoes in Central America, and that the larvæ were transmitted by the mosquitoes. Surcouf considers that it is unlikely that a large fly should lay its eggs on a mosquito. Rincones of Caracas thinks the eggs are deposited on wet leaves in damp situations frequented by the mosquito, *Janthinosoma lutzi*, to which they stick. The packets of eggs are enclosed in a strongly adherent cement substance, which becomes soft and sticky when placed in water. If such a packet comes into contact with a mosquito it sticks to it, and in a short time the larvæ hatch out. Surcouf thinks that these larvæ enter the skin through the punctures made by the mosquito. Tovar of Maturin, Venezuela, placed mosquitoes carrying eggs on animals, which soon developed subcutaneous tumours. When excised after 11 days larvæ were found in the tumours, and from one of these larvæ a specimen of *D. cyaniventris* emerged.

Surcouf's observations are corroborated by Zepeda (1913) who noticed white masses of eggs attached to mosquitoes in Nicaragua. In subjects bitten by such mosquitoes characteristic tumours occurred from which the larvæ of *D. cyaniventris* were extracted. In one instance the appearance of the tumour differed, and a larva of *C. macellaria* was extracted from it. Zepeda thinks that the eggs become attached to the mosquitoes when they settle on rotting bananas and other putrefying substances. Knab (1913) doubts Surcouf's explanation of the manner in which the eggs become attached to the mosquitoes, pointing out that the *Janthinosoma* rests with her body well elevated on her legs, and that the eggs are attached in a definite way with the ends from which the larvæ emerge downwards. He thinks that the eggs are not scattered promiscuously, but that the *Dermatobia* captures the mosquito and attaches the eggs to her.

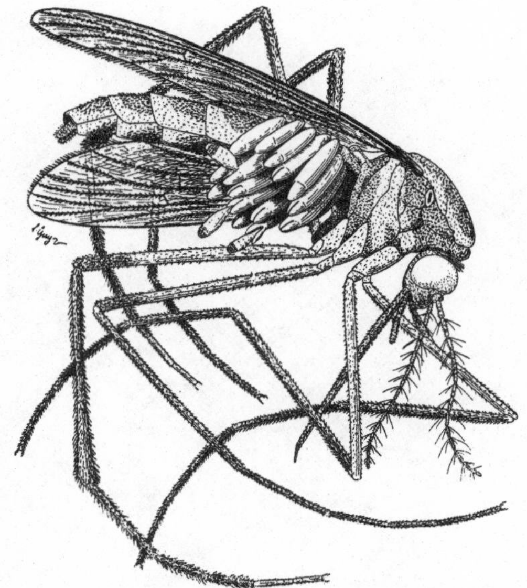

Fig. 1. *Janthinosoma lutzi* ♀ carrying the eggs of *Dermatobia cyaniventris* Macquart (×8). From Surcouf

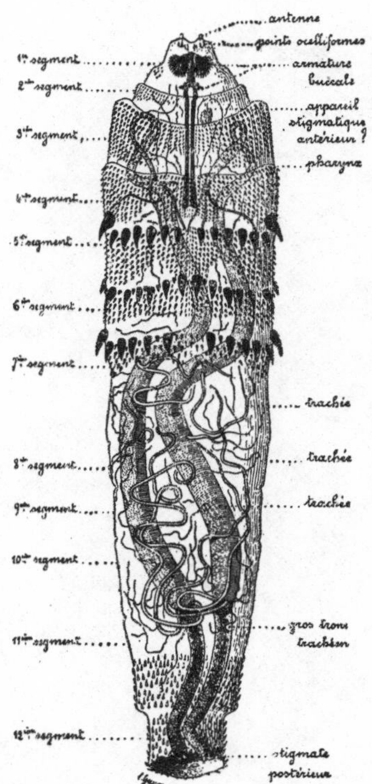

Fig. 2. A larva of *Dermatobia* in an egg carried by *Janthinosoma lutzi* Théobald (×100). From Surcouf.

Hypoderma.

Two cases of cutaneous myiasis due to the larvæ of *Hypoderma bovis* have been described recently. In a case described by Francaviglia (1912) larvæ were found in swellings in the parietal region and sternum of a child, and Balzer, Dantin and Landesmann (1913) obtained larvæ from swellings on the temporal region, shoulder and hip of a girl.

Grünberg (1913) found a larva, belonging to a fly of the genus *Hypoderma*, in the anterior chamber of the eye of a girl. The presence of larval insects in the human eye has been recorded on four occasions. Up to the present about 13 cases of infection in human beings with the larvæ of *H. bovis* have been recorded in Europe.

E. *Intestinal myiasis* (p. 226).

Jones (1913) obtained about 30 living larvæ of *M. domestica* from the stomach of a patient suffering from an hepatic abscess. Another patient, treated by him for irregular attacks of abdominal pain, passed dead larvæ of the house-fly in the stools. Hall and Muir (1913) describe the case of a boy who suffered for ten weeks from indigestion and constipation, and eventually passed an *Eristalis* larva. At least twelve other cases of infection in man with *Eristalis* larvæ have been recorded. Wohl (1913) in Philadelphia records the case of a young man, who was seized with abdominal pain followed by diarrhœa, the motions containing a dozen small larvæ. From these larvæ fed on meat, flies (*Sarcophaga sarraciniæ*, Riley) were reared.

Empusa disease (p. 229).

Gūssow (1913) points out the difficulty of spreading Empusa disease amongst flies by liberating naturally infected individuals, since it is difficult to ascertain whether the latter are really infected, while they are still active. Moreover the disease only occurs in the autumn and there is no record of its causing a virulent epidemic amongst flies at any other time of the year. " In comparison with the enormous masses of flies that may be noticed in a stable, for instance, even as late as October, all of which disappear when the cold weather sets in, comparatively few *Empusa*-infected flies are usually to be found in such places. It is possible that a large number may become infected and die out of doors, but though a considerable number of dead bodies of flies may be discovered lying on the ground, it is a recognized fact that the *Empusa*-infected fly is invariably firmly attached to various substrata in a life-like posture and surrounded by a white halo of spores. It is reasonable to suppose that, if the disease were of an epidemic nature, one should discover far more flies killed by it than is usually the case." He suggests that "it is not unlikely that the fly becomes more susceptible to this disease as it grows older, while newly emerged broods are more or less resistant."

Gūssow has devoted much attention to the life-history of this fungus, and the artificial germination of the spores, but has never succeeded in carrying cultures from spore to spore outside the body of the fly.

Experiments on infecting flies with spores contained in water painted on the abdomen and other parts of the bodies of flies have invariably proved successful. He found also that flies could be infected by being brought into contact with dead flies covered with spores.

After the Empusa began to show externally Gūssow was able to observe the discharge of the spores. "While the flies were still fresh the spore-discharge was easily observed under the microscope, the spores, in a dry atmosphere, being discharged very rapidly and disappearing entirely from the field of vision. In a moist chamber (covered with moist blotting paper) the discharge of the spores continued for four days, as shown by microscopic slides placed in various positions near the body of the fly. The spores were discharged in every direction, but particularly towards either side. This is natural as the conidiophores are specially abundant on the abdomen. We observed spores shot away some seven centimetres from the body."

Gūssow was unable to induce germination of the spores on any medium, 'standard,' 'special' or prepared from extracts of flies. Germination, however, occurred rapidly on slides, but the growth could not be continued. He has been unable to verify Hesse's claims (p. 232), and concludes his paper in the following words: "It is very doubtful whether any practical and economic use of this fungus can be made before the whole life-history is known, and notwithstanding repeated researches, no investigator would seem, thus far, to have made any important addition to our knowledge since the publication of Brefeld's work on the subject."

An interesting photograph accompanies this paper showing numerous proboscis marks on a deposit of empusa spores. This possible mode of infection has not been previously recorded.

Buchanan (1913), in a paper illustrated by numerous excellent photographs of the growth of empusa in the body of the fly, shows that bacteria present on the surface of the flies may be carried on the discharged spores. "A diseased fly was fixed head downwards upon nutritive agar in the centre of a Petri plate. In the course of a few days a zone of colonies appeared around the fly within the area bestrewn by the conidia." Most of the colonies in the experiments proved to be due to organisms of the colon group.

It is very improbable that this potential means of spreading bacterial infection is an important one.

(A.) *External parasites of adult flies. Mites* (p. 233).

Under the name of *Macrocheles muscæ* Ewing (1913) has described a new parasite of the house-fly from New York and Oregon. The female of this mite attaches itself by its cheliceræ to the ventral body wall of the fly, with its anterior end towards the head of the fly.

(B.) *Internal parasites of adult flies.* (1) *Flagellates* (p. 236).

Chatton (1912, A) has found numerous specimens of *Leptomonas legerorum* in *Sphærocera subsultans*, and another species in *Limosina thalammeri*. He has also described a species, *L. roubaudi*, from the malpighian tubules of *P. confusa*.

Chatton and Leger (1913) also announce the finding of *Trypanosoma muscæ domesticæ* in the malpighian tubules of house-flies in Corsica.

The relationship of the various flagellates found in flies to each other and to their hosts has been much discussed recently. The subject is of great interest, but is beyond the scope of this work, and readers who are interested are referred to the papers of Alexeieff (1912, 1913), Cardamatis (1912), Chatton (1912, 1913, A, B, C), Hindle (1912), Patton (1912), Prowazek (1913), Sinton (1912), and Wenyon (1913).

Dunkerly (1912) once found a *Prowazekia* (sp. ?) in the rectum of *F. canicularis.*

(c) *Microsporidia.*

Flu (1911) has published a description of a microsporidian parasite, which he named *Octosporea muscæ domesticæ*, found in house-flies, and Chatton and Krempf (1912) have discovered a similar parasite in *D. confusa.* Dunkerly (1912) has also noticed the spores of a microsporidian, *Thelohania ovata*, in the rectum of a single specimen of *F. scalaris.* Cardamatis (1912, B) found stages of a microsporidian in the intestines of flies allowed to feed on material obtained from an oriental sore. At present the significance of these discoveries is unknown.

(2) *Nematoda. Habronema muscæ.*

Johnston (1913) has recently found the larval form of this parasite in *Stomoxys calcitrans* and *M. domestica* in Sydney and Brisbane, Australia. The larval form does not seem to have been previously recorded from Australia.

C. *Parasites of the larvæ* (p. 242).

Richardson (1913) described a pteromalid parasite, *Spalangia muscidarum*, which he reared from the pupæ of *M. domestica* and *S. calcitrans* in Texas. Pinkus (1913) reared the same parasite from the pupæ of house-flies near Boston and Washington, and from those of *Stomoxys* in Texas, Kansas and Louisiana.

This parasite seems to have a wide distribution, and Pinkus found that it would readily oviposit in many species of dipterous pupæ. He observed that the period of development varied with the host, and with the temperature. At a temperature of 56–58° F. 84 days were required for development in *Stomoxys*, 100 days in *Lyperosia irritans*, and 106 in *Musca domestica*. The parasites can be bred artificially with ease, and the period of emergence can be retarded by keeping the infected pupæ at 50–55° F. Pinkus therefore thinks that it could be made use of in destroying flies, especially *Stomoxys*, by liberating specimens near places where the stable-fly is known to be breeding.

Enemies of flies (p. 245).

Adult flies. (*a*) *Invertebrate enemies.*

Hewitt (1914) states that in Canada the yellow dung-fly (*Scatophaga stercoraria*, see p. 37) destroys numerous other diptera, especially muscid flies. It has been seen capturing *M. domestica*, *C. erythrocephala*, *S. calcitrans*, *F. canicularis*, *P. rudis* and others. The preference of *Scatophaga* for muscid flies is noticeable.

Larvæ.

Portchinsky (1913) in Russia describes his studies on the relationship of the dung-feeding larvæ of *Hydrotæa dentipes*, an Anthomyid fly, to those of *M. domestica*. The former rapidly destroy the larvæ of *M. domestica*, *S. calcitrans* and *L. cæsar*. "The importance of *H. dentipes* as destroyers of the larvæ of *M. domestica* and of *S. calcitrans* is very great; and they also present the following advantageous characteristics; they are very fertile, laying 170–200 eggs, maturing at about the same time; their larvæ can travel very rapidly, and whether living in large companies, or single (when grown up), never eat each other, even when hungry; the larvæ are omnivorous feeders and will live on all materials serving as breeding-places for the larvæ of *M. domestica*; the flies do not trouble men and never visit human dwellings; and they can be readily reared in captivity."

Measures against adult flies (p. 249).

Some diversity of opinion seems to exist in regard to the degree of success which can be attained by the use of formalin for killing adult flies (p. 250). While some have found the method efficacious, others have found it useless. Houston (1913) who found it useless to expose formalin in shallow dishes, sprinkled a mixture of formalin, milk and water about rooms. The flies readily drank from the tiny pools, and the method proved highly successful in the jail kitchen at Rajkot.

Berlese (1913) found it necessary to take special measures against house-flies at S. Vincenzo in Italy. He found that many of the flies left the house during part of the day, and rested on the under surfaces of leaves near the house. In order to destroy the flies outside and their larvæ he prepared a mixture of 10 parts of treacle, 2 parts of arsenite of potash and 100 parts of water, and sprayed all rubbish and manure heaps in the neighbourhood as well as the trees, taking special care that the solution reached the under sides of the leaves. The operation was performed every ten days, and after rain. He also caused a number of cylindrical metal dust-bins to be distributed about the village, so placed as to be out of reach of the children, and the surfaces of these were regularly sprayed. By these measures Berlese " succeeded in each of two years in almost totally destroying the flies in the village during the period of his residence. Three days after the commencement of operations the reduction was so great that instead of having his meals interrupted and even prevented by veritable clouds of flies they were reduced to two or three, and the same occurred in other houses in the village. It is suggested that if the method were systematized, it would be possible to adopt it as a thoroughly practical means of ridding even large places of the pest."

BIBLIOGRAPHY

The names of the authors quoted in this book are arranged in alphabetical order, and for the convenience of those who wish to refer to the literature relating to special aspects of the subject, the aspect chiefly dealt with in each paper is indicated by a letter in dark type placed at the end of the reference. **A** = anatomy of insects, **B** = bacteriology, **D** = descriptions of insects, **E** = epidemiology, **G** = general remarks, **L** = life-history, **M** = myiasis, **O** = parasitic ova, **P** = parasites or diseases of flies, **S** = sanitary preventive measures.

Ainsworth, R. B. (v. 1909). The house-fly as a disease carrier. *Journ. Roy. Army Med. Corps*, XII. 485–498. **E.S.**

Albert, H. (1905). Rôle of insects in transmission of disease. *New York Med. Journ.*, LXXXI. 220–225. **G.**

Alcock, A. (1911). *Entomology for Medical Officers.* Gurney and Jackson, London. **G.**

Aldridge, A. R. (1904). The spread of the infection of enteric fever by flies. *Journ. Roy. Army Med. Corps*, III. 649–651. **E.S.**

—— (1907). House-flies as Carriers of Enteric Fever Infection. *Journ. Roy. Army Med. Corps*, IX. 558–571. **E.**

Alessandrini, G. and Sampietro, G. (1912). Sulla Vitalità del Vibrione Colerigeno nel Latte e nelle Mosche. *Ann. d' Igiene Sperimentale*, XXII. pp. 623–650. **B.**

Alessi (1888). *Arch. per le Scienze med.*, XII. 279. (Quoted by Celli, 1888.)

Alexander, D. M. (1912). Report on the Prevalence and Characters of Non-lactose Fermenting and Non-liquefying Ærobic Bacilli in the Fæces of Young Children under normal Conditions and in Epidemic Diarrhœa during 1911. *41st Ann. Report of the Local Government Board, Supplement containing the Report of the Medical Officer for* 1911–12, App. B, 288–303. **B.**

—— (1913). Report on the Prevalence and Characters of Bacilli occurring in the Fæces of Young Children under Normal Conditions and in Epidemic Diarrhœa during 1912. *42nd Ann. Report of the Local Government Board, Supplement containing the Report of the Medical Officer for* 1912–13, App. B, 384–400. **B.**

Alexeieff, A. (1912). Sur la Revision du Genre *Bodo*, Ehrbg. *Arch. f. Protistenk.*, XXVI. 413, 419. **P.**

Alexeieff, A. (1913). Introduction à la Revision de la Famille *Herpetomonadidæ* (= *Trypanosomidæ* Dofflein, 1911). *Arch. f. Protistenk.*, XXIX. 313–441. **P.**

Allen, S. G. (1907). The "allies" of enteric fever in India. *Journ. Roy. Army Med. Corps*, VIII. 44–49. **E.**

Anderson (1908). The differentiation of outbreaks of typhoid fever due to infection by water, milk, flies and contacts. *New York Med. Record*, LXXIV. No. 22. **G.**

André (1908). *6th Internat. Cong. on Tuberc., Wash.*, I. 162. (Quoted by Chapin, 1912, p. 422.) **B.**

Andrewes, F. W. Quoted by Austen, 1912, 13. **M.**

Anthony (1874). The suctorial organs of the blow-fly. *Monthly Micros. Journ.*, XI. p. 242. **A.**

Armstrong, D. B. (17. I. 1914). The House-Fly and Diarrhœal Disease among Children. *Journ. Amer. Med. Assoc.*, LXII. 200, 201. **E.**

Armstrong, H. E. (1908). House-Flies and Disease: the Duty of Sanitary Authorities in relation thereto. *San. Rec. London*, N.S. XLII. 542–545. **G.S.**

Arnold, B. M. (1906). See "Report on the Health of the City of Manchester for 1906" by J. Niven.

Austen, E. E. (VI. 1904). The house-fly and certain allied species as disseminators of enteric fever among troops in the field. *Journ. of Roy. Army Med. Corps*, II. 651–668. **D.E.**

—— (1906). Synonymic notes on *Musca marginalis*, Wied., and the Genus, *Pycnosoma*, Br. and von Berg. *Ann. and Mag. Nat. Hist.*, Series VII, XVII. 301. **D.**

—— (1907). *Proc. Entomol. Soc. of London*, XLIII.–XLVII. **D.**

—— (1908). The Tumbu-fly (*Cordylobia anthropophaga*, Grünberg). *Journ. Roy. Army Med. Corps*, X. 18–24. **D.**

—— (1909, A). Notes on the Examination of Batches of Flies received from various centres in London during the Summer and Autumn of 1908. *Reports to the Local Government Board on Public Health and Medical Subjects*, New Series, No. 5, 4. **D.**

—— (1909, B). Blood-sucking and other Flies known or likely to be concerned in the Spread of Disease. *A System of Medicine*, Allbutt, C. and Rolleston, H. D., vol. II. pt. 2, 169–186. **G.**

—— (1910, A). A new Indian Species of Musca. *Ann. and Mag. Nat. Hist.*, Series VIII, V. 114–116. **D.**

—— (1910, B). Some Dipterous Insects which cause Myiasis in Man. *Trans. Soc. Trop. Med. and Hygiene*, III. 215–242. **M.**

—— (1910, C). A new species of Cordylobia, a genus of African diptera (Family Tachinidæ, subfamily Calliphorinæ), the larvæ of which are subcutaneous parasites in man and other mammals. *Bull. Entomol. Research*, I. 79–81. **M.**

—— (1911). Memorandum on the Result of Examinations of Flies, etc., from Postwick Village and refuse deposit; with a note on the occurrence of the Lesser House Fly at Leeds. *Reports to the Local*

Govern. Board on Public Health and Medical Subjects, New Series, No. 53, 11–12. **G.**

Austen, E. E. (1912). British Flies which cause Myiasis in Man. *Reports to the Local Government Board on Public Health and Medical Subjects*, New Series, No. 66, 5–15. **M.**

Bachmann (1898). Ein Fall von lebenden Fliegen-larven im menschlichen Magen. *Deutsche med. Wochenschr.*, XXIV. 193–194. **M.**

Bacot, A. W. (1911). The persistence of *Bacillus pyocyaneus* in pupæ and imagines of *Musca domestica* raised from larvæ experimentally infected with the bacillus. *Parasitology*, IV. 68–74. **B.**

Bahr, P. H. (1912). Dysentery in Fiji during the year 1910. *Journ. London School Trop. Med.*, Suppl. No. 2. **B.**

—— (1914). A study of Epidemic Dysentery in the Fiji Islands. *Brit. Med. Journ.*, I. pp. 294–296. **B.**

Ballard, E. (1889). Diarrhœa and Diphtheria. *Suppl. Report Med. Officer of Local Government Board* (1887).

Balzer, F., Dantin and Landesmann. Un Cas de Myiase rampante due à l'*Hypoderma bovis*. *Bull. Soc. Française de Dermatol. et de Syphiligraphie*, XXIV. 219–226. (Review in *Trop. Dis. Bull.*, II. p. 526.) **M.**

Bancroft. E. (1769). *An essay on the Natural History of Guiana in South America.* London, 385–386. (Quoted by Howard, 1911, 166.) **M.**

Banks, N. (1912). The Structure of Certain Dipterous Larvæ with Particular Reference to those found in Human Foods. *U.S. Dept. of Agricult. Bureau of Entomology*, Technical Series, No. 22. **L.**

Barrows, W. M. (1907). The reactions of the Pomace Fly (*Drosophila ampelophila* Loew) to odorous substances. *Journ. Exp. Zool.*, IV. 515–537. **L.**

Berlese, A. (1913). La distruzione della Mosca domestica. '*Redia,*' VIII. 462–472. (Rev. in *Review of Applied Entom.*, I. B., 68.) **S.**

Bernstein, J. (1910). Summary of Literature relating to the Bionomics of the Parasitic Fungus of Flies, *Empusa muscæ* (Cohn), with Special Reference to the Economic Aspect. *Reports to the Local Government Board on Public Health and Medical Subjects*, New Series, No. 40, 41–45. **P.**

Berry (1892). Conjunctivitis set up by Flies. *Brit. Med. Journ.*, II. 1114. **E.**

Bertarelli, E. (1910). Verbreitung des Typhus durch die Fliegen. Fliegen als Trägerinnen spezifischer Bacillen in den Häusern von Typhuskranken. *Central. f. Bakt.*, Abt. Orig., LIII. 486–495. **B.**

Beyer, H. G. (1910). The dissemination of disease by the fly. *New York Med. Journ.*, XCI. 677–685. **G.**

Bigot, J. M. F. (1887). Diptères nouveaux ou peu connus. *Bull. Soc. Zool.*, France, XII. 581–617. (Quoted by Hewitt, 1909.)

Billings (1898). *Twentieth Century Practice of Medicine*, XV. (Cited by Dickinson, 1907.) **B.**

Blake (1872). *Arch. for Ophthalmology and Otology*, II. (Cited by Wohl, 1913.) **M.**

Blanchard, R. (1896). Contributions à l'étude des Diptères parasites (1). *Ann. Soc. Entom. de France*, LXV. 641–683. **M.**

Blankmeyer, H. C. (1907). Infection with fly-larvæ, *Anthomyia canicularis*. *Journ. Amer. Med. Assoc.*, XLVIII. 1505. **M.**

Blenkinsop, A. P. (1908). Observations on Tumbu-fly disease. *Journ. Roy. Army Med. Corps*, X. 16, 17. **M.**

Brefeld, O. (1873). Untersuchungen über die Entwickelung der *E. muscæ* und *E. radicans*. *Abh. d. Naturf. Gesellsch.*, XII. 1–50. **P.**

Bruce, David (XII. 1895). Tsetse-Fly Disease or Nagana in Zululand. Preliminary Report (Bennett and Davis, Field Street, Durban).

Buchanan, R. M. (27. VII. 1907). The carriage of infection by flies. *Lancet*, II. 216–218. **B.**

—— (22. XI. 1913). *Empusa muscæ* as a carrier of bacterial infection from the house-fly. *Brit. Med. Journ.*, II. 1369–1372. **P.**

Buchanan, W. T. (1897). Cholera diffusion and flies. *Indian Med. Gazette*, 86–97. **E.**

Budd, W. (1862). Observations in the Occurrence (hitherto unnoticed) of Malignant Pustule in England. *Lancet*, II. 164–165. **G.**

Calandruccio, S. (1906). Ulteriori ricerche sulla *Tænia nana*. *Boll. Accad. Gioenia, Catania*, LXXXIX. 15–19. (Quoted by Nicoll, 1911.) **M.**

Cameron, J. S. (1914). House-flies. *Journ. Roy. San. Inst.*, XXXV. 172–181. **G.**

Cardamatis, J. P. (1912, A). Des Flagellaires dans la Mouche Domestique. Identité de la Leptomonade et de l'Herpétomonade. Nouveau Mode de Multiplication de l'Herpétomonade de la *Musca domestica*. *Centralbl. f. Bakt.*, Orig. LXV. 66–76. **M.**

—— (1912, B). De quelques Microsporidies chez la Mouche Domestique. *Centralbl. f. Bakt.*, Orig. LXV. 77–79. **M.**

Carpenter, G. H. (1902). Insects infesting domestic animals. *Econ. Proc. R. Dublin Soc.*, I. 132. (Quoted by Froggatt, 1913.) **M.**

Carter, H. J. (1861). On a bi-sexual nematoid worm which infects the common house-fly (*Musca domestica*) in Bombay. *Ann. Mag. Nat. Hist.*, Ser. III, VII. 29–33. **P.**

Carter, H. F. and Blacklock, B. (I. 1913). External myiasis in the monkey. *Brit. Med. Journ.*, I. 72. **M.**

Castellani, A. (1907). Experimental investigations on *Frambœsia tropica* (Yaws). *Journ. Hygiene*, VII. 558–569. **B.**

Cattle, C. H. (VII. 1906). A case in which large quantities of Dipterous Larvæ were passed *per anum*. *Brit. Med. Journ.*, II. 77. **M.**

Celli, A. (1888). Trasmissibilità dei germi patogeni mediante le dejecione delle mosche. *Bull. d. Soc. Lancisiana d. ospedali di Roma*, I. 1. (Quoted by Nuttall and Jepson, 1909, 27.) **O.**

Chantèmesse, A. and Borel, F. (1906). *Mouches et choléra*, Baillière et Fils. **B.**

Chapin, C. V. (1912). *The Sources and Modes of Infection*, 2nd ed. John Wiley and Sons, New York. **G.**

Chatton, E. (1909). Sur un trypanosomide nouveau d'une Nyctéribie, et sur les relations des formes *Trypanosoma, Herpetomonas, Leptomonas* et *Crithidia*. *Compt. Rend. Soc. Biol.*, LXVII. 42. **P.**

—— (1912, A). *Leptomonas* de deux *Borborinæ* (Muscides). Evolution de *L. Legerorum*, n. sp. *Compt. Rend. Soc. Biol.*, LXXIII. 286–289. **P.**

—— (1912, B). *Leptomonas Roubaudi*, n. sp., Parasite des Tubes de Malpighi de *Drosophila confusa* Staeger. *Compt. Rend. Soc. Biol.*, LXXIII. 289–291. **P.**

—— (1913, A). Position Systématique et Signification Phylogénique des Trypanosomes Malpighiens des Muscides. Le Genre *Rhynchoidomonas* Patton. *Compt. Rend. Soc. Biol.*, LXXIV. 551–553. **P.**

—— (1913, B). L'Ordre, la Succession et l'Importance Relative des Stades, dans l'Evolution des Trypanosomides, chez les Insectes. *Compt. Rend. Soc. Biol.*, LXXIV. 1145–1147. **P.**

Chatton, E. and Alilaire, E. (1908). Co-existence d'un *Leptomonas* (*Herpetomonas*) et d'un *Trypanosoma* chez un muscide non vulnérant, *Drosophila confusa*, Staeger. *Compt. Rend. Soc. Biol.*, LXIV. 1004. **P.**

Chatton and Krempf (1911). *Bull. de la Soc. Zool. de France*, XXXVI. 172–179. (Cited by Dunkerly, 1912.) **P.**

Chatton, E. and Leger, M. (1913). L'Autonomie des Trypanosomes propres aux Muscides démontrée par les Elevages purs Indéfinis. *Compt. Rend. Soc. Biol.*, LXXIV. 549–551. **P.**

Chevrel, R. (1909). Sur la myiase des voies urinaires. *Arch. de Parasitol.*, XII. 369–450. **M.**

Cobb, J. O. (25. III. 1905). Is the common house-fly a factor in the spread of tuberculosis? *American Medicine*, IX. 475–477. **B.**

Cobbett, L. (1907). *Royal Commission on Tuberculosis*. Second Interim Report, 1028. **B.**

Cochrane, E. W. W. (1912). A small epidemic of typhoid fever in connection with specifically infected flies. *Journ. Roy. Army Med. Corps*, XVIII. 271–276. **B.E.**

Cohn, F. (1855). *E. muscæ und die Krankheit der Stubenfliegen. Ein Beitrag zur Lehre von den durch parasitische Pilze characterisirten Epidemieen.* Breslau. **P.**

Copeman, S. M. (1906). Report to the Local Government Board on the General Sanitary circumstances and administration of the County Borough of Wigan, with especial reference to Infantile Mortality and to endemic prevalence of Enteric Fever and Diarrhœa. 18. **E.**

—— (1909). Memorandum by Dr Copeman on Investigation into Possible Carriage of Infection by Flies. Suggested "Plan of Campaign" in Urban Districts. *Reports to the Local Government*

Board on Public Health and Medical Subjects, New Series, No. 16, 1–4. **G.**

Copeman, S. M. (1910). Note as to work in hand, but not yet published; and as to proposed further work in reference to Flies as Carriers of Infection. *Reports to the Local Government Board on Public Health and Medical Subjects*, New Series, No. 40, 45–48. **G.**

—— (1913). Hibernation of house-flies. *Reports to the Local Government Board on Public Health and Medical Subjects*, New Series, No. 85, 14–19. **L.**

Copeman, S. M., Howlett, F. M., and Merriman, G. (1911). An Experimental Investigation on the Range of Flight of Flies. *Reports to the Local Government Board on Public Health and Medical Subjects*, New Series, No. 53, 1–9. **G.**

Coplin, W. M. L. (10. VI. 1899). The Propagation of Diseases by means of Insects, with special consideration of the common domestic types. *Philadelphia Med. Journ.* **G.**

Cordes, L. (1903). Results of the examination of 51 cases of gastro-intestinal disturbance in infants. *Proc. New York Path. Soc.*, N.S. III. 147. **B.**

Corkery, M. P. (XII. 1909). Enteric fever in India—a probable factor. *Journ. Roy. Army Med. Corps*, XIII. 687–689. **B.**

Cox, G. L., Lewis, F. C. and Glynn, E. E. (1912). The numbers and varieties of bacteria carried by the common house-fly in sanitary and insanitary city areas. *Journ. of Hygiene*, XII. 290–319. **B.**

Craig, C. F. (1899). The rôle of insects in the propagation of disease. *Philadelphia Med. Journ.*, III. 1381. **G.**

Daniels, C. W. (1904). Observations on the Diseases of British Malaya. *Studies from the Institute for Medical Research, Federated Malay States*, III. p. 56. **B.**

Darling, S. T. (1912). Experimental infection of the mule with *Trypanosoma hippicum* by means of *Musca domestica*. *Journ. Exp. Med.*, XV. 365–366. **B.**

—— (1913, A). The part played by flies and other insects in the spread of infectious diseases in the tropics, with special reference to ants and to the transmission of *Tr. hippicum* by *Musca domestica*. *Trans.* XV*th Internat. Congr. Hyg. and Demog., Washington.* **B.**

—— (1913, B). The immunization of large animals to a pathogenic trypanosome (*Trypanosoma hippicum* Darling) by means of an avirulent strain. *Journ. Exp. Med.*, XVII. 582–586. **B.**

Davaine, C. (1870). Études sur la contagion du charbon chez les animaux domestiques. *Bull. de l'acad. de Méd.*, Paris, XXXV. 215–235. **B.**

Deaderick, W. H. (XI. 1908). Notes on Intestinal Myiasis. *Arch. f. Schiffs- und Tropen-Hygiene*, XII. 726–729. **M.**

de Moura, C. (1913). Myiase do Seio. *Revista Med. de S. Paula*, XVI. 1. (Rev. in *Trop. Dis. Bull.*, II. 530.) **M.**

Devecchi, B. and Randone, F. (1912). Alcane Osservazioni bacteriologiche e statische praticate durante l' epidemia Colerica nella provincia di Siracusa. *Pathologica*, p. 347. (Quoted by Greig, VII. 1913, B.) **B.**

Dickinson, G. K. (1907). The House-fly, and its Connection with Disease Dissemination. *Medical Record*, LXXI. 134–139. **G.**

Dixon, S. G. (1911). The Common Fly. *Pennsylvania Health Bull.*, No. 23. **G.**

Drew, H. V. (1906). A case of invasion by dipterous larvæ. *Brit. Med. Journ.*, II. 1066. **M.**

Dunkerly, T. S. (1911). On Some Stages in the Life-History of Leptomonas muscæ domesticæ, with some remarks on the Relationships of the Flagellate Parasites of Insects. *Quart. Journ. Microscop. Sci.*, LVI. 645–656. **P.**

—— (1912). On the occurrence of Thelohania and Prowazekia in Anthomyid flies. *Central. f. Bakt.*, Orig. LXII. 136–140. **P.**

Duprey, A. J. B. (1906). The Mosquito worms of Trinidad and their real nature. *Journ. of Trop. Med.*, IX. 22–23. **M.**

du Salle, M. L. (1857). *Compt. Rend. l'Acad. Sci.*, XLV. 600. (Cited by Wohl, 1913). **M.**

Dutton, J. E., Todd, J. A. and Christy, C. (IX. 1904). The Congo floor maggot. *Brit. Med. Journ.*, II. 664–666. Also in Reports of the Trypanosomiasis expedition to the Congo 1903–1904. *Liverpool School of Tropical Medicine*, Mem. XIII. 49–54. **M.**

Dutton, W. F. (1909). Blue-bottle flies as carriers of infection. *Journ. Amer. Med. Assoc.*, LIII. 1561. **B.**

Duval, C. W. and Schorer, E. H. (1903). Results of the examination of 79 cases of Summer Diarrhœa. *Proc. New York Path. Soc.*, N.S. III. 144–146. **B.**

Ebeling, E. (1913). Beobachtungen über die Y-Ruhr, gelegentlich einer Epidemie beim X. Armeekorps im Sommer 1911 und bei Nachuntersuchungen in den Jahren 1912 und 1913. *Zeitschr. f. Hyg. u. Infektionskrankh.*, LXXIV. p. 447. **B.**

Esten, U. N. and Mason, C. J. (1908). Sources of Bacteria in Milk. *Storrs. Agri. Exp. Sta. Bull.*, No. 51, 65–109. (Cited by Hermes, 1911, 527.) **B.**

Ewing, H. E. (1913). A New Parasite of the House-fly (Acarina, Gamasoidea). *Entom. News, Philadelphia*, XXIV. 452–456. (Rev. in *Review of Applied Entom.*, II. 6.) **P.**

Faichnie, N. (1909). Fly-borne enteric fever; the source of infection. *Journ. Roy. Army Med. Corps*, XIII. 580. **B.E.**

—— (1909). *Bacillus typhosus* in flies. *Journ. Roy. Army Med. Corps*, XIII. 672. **B.E.**

Farrar, R. (1905). Reports of Medical Inspectors of the Local Government Board. No. 216, 9. **E.G.**

Felt, E. P. (1910). Methods of controlling the house-fly and thus preventing the dissemination of disease. *New York Med. Journ.*, XCI. 685–687. **S.**

—— (1910). Observations on the House-fly. *Journ. of Economic Entomology*, III. 34. **G.**

Ficker, M. (1903). Typhus und Fliegen. *Arch. f. Hyg.*, XLVI. 274–283. **B.**

Field, F. E. (1913). Myiasis; with special reference to some varieties treated at the Georgetown Hospital. *Brit. Guiana Med. Ann.* for 1911, 60–64. **M.**

Firth, R. H. and Horrocks, W. H. (1902). An inquiry into the influence of soil, fabrics and flies in the dissemination of enteric infection. *Brit. Med. Journ.*, I. 936–943. **B.E.**

Flexner, S. (1912). The mode of infection in epidemic poliomyelitis. *Journ. Amer. Med. Assoc.*, LIX. 1371–1372. **B.**

Flexner, S. and Clark, P. F. (1911). Contamination of the fly with poliomyelitis virus. *Journ. Amer. Med. Assoc.*, LVI. 1717–1718. **B.**

Flu, P. C. (1911). Studien über die im Darm der Stubenfliege, *Musca domestica*, vorkommenden protozoären Gebilde. *Central. f. Bakt.*, LVII. 522–534. **P.**

Flügge, C. (1893). Die Verbreitungsweise und Verhütung der Cholera auf Grund der neueren epidemiologischen Erfahrungen und experimentellen Forschungen. *Zeitschr. f. Hygiene*, XIV. 122–202. **B.**

Forman, R. H. (1906). Indian enteric and latrines. *Journ. Roy. Army Med. Corps*, VII. 304–305. **G.**

Francaviglia, M. C. (1912). Altro Caso di Myiasis nell' Uomo per Larva cuticolare d' *Hypoderma bovis* (De Geer). *Policlinico*, XIX. 1593–1595. **M.**

Francis, C. F. (1893). Cholera caused by a Fly (?). *Brit. Med. Journ.*, II. 65. **B.**

Franklin, G. D. (1906). Some observations on the breeding grounds of the common house-fly. *Indian Med. Gaz.*, 349. **L.**

Fraser (1902). Epidemic diarrhœa in Portsmouth in relation to flies. (Quoted at length by Hewlett, 1905, p. 505.)

Froggatt, W. W. (1905). The Sheep Maggot Fly, with notes on other common flies. *Agricult. Gaz. of N.S. Wales.* Miscell. Public., No. 809. **M.**

—— (1911). The Nasal Fly of Sheep (*Œstrus ovis*) in Australia. *Agricult. Gaz. of N.S. Wales*, 223–227. **M.**

—— (1913). *The Sheep Maggot-Fly Pest in Australia.* Cooper Lab. for Economic Research, 10–48. **M.**

Fuller, C. (1901). *The Agricult. Journ. of Natal*, IV. 656–658. (Quoted by Theobald, 1906.) **M.**

Galli-Valerio, B. (1905). Notes de parasitologie et de technique parasitologique. *Centralbl. f. Bakt.*, Orig. XXXIX. 230–247. (Flies p. 242.) **B.**

Galli-Valerio, B. (1910). L'état actuel de nos connaissances sur le rôle des mouches dans la dissémination des maladies parasitaires et sur les moyens de lutte à employer contre elles. *Central. f. Bakt.*, Orig. LIV. 193–209. **B.**

Gann, T. W. F. (I. 1902). Beef worm in the orbital cavity. *Lancet*, I. 19–21. **M.**

Ganon (1908). (Cholera and Flies.) *Geneesk. Tijdschr. v. Nederl. Indie*, XLVIII. 2. (Quoted in *Journ. Trop. Med.*, 15. V. 1909.) **B.**

Garrood, J. R. (1910). Note on a case of intestinal myiasis. *Parasitology*, III. 315–318. **M.**

Gayon, J. P. (1903). A note concerning the transmission of Pathogenic Fungus by Flies and Mosquitoes. *Public Health*, XXVIII. 116–117. **P.**

Gedoelst, L. (1905). Contribution à l'étude des larves cuticoles de Muscides Africaines. *Arch. de Parasit.*, IX. 568–592. **M.**

Generali, G. (1886). Una larva di nematode della mosca commune. *Atti Soc. d. Nat. di Modena, Rendic.*, Ser. 3, II. 88–89. (Quoted by Hewitt, 1909.) **P.**

Giles, C. M. (1906). The anatomy of biting flies of the Genus Stomoxys and Glossina. *Journ. Trop. Med.*, IX. 99.

Gilruth, J. A. (1908). Bull. No. 12. *Dept. Agric. New Zealand.* **M.**

Girault, A. A. and Sanders, G. E. (1909). *Psyche*, 119–132. (Quoted by Howard, 1911, p. 90.)

Graham-Smith, G. S. (1909). Preliminary Note on Examination of Flies for the presence of Colon Bacilli. *Reports to the Local Government Board on Public Health and Medical Subjects*, New Series, No. 16, 9–13. **B.**

—— (1910). Observations on the Ways in which artificially infected Flies (*Musca domestica*) carry and distribute Pathogenic and other Bacteria. *Reports to the Local Government Board on Public Health and Medical Subjects*, New Series, No. 40, 1–40. **B.**

—— (1911). Further observations on the Ways in which artificially infected Flies (*Musca domestica* and *Calliphora erythrocephala*) carry and distribute Pathogenic and other Bacteria. *Reports to the Local Government Board on Public Health and Medical Subjects*, New Series, No. 53, 31–48. **B.**

—— (1912, A). Some observations on the anatomy and function of the oral sucker of the Blow-fly (*Calliphora erythrocephala*). *Journ. of Hygiene*, XI. 390–408. **A.**

—— (1912, B). An Investigation of the Incidence of the Micro-organisms known as Non-Lactose-Fermenters in Flies in Normal Surroundings and in Surroundings associated with Epidemic Diarrhœa. *41st Ann. Report of the Local Government Board, Supplement containing the Report of the Medical Officer for* 1911-12. App. B, 304–329. **B.**

—— (1912, C). An investigation into the Possibility of Pathogenic Micro-organisms being taken up by the Larva and subsequently distributed by the Fly. *41st Ann. Report of the Local Government*

Board, Supplement containing the Report of the Medical Officer for 1911–12. App. B, 330–335. **B.**

Graham-Smith, G. S. (1913). Further observations on Non-Lactose Fermenting Bacilli in Flies, and the Sources from which they are derived, with special reference to Morgan's Bacillus. *Reports to the Local Government Board on Public Health and Medical Subjects*, New Series, No. 85, 43–46. **B.**

Grassi, B. (1883). Les méfaits des mouches. *Arch. ital. de biol.*, IV. 205–208. (Quoted by Nicoll, 1911.) **O.**

Gratton, H. W. and Harvey, D. (1911). An inquiry into a small epidemic of paratyphoid fever in a Camp in India. *Journ. Roy. Army Med. Corps*, XVI. 9–19.

Greig, E. D. W. (VII. 1913, A). An investigation of an epidemic of cholera caused by a "carrier." *Indian Journ. of Medical Research*, vol. I. **B.**

—— (VII. 1913, B). An investigation of cholera convalescents and contacts in India. *Indian Journ. of Medical Research*, vol. I. **B.**

—— (VII. 1913, C). An investigation on the occurrence of the cholera vibrio in the biliary passages. *Indian Journ. of Medical Research*, vol. I. **B.**

—— (VII. 1913, D). Preliminary Note on the occurrence of the Comma Bacillus in the urine of cases of cholera. *Indian Journ. of Medical Research*, vol. I. **B.**

—— (1913, E). Recent research on Cholera in India. *Indian Medical Gazette*, XLVIII. **B.**

Griffith, A. (1908). Life history of house-flies. *Pub. Health*, XXI. 122–127. **G.**

Grube (1853). *Archiv f. Naturgeschichte*, XIX. 282. (Cited by Wohl, 1913.) **M.**

Grünberg, K. (1913). Ein neuer Fall des Vorkommens der Larve der Rinderdasselfliege im Menschlichen Auge. *Sitz. Gesell. Naturf. Freude*, 298–304. (Cited in *Review of Applied Entom.*, II. p. 6.) **M.**

Güssow, H. T. (1913). *Empusa muscæ* and the extermination of the house-fly. *Reports to the Local Government Board on Public Health and Medical Subjects*, New Series, No. 85, 11–14. **P.**

Hadwen, S. (1912). Warble Flies. *Bull.* 16, *Dept. of Agriculture, Canada.* Health of Animals Branch. **M.**

Hagen, A. (1879). On the larvæ of insects discharged through the urethra. *Proc. Bost. Soc. Nat. Hist.*, XX. 107–118. **M.**

Hall, M. C. and Muir, J. T. (1913). A critical study of a case of myiasis due to *Eristalis*. *Arch. Internat. Med.*, XII. 193–202. **M.**

Hamer, W. H. (1908). Nuisance from flies. *Report of Public Health Committee of London County Council*, Nos. 1138, 1202. **G.**

Hamerton, A. E. (1908). Introduction to methods of study of the morbid histology of disease-carrying insects. *Journn. Roy. Army Med. Corps*, XI. 243–249. **A.**

Hamilton, A. (1903). The fly as a carrier of typhoid; an inquiry into the part played by the common house fly in the recent epidemic of typhoid fever in Chicago. *Journ. of Amer. Med. Assoc.*, XL. 576. (Cited by Dickinson, 1907.) **B.**

—— (1904). The common house fly as a carrier of typhoid fever. *Journ. Amer. Med. Assoc.*, XLII. 1034.

Harrison, J. H. H. (1908). A case of Myiasis. *Journ. Trop. Med.*, XI. 305. **M.**

Hayward, E. H. (1904). The Fly as a Carrier of Tuberculous Infection. *New York Med. Journ.*, LXXX. 643–644. **B.**

Heckenroth, F. and Blanchard, M. (1913). Note sur la Présence et l'Endémicité d'une Myiase furonculeuse au Congo français. *Bull. Soc. Path. Exot.*, VI. 350, 351. **M.**

Hermes, W. B. (1907). An ecological and experimental study of *Sarcophagidæ* with relation to Lake Beach debris. *Ohio State Univ. Contributions from the Dept. of Zoology and Entomology*, No. 24, 45–83. **L.**

—— (1909). Medical entomology, its scope and methods. *Journ. of Economic Entomology*, II. 265–268. **G.**

—— (1910). Fight the fly. *Bull. Berkeley (Cal.) Board of Health.* **G.**

—— (1911). The photic reactions of the sarcophagid flies, especially *Lucilia cæsar* Linn. and *Calliphora* Linn. *Journ. of Exp. Zool.*, X. 167–226. **G.**

—— (1911). The house-fly in its relation to public health. *Univ. of California publications, Bull.* Nos. 215, 513–548. **G.**

Hervieux (16. VI. 1904). Report on carriage of smallpox by flies, read to the Academy of Medicine, Paris, June 5th, 1904. *Lancet*, I. 1761. **B.**

Hesse, E. (29. XI. 1912). The parasitic fungus of the House-fly. *Shrewsbury Chronicle.* **P.**

Hewitt, C. G. (1907). The Structure, Development and Bionomics of the House-fly, *Musca domestica* L. Part I. The Anatomy of the Fly. *Quart. Journ. Micr. Sci.*, LI. 395–448. **A.**

—— (1908). The Structure, etc. Part II. The Breeding Habits, Development and Anatomy of the Larva. *Quart. Journ. Micr. Sci.*, LII. 495–545. **A.L.**

—— (1908). The Biology of House-flies in relation to the Public Health. *Journ. Roy. Inst. Pub. Health*, XVI. 596–608. **G.**

—— (1909). The Structure, etc. Part III. The Bionomics, Allies, Parasites and the Relations of *M. domestica* to Human Disease. *Quart. Journ. Micr. Sci.*, LIV. 347–414. **P.**

—— (1910). *The House-fly. A Study of its Structure, Development, Bionomics and Economy.* Biological Series, No. 1. Manchester Univ. Press. **G.**

—— (1910). House-flies and disease. *Nature*, LXXXIV. 73–75. **G.**

Hewitt, C. G. (1912, A). Observations on the Range of Flight of Flies. *Reports to the Local Government Board on Public Health and Medical Subjects*, New Series, No. 66, 1–5. **G.**

—— (1912, B). An Account of the Bionomics and the Larvæ of the Flies *Fannia* (*Homalomyia*) *canicularis* L. and *F. scalaris* Fab., and their relation to Myiasis of the Intestinal and Urinary Tracts. *Reports to the Local Government Board on Public Health and Medical Subjects*, New Series, No. 66, 15–22. **L.M.**

—— (1912, C). *Fannia* (*Homalomyia*) *canicularis* Linn. and *F. scalaris* Fab. An Account of the Bionomics of the Larvæ and their relation to Myiasis of the Intestinal and Urinary Tracts. *Parasitology*, v. 161–174. **L.M.**

—— (1912, D). *House-flies and how they spread disease.* Cambridge Univ. Press.

—— (1914). On the Predaceous Habits of *Scatophaga*: a new enemy of *Musca domestica*. *Canadian Entomologist*, XLVI. 2. (Rev. in *Review of Applied Entom.*, II. 56.) **P.**

Hewlett, H. T. (1905). The ætiology of epidemic diarrhœa. *Journ. of Preventive Med.*, XIII. 496–507. **B.**

Hindle, E. (1912). What is the Genus *Leptomonas*, Kent? *Parasitology*, v. 128–134. **P.**

—— (1913). Note on the Colour-preference of Flies. *Reports to the Local Government Board on Public Health and Medical Subjects*, New Series, No. 85, 41–43. **L.**

—— (1914, A). The Flight of the House-Fly. *Proc. Camb. Phil. Soc.*, XVII. 310–313. **L.**

Hindle, E. and Merriman, G. (1913). The Range of Flight of *Musca domestica*. *Reports to the Local Government Board on Public Health and Medical Subjects*, New Series, No. 85, 20–41. (Also reprinted in *Journ. Hygiene*, XIV. 23–45.) **L.**

Hirsch, A. (1886). *Handbook of Geographical and Historical Pathology*, Vol. III. New Sydenham Soc. London. **G.**

Hirsch, C. T. W. (1896). An account of two cases of Coko or Frambœsia. *Lancet*, II. 173–175. **B.**

Hodge, C. F. (1910). A practical Point in the Study of the Typhoid or Filth Fly. *Nature Study Review*, VI. 195–199. (Quoted by Howard, 1911, 212.) **G.S.**

—— (1913). The Distance House-Flies, Bluebottles and Stable-Flies may travel over water. *Science*, XXXVIII. 512–513. **L.**

Hofmann, E. (1888). Ueber die Verbreitung der Tuberculose durch Stubenfliegen. *Correspondenzbl. d. ärztl. Kreis- u. Bezirksvereine im Königr. Sachsen.*, XLIV. 130–133. **B.**

Hope, F. (1840). On the Insects and their Larvæ occasionally found in the Human Body. *Trans. Entom. Soc. Lond.*, II. **M.**

Houston, W. M. (1913). Formalin against flies. *Indian Med. Gaz.*, 84. **S.**

Howard, C. W. and Clark, P. F. (1912). Experiments on insect transmission of the virus of poliomyelitis. *Journ. Exp. Med.*, XVI. 850–859. **B.**

Howard, L. O. (1896). The Cheese Skipper. *Bull.* 4, n.s., *Division of Entomology, U.S. Dept. Agric.*, 102–104. **A.**

—— (1896). The Fruit Flies or Vinegar Flies. *Bull.* 4, n.s., *Division of Entomology, U.S. Dept. Agric.*, 109–111. **A.**

—— (1900). A Contribution to the Study of the Insect Fauna of Human Excrement. *Proc. Washington Acad. of Sciences*, II. 541–604. **L.**

—— (1911). *The House-fly, Disease Carrier*. Fred. A. Stokes Co., New York. **G.**

Howard, L. O. and Marlatt, C. L. (1896). House-flies. *Bull.* 4, n.s., *Division of Entomology, U.S. Dept. Agric.*, 43–47. **G.**

Howe, L. (1888). (Egyptian Ophthalmia.) *7th Internat. Congr. of Ophthalmol., Wiesbaden*, Becker u. Hess., 323. (Quoted by Howard, 1911, p. 168.) **B.**

Hutchinson (28. II. 1914). The Migratory Habit of House-fly Larvæ as indicating a favorable remedial measure. An account of progress. *Bull.* 14, *U.S. Dept. Agricult.* **L.**

Hutt, C. W. (1914). A Study of Summer Diarrhœa in Warrington in 1911. *Journ. of Hygiene*, XIII. 422–432. **E.**

International Sanitary Conference, Paris (1911). *Bull. de l'offic. intern. d'Hyg.*, 1912, IV. No. 2. **B.**

Jackson, D. D. (1907). Rep. to Committee on Pollution of the Merchants' Ass. of N. York, 16 (cited by Chapin, 1912).

Jenyns, L. (1839). Notice of a Case in which the Larvæ of a Dipterous Insect, supposed to be *Anthomyia canicularis*, Meig., were expelled in large quantities from the human intestines; accompanied by a description of the same. *Trans. Entomol. Soc. London*, II. 152–156. (Quoted by Austen, 1912, B.) **M.**

Jepson, F. P. (1909). Some Observations on the Breeding of *Musca domestica* during the Winter Months. *Reports to the Local Government Board on Public Health and Medical Subjects*, New Series, No. 5, 5–8. **L.**

—— (1909). Notes on Experiments in Colouring Flies, for purposes of Identification. *Reports to the Local Government Board on Public Health and Medical Subjects*, New Series, No. 16, 4–9. **G.**

Johnson, W. B. (1892). *Ophthalmological Record*, I. 274. (Cited by Wohl, 1913.) **M.**

Johnston, T. H. (1913). Notes on some Entozoa. *Proc. Roy. Soc. Queensland*, XXIV. 63–91. (Rev. in *Review of Applied Entom.*, I. B. 165.) **P.**

Jones, G. I. (1913). Hepatic abscess (non-amebic) and gastro-intestinal myiasis. *Journ. Amer. Med. Assoc.*, LXI. 1457. **M.**

Jones, F. W. C. (1907). Notes on enteric fever prevalent in India. *Journ. Roy. Army Med. Corps*, VIII. 22–34. **E.**

Judd, G. S. (1876). Larvæ discharged from the Lower Intestine of a Boy. *Amer. Nat.*, X. 374. (Quoted by Hewitt, 1912, B.) **M.**

Keilin, D. (1909). Sur le parasitisme de la larve de *Pollenia rudis* Fab. dans *Allolobophora chlorotica* Savigny. *Compt. rend. Soc. Biol.*, LXVII. 201.

Keyt, F. T. (II. 1900). A case of " beef-worm " (*Dermatobia noxialis*) in the orbit. *Brit. Med. Journ.*, 316. **M.**

Kimball, J. P. (1893). Maggots in the nose successfully treated by injections of chloroform. *New York Med. Journ.*, LVII. 273–275. (Quoted by Wohl, 1913.) **M.**

King, E. E. (1908). Report on economic entomology. *Third Report Wellcome Research Labs.*, 215–218. **M.**

Klein, E. (17. X. 1909). " Flies " as carriers of *Bacillus typhosus*. *Brit. Med. Journ.*, 1150–1151. **B.**

Knab, F. (1913). The Life-History of Dermatobia Hominis. *Amer. Journ. Trop. Dis. and Prev. Med.*, I. 464–467. **M.**

Krontowski, A. (1913). Zur Frage über die Typhus- und Dysenterie verbreitung durch Fliegen. *Central. f. Bakt.*, Orig. LXVIII. 586, 590. **B.**

Kuznezo (1893). Review in *Central. f. Bakt.*, XXV. 236. **M.**

Lallier, P. (1897). Tableau des larves de Diptères évacuées par l'urethra. *Thesis*, Paris. (Quoted by Hewitt, 1912.) **M.**

Laveran, A. (1880). Contribution à l'étude du bouton de Biskra. *Ann. de Dermatologie*, 2 S. I. 173–179. **B.**

Lawrence, S. M. (I. 1909). Dangerous dipterous larvæ. *Brit. Med. Journ.*, 88. **M.**

Lebœuf, A. (1912). Recherches Expérimentales sur le Valeur du Rôle que peuvent jouer certains Insectes Hématophages dans la Transmission de la Lèpre. *Bull. Soc. Path. Exot.*, V. 667, 686. **B.**

—— (1912). Dissémination du Bacille de Hansen par la Mouche domestique. *Bull. Soc. Path. Exot.*, V. 860–868. **B.**

—— (1913). Notes sur l'Epidémiologie de la Lèpre dans l'Archipel-Calédonien. *Bull. Soc. Path. Exot.*, VI. 551–556. **B.**

Ledingham, J. C. G. (III. 1911). Addendum to Bacot's (1911) paper. **B.**

—— (X. 1911). On the survival of specific microorganisms in pupæ and imagines of *Musca domestica* raised from experimentally infected larvæ. Experiments with *B. typhosus*. *Journ. of Hygiene*, XI. 333–340. **B.**

Léger, L. (1902, A). Sur la structure et de la mode de multiplication des flagellés du genre *Herpetomonas*, Kent. *Compt. rend. Acad. Sc.*, CXXXIV. 781. **P.**

—— (1902, B). Sur un flagellé parasite de l'Anopheles maculipennis. *Compt. Rend. de la Soc. de Biol.*, 354. **P.**

Léger, L. (1903). Sur quelques Cercomonadines nouvelles ou peu connues parasites de l'intestin des Insectes. *Arch. f. Protistenk.*, II. 180. **P.**

Lelean, P. S. (I. 1904). Notes on Myiasis. *Brit. Med. Journ.*, I. 245–246. **M.**

Léon (1908). *Bull. d. Méd. et Naturalistes.* Jassy, 1908, Nos. 9 and 10. (Quoted by Galli-Valerio, 1910.) **M.**

Levy, E. C. and Tuck, W. T. (1913). The maggot-trap—a new weapon in our warfare against the typhoid fly. *Amer. Journ. Pub. Health*, V. 657–660. (Quoted by Hutchinson, 1914.) **L.**

Lewis, C. J. (1911). Report on the results of an Examination of the Fæces of Children with Special Reference to the Occurrence of Bacilli which neither Liquefy Gelatin nor Ferment Lactose. *40th Annual Report of Local Government Board, Supplement containing the Report of the Medical Officer for* 1910–11. App. B, 314–346. **B.**

—— (1912). Report on the Prevalence and Characters of Non-lactose Fermenting and Non-liquefying Ærobic Bacilli in the Fæces of Young Children under normal conditions and in Epidemic Diarrhœa during 1911. *41st Annual Report of the Local Government Board, Supplement containing the Report of the Medical Officer for* 1911–12. App. B, 265–287. **B.**

—— (1913). Report on the Agglutination Reactions of Morgan's Bacillus. *42nd Annual Report of the Local Government Board, Supplement containing the Report of the Medical Officer for* 1912–13. App. B, 375–383. **B.**

Lindsay, T. W. (1902). Myiasis—The *Lucilia macellaria*—The screw-worm. *Journ. of Trop. Med.*, V. 220. **M.**

Lord, F. T. (15. XII. 1904). Flies and Tuberculosis. *Boston Med. and Surg. Journ.*, CLI. 651–654. **B.**

Lowne, B. T. (1895). *The Anatomy, Physiology, Morphology and Development of the Blow-fly* (*Calliphora erythrocephala*). R. H. Foster, London. **A.**

Lubbock, Sir John (1871). The fly in its sanitary aspect. *Lancet*, II. 270. **G.**

McCampbell, E. F. and Cooper, H. J. (1909). Myiasis intestinalis due to infection with three species of dipterous larvæ. *Journ. Amer. Med. Assoc.*, LIII. 1160–1162. **M.**

MacDougall, R. T. (1909). Sheep Maggot and Related Flies. *Trans. Highland Agric. Soc.*, XXI. 135–174. **M.**

Mackinnon, D. L. (1910). Herpetomonads from the alimentary tract of certain Dung flies. *Parasitology*, III. 255. **P.**

Macrae, R. (1894). Flies and Cholera Diffusion. *Ind. Med. Gaz.*, 407–412. **B.**

Maddox, R. L. (1885). Experiments on feeding some insects with the curved or "comma" bacillus, and also with another bacillus (*subtilis*?). *Journ. Roy. Microsc. Soc.*, Ser. 2, V. 602–607, 941–952. **B.**

Major, H. S. (1913). The Maggot Fly Pest in Sheep. *Agric. Gaz. N.S.W., Sydney,* XXIV. 645–652. **M.**

Marlatt, C. L. (1894). The House Centipede. *Bull.* 4, n.s., *Division of Entomology, U.S. Dept. Agric.*, 47–50. **P.**

Marshall, G. A. K. (1902). *Trans. Entomol. Soc. of London,* 540. (Quoted by Austen, 1908.) **M.**

Martin, C. J. (4. I. 1913). The Horace Dobell Lectures on insect porters of bacterial infections. *Brit. Med. Journ.*, I. 1–8. **G.**

Miller, R. T. (1910). Myiasis dermatosa due to ox-warble flies. *Journ. Amer. Med. Assoc.*, LV. 1978–1979. **M.**

Minett, E. P. (1912). The Question of Flies as Leprosy Carriers. *Journ. of London School of Trop. Med.*, I. 31–35. **B.**

Mitzmain, M. B. (1913). The Bionomics of *Stomoxys calcitrans* Linnæus; A Preliminary Account. *Philippine Journ. of Science*, B. VIII. 28–48. **L.**

Moore, W. (3. VI. 1893). Diseases probably caused by flies. *Brit. Med. Journ.*, I. 1154. **G.**

Morgan, H. de R. (1906). Upon the Bacteriology of Summer Diarrhœa in Infants. *Brit. Med. Journ.*, 908–912. **B.**

—— (1907). Upon the Bacteriology of Summer Diarrhœa in Infants. *Brit. Med. Journ.*, 16–19. **B.**

—— (1911). The differentiation of the mannite fermenting group of *B. dysenteriæ* with special reference to strains isolated from various sources in this country. *Journ. of Hygiene*, XI. 1–23. **B.**

—— (30. XI. 1912). A Parasitic Mould of the House Fly. *Brit. Med. Journ.*, II. 1582. **P.**

Morgan, H. de R. and Ledingham, J. C. G. (1909). The Bacteriology of Summer Diarrhœa. *Proc. Roy. Soc. Med.*, II. (Epidem. Sect.) 133–158. **B.**

Morgan, J. C. and Harvey, D. (1909). An experimental research on the viability of the *Bacillus typhosus* as excreted under natural conditions by the "chronic carrier." *Journ. Roy. Army Med. Corps*, XII. 587–598. **B.**

Morris (XI. 1912). *Louisiana Bull.*, No. 156. Agricul. Exp. Station. (Abstract in *Journ. Comp. Path.* (1913), XXVI. 95.) **M.**

Munsen, E. (1901). *The Theory and Practice of Military Hygiene.* Baillière, Tindall and Cox, London. **G.**

Nash, J. T. C. (31. I. 1903). The etiology of summer diarrhœa. *Lancet*, I. 330. **B.**

—— (1903). The seasonal incidence of typhoid fever and of diarrhœa. The seasonal consumption of shell-fish, and the seasonal prevalence of flies as regards the latter (diarrhœa). *Trans. Epidemiol. Soc. London*, n.s., XXII. 110–138. **E.**

—— (II. 1904). Some points in the prevention of epidemic diarrhœa. *Lancet*, I. 892. **E.**

Nash, J. T. C. (1909). House-flies as carriers of disease. *Journ. of Hygiene*, IX. 141–169. **G.**

Neiva, A. and Gomes de Faria (1913). Myiasis humana, verursucht durch Larven von *Sarcophaga pyophila*, n. sp. *Mem. Inst. Oswaldo Cruz*, V 16–22. (Review in *Trop. Dis. Bull.*, II. 529.) **M.**

Newsholme, A. (1903). *Ann. Report on the Health of Brighton*, 21. **E.**

—— (1906). Domestic infection in relation to epidemic diarrhœa. *Journ. of Hygiene*, VI. 139–148. **E.**

—— (1910). A Report on Infant and Child Mortality. *Supplement to the Report of the Medical Health Officer in the 39th Annual Report of the Local Government Board.* **E.**

Newstead, R. (1906). On the Life-history of *Stomoxys calcitrans* Linn. *Journ. Econ. Biol.*, I. 157–166. **A.**

—— (1907). *Preliminary Report on the Habits, Life-cycle and Breeding Places of the Common House-fly* (Musca domestica *Linn.*), *as observed in the City of Liverpool, with Suggestions as to the best means of Checking its Increase.* C. Tinling and Co., Liverpool. **L.**

—— (1909). *Second Interim Report on the House-Fly, as observed in the City of Liverpool.* C. Tinling and Co., Liverpool. **L.**

Nicholas, G. E. (1873). The fly in its sanitary aspect. *Lancet*, II. 724. **G.**

Nicholls, L. (1911). St Lucia. Laboratory report for the half year ending Sept. 30th, 1911. *Report to the Advisory Committee of the Trop. Dis. Research Fund*, App. VI. No. 14, 199. **G.**

—— (1912). The transmission of pathogenic micro-organisms by flies in Saint Lucia. *Bull. of Entomolog. Research*, III. 81. **B.**

Nicholson, T. L. (1910). Myiasis, a report of three cases of primary rectal infection. *Journ. Amer. Med. Assoc.*, LIV. 1687–1688. **M.**

Nicoll, W. (1911). On the Part played by Flies in the Disposal of the Eggs of Parasitic Worms. *Reports to the Local Government Board on Public Health and Medical Subjects*, New Series, No. 53, 13–30. **O.**

—— (1912). On the varieties of *Bacillus coli* associated with the House-fly (*Musca domestica*). *Journ. of Hygiene*, XI. 381–389. **B.**

Niven, J. (1910). Summer Diarrhœa and Enteric Fever. *Proc. Roy. Soc. of Med.*, III. (Epidem. Sect.) 131–216. **E.**

Noc, F. (1912). Remarques et Observations sur le Rôle des Moustiques dans la Propagation de la Lèpre. *Bull. Soc. Path.*, V. 787–789. **B.**

Novy, F. G., MacNeal, W. J. and Torrey, H. N. (1907). The Trypanosomes of Mosquitoes and other insects. *Journ. of Inf. Dis.*, IV. 223–276. **P.**

Nuttall, G. H. F. (IX. 1899). The part played by insects, arachnids, and myriapods in the propagation of infective diseases of man and animals. *Brit. Med. Journ.*, II. 642–644.

—— (X. 1899). On the rôle of insects, arachnids and myriapods as carriers in the spread of bacterial and parasitic diseases of man and animals. A critical and historical study. *Johns Hopkins Hosp. Reports*, VIII. I. **G.**

—— (XI. 1899). The rôle of insects, arachnids, and myriapods in the propagation of infective diseases of man and animals. *Journ. Trop. Med.*, II. 107–110.

Nuttall, G. H. F. (1899). Die Rolle der Insekten, Arachniden (*Ixodes*) und Myriapoden als Träger bei der Verbreitung von durch Bakterien und thierische Parasiten verursachten Krankheiten des Menschen und der Thiere. *Hyg. Rundschau*, IX. 209, 275, 393, 503, 606. **G.**

Nuttall, G. H. F. and Jepson, F. P. (1909). The part played by *Musca domestica* and allied (Non-biting) Flies in the Spread of Infective Diseases: A Summary of our present knowledge. *Reports to the Local Government Board on Public Health and Medical Subjects*, New Series, No. 16, 13–41. **G.**

O'Brien, R. A. (1911). Report on an Investigation of the Bacterial Contents of the Fæces of Young Children. *40th Annual Report of the Local Government Board, Supplement containing the Report of the Medical Officer for* 1910–11, App. B, 367–373. **B.**

Odlum, W. H. (1908). Are flies the cause of enteric fever? *Journ. Roy. Army Med. Corps*, X. 528–530. **G.**

Olive, E. W. (1906). Cytological studies on the Entomophthoreæ. I. The Morphology and Development of *Empusa*. *Bot. Gaz.*, XLI. 192. (Quoted by Bernstein, 1910.)

Orr, T. (1911). Report on an Investigation into the presence of certain Intestinal Bacteria in the Fæcal Excreta of Infants. *40th Annual Report of the Local Government Board, Supplement containing the Report of the Medical Officer for* 1910–11, App. B, 374–386. **B.**

Orton, S. T. (1910). Experiments on the transmission of bacteria by flies with special relation to an epidemic of bacillary dysentery at the Worcester State Hospital. *Boston Med. and Surg. Journ.* (Quoted by Howard, 1911, p. 155.)

Palmer, J. F. (1901). Quoted by Austen (1912, p. 12). **M.**

Park, W. H., Collins, K. R. and Goodwin, M. E. (1903). Results of an investigation upon the etiology of Dysentery and Acute Diarrhœa. *Proc. New York Path. Soc.*, n.s. III. 148–159. **B.**

Patton, W. S. (13. VII. 1907). Preliminary note on the life-cycle of a species of Herpetomonas found in *Culex pipiens*. *Brit. Med. Journ.*, 178. **P.**

—— (1909). A critical review of our present knowledge of the hæmoflagellates and allied forms. *Parasitology*, II. 91–143. **P.**

—— (1908). The life-cycle of a species of Crithidia parasitic in the intestinal tract of *Gerris fossarum* Fabr. *Arch. f. Protistenk.*, XII. 131. **P.**

—— (1909). Herpetomonas lygæi. *Arch. f. Protistenk.*, XIII. 1–18. **P.**

—— (1909). The Life-Cycle of a Species of Crithidia parasitic in the intestinal tracts of *Tabanus hilarius* and *Tabanus sp.* *Arch. f. Protistenk.*, XV. 333. **P.**

Patton, W. S. (1912). Studies on the Flagellates of the Genera *Herpetomonas*, *Crithidia*, and *Rhynchoidomonas*. No. I. The Morphology and Life-History of *Herpetomonas culicis*, Novy, MacNeal, and Torrey. *Sci. Mems. by Officers of the Med. and Sanit. Depts., Govt. of India*, New Ser. No. 57, 1–21. (Review in *Trop. Dis. Bull.*, II. 48.) **P.**

Patton, W. S. and Cragg, F. W. (1912, A). The Genus *Pristirhynchomyia*, Brunetti, 1910. *Ann. Trop. Med. and Parasitol.*, V. 509–514. **A.**

—— (1912, B). The Life-History of *Philæmatomyia insignis*, Austen. *Ann. Trop. Med. and Parasitol.*, V. 515–520. **A.L.**

—— (1913, A). On Certain Hæmatophagous Species of the Genus Musca, with Descriptions of Two New Species. *Indian Journ. Med. Research*, I. **A.L.**

—— (1913, B). A New Species of Philæmatomyia, with some remarks on the Genus. *Indian Journ. Med. Research*, I. **A.L.**

—— (1913, C). *A Textbook of Medical Entomology*. Christian Literature Society for India, London. **A.G.**

Peters, O. H. (1910). Observations upon the natural history of epidemic diarrhœa. *Journ. of Hygiene*, X. 602–777. **E.**

Piana, G. P. (1896). Osservazioni sul Dispharagus nasutus, Rud. dei polli e sulle larve Nematoelmintiche delle mosche e dei Porcellioni. *Atti della Soc. Ital. d. Sci. Nat.*, XXXVI. 239–262. (Quoted by Hewitt, 1909.)

Pieter, H. (1912). Un Cas de Myase Vulvo-Vaginale. *Rev. de Méd. et d'Hyg. Trop.*, IX. 176–177. **M.**

Pinkus, H. (1913). The Life-History and Habits of *Spalangia muscidarum*, Richardson ; a parasite of the Stable-Fly. *Psyche*, XX. 149–158. **P.**

Pirajá da Silva, M. (1912). Nouveaux cas de myase dus à *Chrysomyia macellaria* Fabricius, à Bahia. *Arch. de Parasitol.*, XV 425–430. **M.**

Poore, G. V. (1901). Flies and the science of scavenging. *Lancet*, I. 1389–1391. **G.**

Portchinsky, J. A. (1913, A). Review in *Review of Applied Entomol.*, I. B. 134. **P.**

—— (1913, B). Review in *Review of Applied Entomol.*, I. B. 149. P.

Porter, A. (1912). Some remarks on the genera *Crithidia*, *Herpetomonas* and *Trypanosoma*. *Parasitology*, IV. 22. **P.**

Prowazek, S. (1904). Die Entwicklung von Herpetomonas, einem mit den Trypanosomen verwandten Flagellaten. *Arb. a. d. Kais. Gesundheitsamte*, XX. 440–452. **P.**

—— (1913). Notiz sur *Herpetomonas*—Morphologie sowie Bemerkung zu der Arbeit von Wenyon. *Arch. f. Protistenk.*, XXXI. 37–38. **P.**

Quill, R. H. (1900). Report on an outbreak of enteric fever at

Diyatalawa Camp, Ceylon, among the 2nd King's Royal Rifles during the period they acted as guard over Boer prisoners of war. *Army Med. Dept. Report for the Year* 1900, 452, Appendix 4. **E.**

Quill, R. H. (1905). The spread of enteric fever by latrine infection. *Journ. Roy. Army Med. Corps*, IV. 809–810. **E.**

Raimbert, A. (1869). Recherches expérimentales sur la transmission du charbon par les mouches. *Compt. rend. d. l'Acad. de Sc.*, LXIX. 805–812. (Quoted by Nuttall, 1899.) **B.**

Ransom, B. H. (1911). The Life-history of a Parasitic Nematode (*Habronema muscæ*). *Science*, N.S. XXXIV. 690–692. (Quoted by Hewitt, 1912.) **P.**

—— (1913). The Life-History of *Habronema muscæ* (Carter), a Parasite of the Horse transmitted by the House-Fly. *U.S. Dept. Agric. Bureau of Animal Industry*, Bull. 163. **P.**

Reed, W., Vaughan, V. M. and Shakespeare, E. O. (1899). *Report on the Spread of Typhoid Fever in the United States Military Camps during the Spanish-American War of* 1898 *to the Surgeon-General of the U.S. Army*, Washington. **E.**

Richardson, C. H. (1913). An undescribed Hymenopterous Parasite of the House-Fly. *Psyche*, XX. 38–39. **P.**

Rieley, S. D. and Howlett, F. M. (1914). A Few Observations on Myiasis (Screw-Worm Disease) in Behar. *Indian Med. Gaz.*, XLIX. 8–10. **M.**

Robertson, A. (1908). Flies as carriers of contagion in Yaws (*Frambœsia tropica*). *Journ. of Trop. Med. and Hygiene*, XI. 213. **B.**

Rodhain, J. and Bequaert, J. (1913). Nouvelles observations sur *Auchmeromyia luteola*, Fab., et *Cordylobia anthropophaga*, Grünb. *Revue Zoologique Africaine*, II. 145–154. (Review in *Rev. of Applied Entomol.*, I. B. 91.) **M.**

Rodhain, J., Pons, C., Vandenbranden, F. and Bequaert, J. (1913). *Rapport sur les Travaux de la Mission Scientifique du Katanga, Oct.* 1910 *à Sept.* 1912. Brussels. (Review in *Trop. Dis. Bull.*, II. 530.)

Rosenau, Lumsden and Kastle (1909). Report No. 3 on origin and prevalence of Typhoid Fever in the District of Columbia. *Bull.* 52, *Hyg. Lab. U.S. Pub. Health and Mar. Hosp. Service, Washington*, p. 30. (Quoted by Martin, 1913.)

Rosenbusch, F. (1909). Über eine neue Encystierung bei *Crithidia muscæ-domesticæ*. *Central. f. Bakt.*, LIII. 387–393. **P.**

Ross, E. H. (1913). *The Reduction of Domestic Flies*. John Murray, London. **G.**

Ross, R. (1898). Report on the cultivation of Proteosoma Labbé in Grey Mosquitoes. Calcutta. (Office of the Superintendent of Government Printing, India.)

Ross, S. M. (1911). Report upon the Examination of Infants' Fæcal Excreta for Bacilli which do not ferment Lactose. *40th Annual*

Report of the Local Government Board, Supplement containing the Report of the Medical Officer for 1910–11, App. B, 347–366. **B.**

Roubaud, E. (1908). Sur un nouveau flagellé parasite, de l'intestin des Muscides, au Congo français. *Compt. rend. soc. Biol.*, LXIV. 1106. **P.**

—— (1908). *Leptomonas mesnili* n.sp.; nouveau flagellé à formes trypanosomes de l'intestin de Muscides non piqueurs. *Compt. rend. soc. Biol.*, LXV. 39. **P.**

—— (1913, A). Études biologiques sur les Auchmeromyies. *Bull. Soc. Path. Exot.*, VI. 128–130. **M.**

—— (1913, B). Recherches sur les Auchmeromyies, Calliphorines à larves suceuses de sang de l'Afrique tropicale. *Bull. Scient. de la France et de la Belgique*, XLVII. 105–202. **M.**

Sandilands, J. E. (1906). Epidemic diarrhœa and the bacterial content of food. *Journ. of Hygiene*, VI. 77–92. **B.**

Sandwith, F. M. (1904). *The Practitioner*, LXXII. 15. **G.**

Sangree (1899). *New York Med. Record*, LV. 88. (Quoted by Nuttall and Jepson, 1909.) **B.**

Sawtchenko, J. D. (1892). Le rôle des mouches dans la propagation de l'épidémie cholérique. *Vratch.* (St Petersburg); rev. in *Ann. de l'Inst. Pasteur*, VII. 222. **B.**

Schnee (1853). *Archiv. f. Naturgeschichte*, XIX. (Cited by Wohl, 1913.) **M.**

Sedgwick, W. T. and Winslow, C. E. A. (1902). Statistical studies on the seasonal prevalence of typhoid fever in various countries and its relation to seasonal temperature. *Mem. Am. Acad. Sci.*, XII. 521–577. (Quoted by Howard, 1911.) **E.**

Seicluna, G. C. (1912). *Supplement to the Malta Government Gaz.* 1912, No. 5522. (Review in *Centralbl. f. Bakt.*, Referale VII. p. 296.) **B.**

Sergent, Ed. and Sergent, Et. (1907). La "Thim'ni," myiase humaine d'Algérie, causée par "*Oestrus ovis.*" *Ann. de l'Inst. Pasteur*, XXI. 392–399. **M.**

—— (1913). La "Tamné," myiase humaine des montagnes sahariennes touareg, identique à la "Thimni" des Kabyles, due à *Oestrus ovis. Bull. Soc. Path. Exot.*, VI. 487–488. **M.**

Sharp, D. (1899). Diptera (Chapter VII) of *The Cambridge Natural History*, VI. 438. **A.**

Shipley, A. E. (1905). *The Infinite Torment of Flies.* Cambridge Univ. Press. (Printed privately.) **G.**

Sibthorpe, E. H. (1896). Cholera and Flies. *Brit. Med. Journ.*, II. 700. **B.**

Simmonds, M. (1892). Fliegen und Choleraübertragung. *Deutsche Med. Wochenschr.*, 931. **B.**

Simpson, R. J. S. (1902). Medical History of the South African War. *Journ. Roy. Army Med. Corps*, XV. 3, 257 and 260–261. **E.**

Sinton, J. A. (1912). Some Observations on the Morphology and Biology of *Prowazekia urinaria* (*Bodo urinarius*, Hassall). *Ann. Trop. Med. and Parasit.*, VI. 245–268. **P.**

Skinner, H. (1913). How does the House-Fly pass the Winter? *Entom. News, Philadelphia*, XXIV. 303–304. **L.**

Smith, A. J. (1902). Notes upon several larval insects occurring as parasites in man. *Med. News*, LXXXI. 1060. **M.**

Smith, F. (1903). Municipal Sewerage. *Journ. of Tropical Medicine*, VI. 285, 304, 330, 353, 381. **G.**

—— (1907). House-flies and their ways at Benares. *Journ. Roy. Army Med. Corps*, IX. 150–155 and 447. **L.**

—— (1908). Tumbu-fly disease in Sierre Leone. *Journ. Roy. Army Med. Corps*, X. 14–15. **M.**

Smith, R. I. (1912). The House-fly (*Musca domestica*). *No. Car. Agr. Exp. Sta., Col. Agr. and Mech. Arts, Ann. Rpt.*, XXXIV, 62–69. (Quoted by Hutchinson, 1914.) **G.**

Soltau, A. B. (1910). Note of a case of intestinal infection in man, with the larva of *Homalomyia canicularis*. *Parasitology*, III. 314. **M.**

Spillman and Haushalter (1887). Dissémination du bacilli de la tuberculose par la mouche. *Compt. rend. Acad. Sci.*, CV. 352–353. **B.**

Stein, F. R. (1878). *Der Organismus der Infusionsthiere* III. Abtheilung—*Die Naturgeschichte der Flagellaten oder Geisselinfusiorien*, 154 pp. Leipzig. (Quoted by Hewitt, 1909.)

Stephens, J. W. W. (1905). Two cases of intestinal myiasis. *Thomson—Yates and Johnstone, Lab. Report*, VI. 119–121. **M.**

Stiles, C. W. (1889). Private communication to Nuttall. (Nuttall and Jepson, 1909, 28.) **B.**

—— (1910). The Sanitary Privy : its Purpose and Construction. *Pub. Health Bull.* No. 37, *U.S. Pub. Health and Marine Hospital Service*, 24. (Quoted in detail by Howard, 1911.) **S.**

Stiles, C. W. and Keister, W. S. (1913). Flies as carriers of Lamblia spores. The contamination of food with human excreta. *U.S. Pub. Health Rep.*, XXVIII. 2530–2534. **B.**

Straton, C. H. (1907). The Prevention of Enteric Fever in India. *Journ. Roy. Army Med. Corps*, VIII. 224. **L.**

Strickland, C. (1912). Description of a *Herpetomonas* parasitic in the alimentary tract of the common green-bottle fly, *Lucilia* sp. *Parasitology*, IV. 222. **P.**

Surcouf, J. (1913). La Transmission du Ver Macaque par un Moustique. *Compt. Rend. Acad. Sci.*, CLVI. 1406–1408. **M.**

Swann, J. M. (1910). A report of two cases of external myiasis. *Journ. of Trop. Med.*, XIII. 1–3. **M.**

Swellengrebel, N. H. (1912). Note on the morphology of *Herpetomonas* and *Crithidia*, with some remarks on "physiological degeneration." *Parasitology*, IV. 108–130. **P.**

Swingle, L. D. (1911). The transmission of *Trypanosoma lewisi* by rat fleas (*Ceratophyllus sp.* and *Pulex sp.*), with short descriptions of three new Herpetomonads. *Journ. of Inf. Dis.*, XIII. 125–146. **P.**

Sydenham, T. (1666). *Sydenham's Works*, Syd. Soc. Ed., I. 271. **E.**

Taschenberg (1870). *Gesam. Naturg.*, XXVI. (Cited by Wohl, 1913.) **M.**

Tebbutt, H. (I. 1913). On the influence of the metamorphosis of *Musca domestica* upon bacteria administered in the larval stage. *Journ. of Hygiene*, XII. 516–526. **B.**

Thaxter, R. (1888). The Entomophthoreæ of the United States. *Mem. Bost. Soc. Nat. Hist.*, IV. 133–201. **P.**

Thébault, V. (1901). Hémorrhagie intestinale et affection typhoïde causée par des larves de Diptère. *Arch. de Parasitol.*, IV. 353–361. **M.**

Theobald, F. V. (1904). Swarms of flies bred in House refuse. Second report on Economic Zoology, Pt. II. *Report on Agricultural Zoology to Board of Agriculture*, 125–126. **L.**

—— (1906). Report on Economic Entomology. *Second Report Wellcome Research Labs.*, 83–85. **D.**

Thomson, F. W. (16. X. 1912). The house-fly as a carrier of typhoid infection. *Journ. of Trop. Med. and Hyg.*, XV. 273–6. **B.**

Tizzoni, G. and Cattani, J. (1886). Untersuchungen über Cholera. *Centralbl. f. d. Med. Wissensch.*, XXIV. 769–771. **B.**

Tooth, H. H. and Calverley, J. E. G. (1901). *A Civilian War Hospital; being an account of the work of the Portland Hospital, and of the experience of Wounds and Sickness in South Africa*, 1900. John Murray, London. **G.**

Torrey, J. C. (1912). Numbers and types of Bacteria carried by city flies. *Journ. of Inf. Dis.*, X. 166–177. **B.**

Tsuzuki, J. (1904). Bericht über meine epidemiologischen Beobachtungen und Forschungen während der Choleraepidemie in Nordchina im Jahre 1902. *Arch. f. Schiffs- u. Tropen-Hyg.*, VIII. 71–81. (Quoted by Nuttall and Jepson, 1909.) **B.**

Tulpius, N. (1641). *Observationes medicæ* (Ed. 1672), II. 173–174. (Quoted by Hewitt, 1912.) **M.**

Uffelmann, J. (1892). Beiträge zur Biologie des Cholerabacillus. *Berlin. klin. Wochenschr.*, 1213–1214. **B.**

Vacher, F. (1909). Report of County Medical Officer of Health on "Some recent Investigations regarding the propagation of Disease by Flies." Cheshire County Council. **G.**

Varley, C. (1852). Microscopical observations on a Malady affecting the Common House-fly. *Trans. Micros. Soc. Lond.*, III. 55–57. **P.**

Vaughan (1900). *Journ. Amer. Med. Assoc.*, XXXIV. 1456. (Quoted by Chapin, 1912, p. 425.) **E.**

Veau de Launay (1792). Observations sur des vers rendus avec l'urine. *Observ. de phys. de Rozier*, L. 158. (Quoted by Hewitt, 1912, c.) **M.**

Veeder, M. A. (1898). Flies as spreaders of disease in camps. *New York Med. Record*, LIV. 429–430. **E.**

Verrall, G. H. (1909). *British Flies.* Vol. v. Gurney and Jackson, London. **D.**

von Linstow (1875). Beobachtungen an neuen und bekannten Helminthen. *Arch. f. Naturgesch.*, 183–207. (Quoted by Hewitt, 1909.) **P.**

Walsh, B. D. (1870). Larvæ in the Human Bowels. *Americ. Entom.*, II. 137–141. (Quoted by Hewitt, 1912.) **M.**

Wanhill, C. F. (1909). An investigation into the causes of the prevalence of enteric fever among the troops stationed in Bermuda, giving details of the measures adopted to combat the disease, and shewing the results of these measures, during the years 1904 to 1906. *Journ. of Roy. Army Med. Corps*, XII. 28–45 (flies p. 35). **E.**

Ward, H. B. (1903). Some Points in the Development of Dermatobia hominis. *Studies from the Zool. Lab., Univ. of Nebraska*, No. 58. **M.**

Weaver, G. H., Tunnicliffe, R. M., Heinemann, P. G. and Michael, M. (1905). Summer diarrhœa in Infants. *Journ. of Inf. Dis.*, II. 70–96. **B.**

Welander (1896). *Wein. klin. Wochenschr.*, No. 52. (Quoted by Nuttall and Jepson, 1909, p. 21.)

Wellman, F. C. (1906). Experimental myiasis in goats, with a study of the life-cycle of the fly used in the experiment and a list of some similar noxious diptera. *Journ. of Med. Research*, XIV. 439–446. **M.**

—— (1907). Intestinal Myiasis in Angola. *Journ. Trop. Med.*, XII. 186. **M.**

Wenyon, C. M. (1912). Oriental Sore in Bagdad, together with Observations on a Gregarine in *Stegomyia fasciata*, the Hæmogregarine of Dogs and the Flagellates of House-flies. *Parasitology*, IV. 273–344. **P.**

—— (1913). Observations on *Herpetomonas muscæ domesticæ* and some allied flagellates. With special reference to the structure of their nuclei. *Arch. f. Protistenk.*, XXXI. 1–36. **P.**

Werner, H. (1909). Über eine eingeisselige Flagellatenform im Darm der Stubenfliege. *Arch. f. Protistenk.*, XIII. 19–22. **P.**

Westcott, S. (VIII. 1913). Flies and Disease in the British Army. *Journ. of State Med.*, XXI. 480–488. **G.**

Williston, S. W. (1908). *Manual of North American Diptera.* James T. Hathaway, New Haven. **D.**

Wingate, W. J. (1906). A preliminary list of Durham diptera, with analytical tables. *Trans. Nat. Hist. Soc. of Northumberland and Durham and Newcastle-upon-Tyne*, II. 1–416. **D.**

Wohl, M. G. (1913). Myiasis, or Fly Larvæ as Parasites of Man. With Report of a Case. *New York Med. Journ.*, XCVIII. 1018–1020 **M.**

Wollstein, M. (1903). The dysentery bacillus in a series of cases of infantile diarrhœa. *Journ. Med. Research*, x. 11–20. **B.**

Woodburn, J. L. F. (1913). *Second Prize Essay on 'The Sheep Maggot-Fly Pest in Australia.'* Cooper Lab. for Economic Research, 49–54. **M.**

Woodhouse, T. P. (1908). Notes on the causation and prevention of enteric fever in India, with remarks on its diagnosis and treatment. *Journ. Roy. Army Med. Corps*, x. 616–626. **G.**

Wright, H. M. (1884). *Journ. of the Roy. Micro. Soc.*, Series 2, IV. 1003. (Cited by Lowne, p. 395.) **A.**

Yersin, A. (1894). La peste bubonique à Hongkong. *Ann. Inst. Pasteur*, VIII. 662–667. **B.**

Zepeda, P. (1913). Nouvelle Note concernant les Moustiques qui propagent les Larves de *Dermatobia cyaniventris* et de *Chrysomia macellaria* et peut-être celle de Lund, et de la *Cordylobia anthropophaga*. *Rev. de Méd. et d'Hyg. Trop.*, x. 93–95. **M.**

AUTHORS' INDEX

Showing the pages on which the authors quoted, except the writer, are mentioned

SUBJECT INDEX

Printed in the United States
By Bookmasters